Fluoride Harm

Suppressed Science and Silenced Voices

Fluoride Harm

Suppressed Science and Silenced Voices

A Collection of 21st Century Essays

Editor: Hardy Limeback, BSc, PhD, DDS
Co-Editor: Karen Favazza Spencer, MA

HERON LODGE PRESS

McKellar, Canada

ISBN 978-1-0698022-0-0 (Paperback)
ISBN 978-1-0698022-1-7 (eBook)

Disclaimer: This book is intended for informational purposes only. Although every effort has been made to report facts, the opinions are those of the individual authors. The editors, authors, and publisher do not assume, and hereby disclaim, any liability and make no warranty to any party regarding the use of this book as it is not intended as a substitute for dental, medical, or legal consultation.

Cover Design: Kevin Limeback

EDITOR'S NOTE

This book is dedicated to all the families who have supported the activist in the family, whether a scientist, medical/dental health care provider, journalist, or activist/protester. Most who have voiced their anti-fluoridation positions publicly have suffered the consequences of personal or academic attacks, attempts to discredit them, and 'cancel' them. There have even been attempts to have them dismissed or disciplined by their employer. Some of the recipients of these attacks have lost income, even their jobs. This collection of essays is from just a few of the people who had the courage to speak out against the 'machine'. There are hundreds more.

I was able to get through my hardships brought on by speaking out against fluoridation because of the love and support of my wife Lynne and my two sons Kevin and Kurt.

I personally would like to give special thanks to Karen F. Spencer, who, as my co-editor, has been an intrepid researcher, a brilliant and creative writer, a meticulous copywriter, and friend throughout these last few years. She has opened my eyes to a number of issues drastically affecting the people who fall between the cracks of a failing health care and public health system, both the US and Canada. This book would not have been possible without her involvement.

—Dr Hardy Limeback, BSc, PhD (Biochem), DDS

TABLE OF CONTENTS

"Here's freedom to him who would read;
Here's freedom to him who would write;
None ever feared that the truth should be heard,
But them that the truth would indict."

—Robert Burns (1759-1796)

FOREWORD

By: Dr Joseph Ladapo, MD, PhD

ABOUT: *Dr Ladapo is the author of "Transcend Fear: A Blueprint for Mindful Leadership in Public Health," a Professor at the University of Florida College of Medicine, and Surgeon General of Florida.*

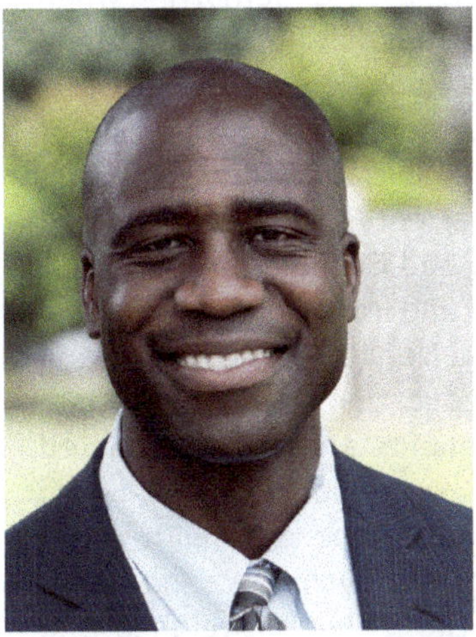

ONE OF THE remarkable things about human history is that change, for better or for worse, has often stemmed from the will of a single individual or small group of individuals. That individual's will—or the collective will of a group propagates across the wider consciousness through the power of manifestation, shaping the beliefs of others and creating the momentum to bring forth into reality what began as an idea or desire. The movement currently underway to end community water fluoridation in the United States reflects this pattern, expanding by the power of its merits and giving us all an opportunity to watch—and possibly participate in—a history-making moment for public health, scientific integrity, and human sovereignty.

I am one of many downstream figures in the movement to end this 80-year practice in the United States. I was moved to act because of the courageous actions of others—nearly all of whom tirelessly and selflessly advocated for the cessation of water fluoridation on the grounds of safety, scientific evidence, or medical freedom. They bravely followed their convictions, often at great personal cost and always while facing derision and contempt from the public health establishment.

As a physician who studied health policy and trained at Harvard Medical School, I was deeply steeped in the traditional, old guard ways of public health. My education—which I now recognize often verged on indoctrination—included teachings about unabated reverence for vaccines, exaltation of water fluoridation, and limiting beliefs about what "good health" meant and how allopathic medicine was the only pathway to attaining it.

Like many Americans, it took the profoundly unethical overreaches of the COVID-19 pandemic and its policymaking—from forced lockdowns to forced masking to forced vaccinations through inhumane leverage—to awaken me from my trance. My awakening continues, and helping to create policy ending community water fluoridation is as much a step in my own personal journey as it is for mankind.

Some of the early scientific work that fueled concerns about the safety of community water fluoridation included studies from China linking high levels of naturally occurring fluoride in water to lower IQs. There was also a 1995 study by Dr. Phyllis J. Mullenix, a researcher at Harvard and chair of a toxicology department, who found that fluoride exposure in rats led to behavior changes that were akin to attention-deficit/hyperactivity disorder (ADHD) in humans. After demurring when senior colleagues strongly cautioned her to abandon her research and not publish these results, she lost her faculty position.

Dr. Mullenix's work undoubtedly inspired many people, and one of those people was Dr. Ashley Malin. An epidemiologist and psychologist at the University of Florida, she led seminal scientific studies examining health impacts of water fluoridation in U.S. and Canadian populations. Her work received international attention and recognition, including from the National Institute of Environmental Health Sciences. She and I ultimately partnered in efforts to provide education to county and city leaders across the state of Florida about benefits and risks associated with water fluoridation. Based on current scientific evidence, which reflects both markedly diminished dental health benefits with water fluoridation compared to the past and neuropsychiatric and other developmental harms, we argued that the risks outweighed the benefits. This conclusion was brought even more sharply into focus by the fact that children and pregnant women were the populations that appear to be most greatly harmed.

As we visited beautiful Florida cities like Clearwater, Fort Meyers, and Miami, we were graced by the presence of many members of Florida's medical freedom movement, including the group Stand for Health Freedom. We also met many members of the local community. Some of them favored the practice of water fluoridation and argued that removing it would be harmful. However, most were fierce advocates for their own health, the health of their families, and their right to consciously choose whether or not to ingest a medical therapy, which water fluoridation undoubtedly is. This last point was, perhaps, the most common theme as we traveled to different cities—many Floridians were simply unwilling to compromise on the issue of personal sovereignty, which demands consent before medical treatment.

Outside of Florida, a dentist named Dr. Rich Fischer, who incidentally had written a 1987 article in *Homeopathy Today* outlining potential health risks of fluoridation, introduced me to the dedicated professional group International Academy of Oral Medicine and Toxicology (IAOMT). From this group, I learned how dentistry can be reimagined to be more harmonious with the body's natural healing processes, while avoiding toxicity from substances like mercury and fluoride.

Other partners in our visits to cities across Florida included Scott Kiley, his wife Jill Kiley, and Justin Robert, all of whom had long advocated for the removal of fluoride from public water systems and were stalwart partners in this cause. Listening to depositions and lectures by Michael Connett, the lawyer who successfully sued the U.S. Environmental Protection Agency (EPA) over their under-regulation of fluoride, was entertaining and invaluable. I will never forget watching footage of officials from the Centers for Disease Control and Prevention, the EPA Chemical Safety and Pollution Office, and the EPA Office of Water being deposed by Michael. They squirmed under oath as they admitted to not having sufficiently studied the safety of water fluoridation. Instead, they seemed to prioritize preserving water fluoridation's status as a public health achievement over the preferences and safety concerns of their community members. I felt as though I was watching replays from the COVID-19 pandemic's greatest (worst) policy hits.

In Bartow, I got to know Mayor Trish Pfeiffer, whose challenges with a chronic immune condition honed her appreciation for the relationship between environment exposures and health outcomes. She led efforts in her city to end water fluoridation, but faced headwinds from her fellow city commissioners, most of whom appeared afraid to veer from "accepted" public health recommendations. This was a pattern that would be repeated across several municipalities in Florida. We encountered it in Miami-Dade County too, but thanks to the indefatigable and inspiring leadership of Commissioner Roberto Gonzalez, the county overrode the mayor's veto and became the largest in modern history to vote to end the practice of water fluoridation. This was the most unlikely of outcomes, but became a reality when a single, intensely pensive commissioner—undoubtedly swayed by the power and virtue of the moment—changed his vote.

The final stage of the movement here in Florida unfolded when Governor Ron DeSantis signed Agriculture Commissioner Wilton Simpson's Florida Farm Bill, which effectively banned the addition of fluoride to public water systems. As of July 1, 2025, cities in Florida can no longer add fluoride to their water. This is a victory for ethical public health, science-based decision-making, and personal sovereignty, because treatment without consent (outside of emergency settings) is an affront to the dignity of human beings.

Our efforts have been successful in Florida, but water fluoridation is one of many issues we face as Americans that involve attacks on individual sovereignty, scientific integrity, and the need to pursue right action even when doing so is unpopular. Other important public health issues that wax similar themes include policies that involve vaccination, food additives and pesticides, and geoengineering, to name a few. Ultimately, our capacity as humans to navigate all of these issues and reach outcomes that best serve humanity will depend on our ability to raise our consciousness, both at the individual and collective level. Only then will we be able to hear what the universe is telling us.

As human beings, we each carry a tremendous amount of stress, tension, and trauma, either through our own experiences or the epigenetic experiences of our ancestors—and most of us carry both. These experiences and the imprints they leave on our bodies, minds, and spirits shape our beliefs, perspectives, and ultimately, our consciousness.

I have been fortunate to have had the opportunity to unburden myself of much of the personal and epigenetic weight I once carried. For me, that journey started with meeting my soulmate, Brianna, in 2005, and then working with a healer and former Navy Seal named Christopher Maher in December 2019. Falling in love created a personal crisis for me, as the purity of love challenged, mercilessly, the corrupt constructs I had consciously and unconsciously created to cope with the stress and trauma I carried within myself. That crisis and the grace of God opened the door to a body of knowledge about how to de-stress and de-tense through specific physical exercises and stretches, mediation, and transmutation that drew on Chinese medicine, meridian theory, and other ancient knowledge. And as I de-stressed and de-tensed, my consciousness rose.

While my path to healing has been and continues to be intense, every step we take to care for our souls—like meditation, yoga, time spent in nature, and time spent engaging in activities we enjoy—helps elevate our consciousness. And as our consciousness rises, it becomes easier to see what old practices and beliefs are out of alignment with our innate connection with divinity and the universe ... and how to resolve all that is incongruous. As the saying goes, we have a lot of work to do. But the more of us that cross this threshold, the sooner we will be able to manifest the future that humanity deserves.

Editor's Biography

By: Dr Hardy Limeback, BSc, PhD, DDS

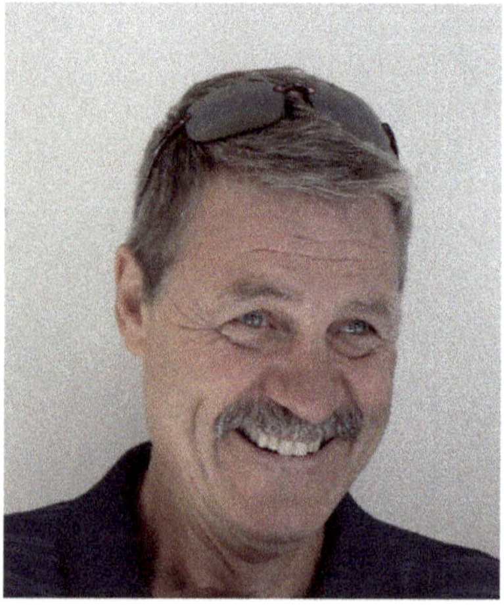

I'm a retired full professor, now Professor Emeritus, at the Faculty of Dentistry, University of Toronto. I was the head of Preventive Dentistry for 18 years. I started with a BSc and PhD in Biochemistry then entered dental school, graduating in 1983, all at the University of Toronto. As a professor I ran my own laboratory studying the proteins responsible for tooth development and the effects of fluoride on teeth and bones. I authored/co-authored over 150 papers, book chapters and abstracts. The last big project I undertook was a textbook in preventive dentistry ('Comprehensive Preventive Dentistry', Wiley-Blackwell, June 2012). My academic service included president of the Canadian Association for Dental Research (1998-99) and member of the 2006 US National Academy of Sciences Subcommittee on Fluoride in Drinking Water. I worked part-time as an associate general dentist, as Chief Dentist for the Metropolitan Toronto Homes for the Aged, then operated and owned my own dental office from 1993-2014. I still practiced dentistry part-time until 2020, then gave up my license. I continue to be engaged with the public on social media and publish scientific papers primarily on calcium phosphates in oral health, with a focus on hydroxyapatite.

Introduction

"The right to search for the truth implies also a duty; one must not conceal any part of what one has recognized to be true."

—Albert Einstein (1879 - 1955)

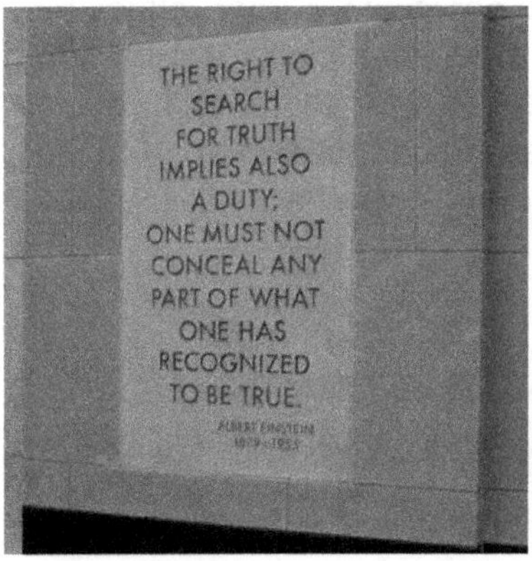

Engraving of an Einstein quote at the entrance of the National Academies of Sciences, Washington DC, USA.

I took the photo as I entered the building to start the three-year review of fluoride in drinking water with the other committee members of the NRC Review (Doull, 2006).

Motivation for this book

DR ROBERT DICKSON MD of Calgary Alberta was inspired by the book *Canary in a Covid World*. He discussed the idea of using a similar format by videoconference with colleagues who were opposed to fluoridation.

Dr Dickson had been battling for decades to keep fluoride out of the drinking water in the Canadian city of Calgary, which now provides fluoridated water to 1.8 million citizens. Success came when Calgary City Council voted to remove fluoride from its drinking water in 2011. Since then, Dr Dickson has been vilified in the province of Alberta by the media, public health officials, and by a lawyer/professor of ethics at the University of Calgary.

After a long legal battle defending himself against complaints made by that group to the College of Physicians and Surgeons of Alberta, the self-regulating body that oversees physicians in Alberta, Dr Dickson still faced a Tribunal Trial in January 2025. He reluctantly conceded to the single charge of professional misconduct after the three major charges were dropped, was levied a hefty fine, and ordered to take a public engagement retraining course. Readers will find his chapter riveting.

I, too, was wrongly accused of spreading misinformation about fluoridation in 1999. The negative outcomes I experienced for daring to speak the scientific and dental truth are described in *my* chapter in this book.

I defended myself against a formal complaint made to the University of Toronto president and the Royal College of Dental Surgeons of Ontario (RCDSO), the college that provides licenses to dentists in Ontario, Canada to practice dentistry. As you will read, I survived that challenge but my career was drastically curtailed.

Chapter contributors to *Fluoride Harm* have very telling accounts of what they experienced as vocal opponents of the long-standing (80-year-old) practice of fluoridation. Only the occasional author relates he or she did not have to pay too high of a personal cost for opposing fluoride use but felt so compelled to speak out for moral and ethical reasons that they spent most of their adult lives dedicated to convincing others that fluoride does more harm than good, especially when added to community drinking water.

Background:

Fluoride is the negative ion (anion) of the atom fluorine, the 13th most abundant element in the earth's crust. It is the most reactive of the halogens (a family of 'salt makers') on the periodic table with chemically-related chlorine, bromine and iodine. Fluorine (which exists only as a diatomic gas, F_2) is the most reactive nonmetal in chemistry because of its extreme electronegativity, and is extremely toxic. It is found mostly in the earth's crust as a relatively insoluble fluorite, CaF_2. The purest grade of fluoride is used to make hydrogen fluoride (HF), from which so many fluorine-containing organic compounds are made. The fluorine-carbon bond is highly stable. This is why so many man-made organic chemicals contain the fluorine atom. In mining, fluorite is called 'fluorspar' and it is added to iron ore as 'flux' to allow molten ore to flow better (the Latin for 'fluor' is *fluere*, meaning 'to flow').

When volcanoes erupt, they spew out fluorine gas (from molten fluorspar). Volcanic smog (vog) can contain harmful gases, including fluorine. Vog should be avoided until the air is clear again (CDC, 2024). The ash contaminates the ground water and increases the fluoride levels, which can pose health risks such as dental and skeletal fluorosis (Tomašek et al., 2022). The Rift Valley in Africa, where there is a string of volcanos, provides a good example of contaminated groundwater leading to endemic fluorosis. People living in a few of the small Italian towns on the slopes of Mt Etna and Mt Vesusius often have what was traditionally known as *denti scritti* or *denti neri* which describes the striations and discoloration of dental fluorosis.

Smokestacks of industry, especially the phosphate industry, are the equivalent of volcanoes in that they also spew harmful fluoride gases. Environmental laws no longer allow polluting industries to scorch nearby plant life (e.g. the grass on nearby farms, in which crippling fluorosis in cattle has been documented), and harming humans nearby. This is summarized nicely by FAN, 2012. Fluoridation water additives are derived from the air-pollution control devices (wet scrubbers) of the phosphate fertilizer plants.

Endemic fluorosis is common in India and China. Groundwater sources for drinking water contain unacceptably high levels of fluoride through increased dissolution of fluorspar and geothermal release of fluoride into the aquifers. This leads to many adverse health effects, not just for mineralized tissues such as bones and teeth, but in soft tissue organs including the brain (Wei et al., 2019). The story of how fluoridation came to be, despite the knowledge that fluoride is very harmful to human health, is summarized by the National Institute for Dental and Craniofacial Research (NIDCR, 2024).

The public health policy of fluoridation, instituted in America at the end of WWII, was initially opposed by the American Dental Association because the idea of medicating people without their consent by adding a drug to their drinking water was regarded as unethical. But there were very powerful people in charge at that time who convinced American legislators that this was necessary to help solve the dental decay crisis in America.

In Chapter 1 David Kennedy summarizes the nefarious means of how people in power not only hid the ill-effects of fluoride from the public but convinced dentists and public health to promote fluoridation in the US, all to protect the atomic bomb program, as well as other industries that were generating fluoride pollution. This was carefully documented in Christopher Bryson's book "The Fluoride Deception".

The first 'clinical trial' conducted in an attempt to show fluoridation reduces dental decay was started in 1945 by Arnold et al., (1953) with Grand Rapids Michigan being the first city in the world to be fluoridated. This was followed by flawed 'clinical trials' and cross-sectional ecological studies that were conducted in other countries such as Canada, Australia, and New Zealand (Sutton, 1960).

Other countries soon followed the American lead and instituted fluoridation. Some conducted their own 'trials', comparing cities that were fluoridated to non-fluoridated in crude unblinded, non-randomized trials. Some countries did not like medicating people through the water supply and offered their citizens a choice of purchasing fluoridated salt. Where the Americans decided fluoridation was a good idea, other English-speaking countries followed (Canada, New Zealand, Australia, Ireland, and England). Some South American countries also favoured fluoridation.

A select handful of European cities experimented with fluoridation of water but those countries either abandoned fluoridation or banned the programs altogether after considering the lack of ethics (individual autonomy vs benefitting all), the lack of evidence for effectiveness and the obvious high cost-to-benefit ratios (Ruggeri, 2025). When fluoridated salt was used as an alternative in processed foods without citizens knowing about it, that was rejected and 'fluoridized' salt was made available in stores so that citizens had a choice. Fluoridating milk was tried (Marthaler, 2013). The general decline of caries in countries that experimented with fluoridated salt and milk, never proved those approaches worked in the background of improvement of overall oral health and the widespread use of fluoride toothpaste. None of these countries had ever experienced the devastation of endemic fluorosis where the teeth and bones are permanently damaged by ingestion of high levels of fluoride in drinking water. Those that did avoided artificial fluoridation altogether.

The World Health Organisation set the upper limit of how much fluoride should be in drinking water at 1.5 mg/L but the USA initially set its upper limit at 2.4 mg/L for Americans, claiming that even with those levels of exposure, the dental fluorosis which previously occurs in about 1% of Americans, would only increase to no more than 10%, would be mild, and was nothing to worry about. The American EPA adjusted that upper limit to 4.0 ppm in 1985 and it remained at this level against internal expert advice (Doull, 2006; Carton, 2006) reaffirming 4.0 ppm as a "safe" upper limit in July 2024. Dental fluorosis, the visible evidence of fluoride overdose while young, now afflicts over half of American teens (Neurath et al., 2019). It is often moderate to severe and requires costly cosmetic dentistry to repair in a significant portion of young adults.

So now 80 years after the first fluoridation trial, the American Dental Association (ADA) has successfully lobbied its colleague health care organizations such as the American Medical Association (AMA), the American Academy of Pediatricians (AAP), the American Public Health Association (APHA), the American Association of Public Health Dentistry (AAPHD), and even the International Association for Dental Research (IADR), to all go along with whatever fluoride recommendations they devise.

The ADA lobbying efforts extended to government agencies, especially the US Human Health Services (HHS) and the organizations that function under its direction: the US Public Health Service (USPHS), the Food and Drug Association (FDA), and the Center for Disease Control (CDC). Other government agencies have also protected fluoridation. For example, the FDA denied that it should be regulating fluoride in the drinking water even though fluoride is consumed as a food in bottled water and added to the food supply; the FDA position is its duty is only to align their bottled-water regulations with the decisions of other agencies regarding drinking water. The EPA colluded with the HHS to protect fluoridation by ignoring evidence of harm even at the current level of 0.7 mg/L.

The decision to lower the 'optimal level' of fluoride in the drinking water by 2015, from the range of 0.7 to 1.2 mg/L to a single maximum of 0.7 mg/L, was made in order to reduce the incidence of dental fluorosis without any real evidence that this change would affect the incidence of either dental fluorosis or cavities.

Regulators in other English-speaking countries, such as Health Canada, have followed the lead of the Americans, sometimes even using American dental experts to help them develop their own recommendations, so that they are not in conflict with the Americans. They all seemingly fell in line with the Americans and also recommended the 0.7 mg/L fluoride in drinking water as their optimal level for, supposedly, preventing tooth decay.

Thus, fluoridation is still practiced in most English-speaking countries. However, as mentioned before, nearly all European countries have either never started it, have abandoned fluoridation or experimented with salt or milk fluoridation. The figure below demonstrates the current state of public health measures of medicating people with fluoride throughout the world (taken from Till et al., 2025, Supplement)

Supplemental Figure 1 A. World map showing percentage of population receiving community water fluoridation or salt fluoridation. Blue shades represent countries with water fluoridation. From lightest to darkest: 0-25%, 26-50%, 51-75%, 76-100%. Purple shading represents countries with salt fluoridation. Population estimates are based on data provided by the British Fluoridation Society, Extent of Water Fluoridation and data reported by Mullane et al (2016). doi:10.1922/CDH_3707O'Mullane31

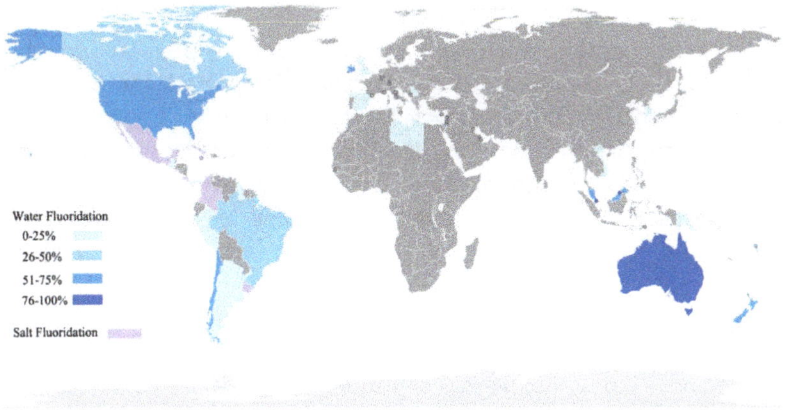

The status quo on the non-consensual drugging of citizens in the service of "public health" has continued for over 3/4 of a century (since 1945). It's been labeled by the CDC as "One of the top 10 public health measures of the 20th century" but as more and more evidence, supported by well-done studies, has been published over the last 25 years, it looks as if the public health promotion of medicating the general public by adding fluoride to the water supply, or in salt, or in milk, is turning out to be one of the top 10 mistakes of the 21st century.

This book is a collection of revealing personal stories. The chapter authors are scientists, doctors, dentists, knowledgeable activists, and victims who have met with personal and professional difficulties in trying to convince the authorities about the harm of fluoride, and why it is ruining our health. Included are the stories of journalists and scientists who have struggled to report the 'other side' of the story.

The authorities refuse to acknowledge that it is *not* an innocent element that is simply added as a dental-decay medication to our tap water by municipalities on the recommendation of public health authorities, which implies it is a nutrient.

It is generally accepted that the product injected into our water supply and food supply is neither a nutrient nor a pharmaceutical grade drug. The EPA did a 'bait and switch' on Americans and other countries followed suit.

Rather than use purified sodium fluoride, which is added to toothpaste, they use contaminated effluent primarily from the aluminum and phosphate fertilizer industries. The EPA even admitted that this was a low-cost solution to their headache of policing corporate fluoride pollution in 1983 (See Appendix I).

Fluoride Harm attempts to cover all fluoride issues, including fluoride compounds used as a pesticides and fungicides. This book is generally not a detailed scientific book intent on critiquing the evidence of the benefit of fluoridation, although doubts about the benefits have been expressed by most of the chapter contributors.

There are 36 chapters written by authors from the US, Canada, the UK, Ireland, New Zealand, and Australia. Supported by scientific evidence and documents, the book is well cited. Each contributor is introduced with a short biography followed by his or her story in their own words in a conversational-style, easy-to-read prose.

Most readers will not be aware of the struggles of the writers of the chapters, what transpired behind the scenes, and how many were unfairly treated.

After reading the book, the reader will understand why there has been so much controversy over the use of fluoride as a medication to treat dental decay. That controversy continues today and, even as this manuscript is being submitted for publication, many changes have occurred in Canada and the USA.

Current Climate

The most impactful changes are as follows:

2024

- In an historic lawsuit against the EPA, a federal judge ruled that fluoridation poses an unreasonable risk because of its potential harm to developing human brains. The EPA appealed.
- The appointment of Robert F. Kennedy Jr. to HHS Secretary who promises to end fluoridation in the US.
- Florida State Surgeon General Dr Joseph Ladapo declared fluoridation was public health "malpractice".

2025

- Utah and Florida banned community water fluoridation.
- Calgary, Alberta, in Canada has reinstituted fluoridation as of June 30, 2025.
- Many more American state legislatures filed bills to ban fluoridation or rescind state fluoridation mandates.
- The US FDA proposed a ban on pediatric fluoride supplements.
- The Make America Healthy Again (MAHA) Report identified fluoride exposure as an environmental threat to health being investigated in an inter-agency initiative.
- Campaigners in Canada, New Zealand, Australia, and the UK work to leverage the US momentum in their countries.

The struggle continues. The truth will show that fluoridation can no longer be considered 'safe and effective'. Fluoride ingestion is dangerous from any source. It must be drastically reduced worldwide in order to reduce the toxic burden on future generations.

How we all got F'd (Fluoridated)

By: Dr David Kennedy, DDS, MIAOMT

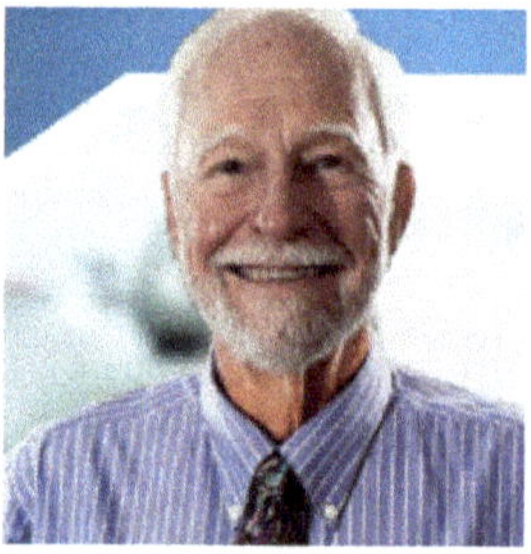

ABOUT: *Dr David Kennedy practiced dentistry for over 30 years. He retired from clinical practice in 2000. He is the Past President of the "International Academy of Oral Medicine and Toxicology" (IAOMT) and has lectured to dentists and other health professionals all over the world on the subjects of preventive dental health, mercury toxicity, and fluoride. Dr Kennedy is internationally recognized as an advocate for safe drinking water and biological dentistry, as well as a leader in the field of preventive dentistry. Dr Kennedy is also a pilot, accomplished author, and director of the award-winning documentary film "Fluoridegate: An American Tragedy."*

CHAPTER 1

"By focusing on fluoridation instead of diet and dentist-access, organized dentistry allowed a national dental health crisis to occur on its watch and created a new one—dental fluorosis."

—Dr David Kennedy, DDS, MIAOMT

I ONCE THOUGHT fluoride was benign and a good thing. It was what I was taught; fluoride use is a platform of the American Dental Association (ADA). I changed my mind after my good friend Roy Kupsinel, MD redlined the false information he saw in the first draft of my book chapter on preventive dentistry and the benefits of fluoride (Kennedy, 1993). He explained that I needed to "rethink my position" and recommended that I read John Yiamouyiannis' book, *Fluoride the Aging Factor* (1983).

Since that time, I've actively opposed fluoridation programs because it is abundantly clear from both toxicological and epidemiological studies that fluoride is not a nutrient; fluoride is dangerous. Consuming fluoride evokes acute illness in many, especially in the endocrine and gastrointestinal systems. It accumulates in bones and organs over time, causing subtle harm throughout the body. Fluoride exposure compromises overall health for the same reason it inhibits cavity-causing oral bacteria—because it is a poison.

Origin Stories

The dental mythology about fluoride began as a coverup. It began because of an unholy alliance between corporate polluters, World War II leadership charged with creating the atomic bomb, and a compliant Public Health Service (FAN, 2012b). It began in order to hide the evidence of deaths and serious harm to Manhattan Project workers, and to thwart litigation from farmers downwind of plants whose crops and animals were sickened and dying because of fluoride pollution (Bryson & Griffiths, 1997; FAN, 2012a; FAN, 2014).

I first learned this history from Clifford T. Honicker (Honicker, 1989), an indefatigable researcher and the first director of the American Environmental Health Studies Project, Inc. (AEHSP). He spoke at a public forum in Worcester, Massachusetts, in 1996. He spoke, in part, about the chief toxicologist of the Manhattan Project, Harold Hodge from the School for Medicine and Dentistry in Rochester, NY, and later at the School of Dentistry at Harvard University. Honicker had personally examined boxes of formerly "Top Secret" documents from World War II that were declassified after fifty years.

Hodge promoted surreptitiously feeding radioactive material to pregnant women and openly feeding large doses of toxic fluoride to Black laborers in the "interest of science." In my opinion, it is not hyperbole to call this man a murderer cut from the same cloth as Josef Menegle. I recorded Honicker's talk but he asked me not to show the video until after two books on the subject were published (Welsome, 1999; Bryson, 2006). That videotape is now archived (Appendix A).

My passion against the dental narrative in favor of any fluoride use ignited when I read the report of three-year-old William Kennerly who died in 1974. After the dental hygienist at the city clinic had swabbed little Billy's teeth with a fluoride gel and then handed him a glass of water, Billy swallowed instead of spit. He immediately began vomiting and sweating. The dentist dismissed the mother's concerns, just like the emergency room staff at Brookdale Ambulatory Pediatric Care Unit who kept mother and child waiting for over two hours, dismissed them. Billy slipped into a coma and died that day.

During the subsequent trial, the dentist and the hygienist testified that they had no idea that fluoride was dangerous. The coroner testified that Billy had enough fluoride in his system to kill eight children. Ultimately, the New York State Supreme Court awarded the family $750,000 (O'Grady, 1977).

As a third-generation dentist, I could not fathom how my profession could condone putting such a dangerous poison in a child's mouth, let alone in drinking water! Young children routinely swallow unsafe amounts of toothpaste (Petrović et al., 2023) and there is no dose control over water consumption! Headaches, stomach aches, irritability, and rashes are frequent results. At first, I thought it was only a matter of education. However, my experience has taught me that fluoridation and fluoride use are maintained by fraud—fraudulent marketing, fraudulent science, and fraudulent politics.

Fraud is only one of the fluoridationist tools; they have others. Fluoridationists also promote scientific ignorance. Dentists are kept ignorant of toxicology. They know nothing about risk assessment, and they do not follow the laws that are designed to protect their dental office employees from the toxic materials used in dentistry, like fluoride and mercury. Instead, they are trained in marketing tricks and gaslighting techniques. Dr. Phyllis Mullenix was the first and last toxicologist to work in a dental research capacity—at Forsyth Dental Research Institute where Hodge often visited her lab (Bryson, 2006).

My Travels

The dental tooth-fairy tale is sustained through funding that has flowed from the government to marketeers. I've been face-to-face with Howard Pollick, the ADA fluoridation spokesperson, many times. He was deposed in an Escondido, CA, case about the source of his salary (Kennedy v. City of San Diego, D072337). It's complicated, but after the "blah, blah, blah," it boiled down to: the government was paying him.

He was paid $500,000 in 1990 by the state of California—taxpayer dollars—to conduct a dental survey that could be used to promote fluoridation. At the time, California was 48th out of the 50 states in percent of the population fluoridated. California had resisted fluoridating the public drinking water because its pesky citizens opposed this intrusion into their health choices more than a hundred times. Communities passed laws against fluoridation and sometimes, as in Los Angeles, reversed city council decisions with a referendum in order to keep this poison out of their drinking water.

Pollick's phony 1990 survey chose wealthy fluoridated San Francisco children who had regular preventive dental care. More than 60% of those children had sealants on vulnerable teeth, a practice I strongly recommend provided that time-release fluoride is not implanted into the child's mouth. Then he chose, for comparison, to use the Head Start children in non-fluoridated Los Angeles who had almost no sealants—only one out of two hundred. Not surprisingly, there was a difference in decay experience between these two very different populations.

Rich kids with two parents who have good dental care had fewer cavities than poor immigrant children whose parents worked all day. Poor children seldom saw a dentist. If they did see a dentist, it was a welfare dentist and only because of a visible problem or acute pain. The results of the improperly designed survey prompted by the California Dental Association was used to pressure the state legislature into passing a state mandate. Paid lobbyists claimed the difference between the two cities was due to the lack of fluoride in LA. Both the Democrats and the Republicans passed the mandatory fluoridation bill, Bill1995 AB733.

Cavities are a function of income and parental education—of good diet, good hygiene, and good dental care. Fluoridation won't address that. Children living in poorer areas will always have more cavities regardless of whether or not there is any amount of fluoride in the public drinking water. And Pollick, like other lobbyists from the dental and sugar industries (Neurath, 2025), knows it.

Pollick was a co-author on a large California Head Start study—this one properly designed, peer-reviewed, and published—that found absolutely no difference in early childhood caries (ECC) between fluoridated and non-fluoridated low-income communities; cultural patterns, such as falling asleep with a bottle of milk or juice, determined ECC experience (Shiboski et al., 2003).

My Battles

Except for a small group of profiteers, fluoridationists seldom engage in debate. I've traveled across this nation over 50 times and often was invited to discuss the validity of fluoridation claims. On very few occasions were fluoride-advocates willing to even show up, unless the city council demanded it. When they do show up, dental fluoridationists accompanied by the occasional duped pediatrician conveniently claim that the efficacy and safety are not debatable because it is government-approved, has been done for decades, and they are the "experts" who only want to "help the poor children." Fluoridationists claim that any semblance of fair debating would give the public the wrong idea that there are unanswered questions about safety and efficacy, and there aren't. "We know it's safe," shout the paid lobbyists, biased dentists, and ignorant shills.

In Modesto, California, the city council insisted on an open discussion, so I flew up from my home in San Diego. The pro-fluoridation side was the military USPHS, and the safe water side was myself and another citizen. After the "blah, blah" presentations, we were allowed to answer questions and discuss the issue. The USPHS nurse claimed that drinking any amount of optimally fluoridated water (1 ppm) gave everyone the ideal amount of fluoride to grow strong teeth that resist decay. This nurse obviously didn't consider that fluoride dosage is a function of the amount consumed.

I pointed out that drinking one liter of water with the so-called 'optimal 'concentration of 1 ppm caused dental fluorosis in children, and higher consumption caused more fluorosis. I gave the example of a newborn baby suffering from diabetes insipidus who experienced excessive thirst because it did not produce enough antidiuretic hormone (ADH). That baby must drink its weight in water every day to stay alive—an enormous fluoride dose of 1 mg/kg.

The flustered USPHS nurse who realized the implications of that dose blurted out that, "Hopefully, that baby will die before it's a problem." What can you say in reply to that sort of stupidity?

That's why the advocates steadfastly for 80 years have refused to debate. They might stand up in a forum or on a soapbox, but they won't actually debate. They can't answer questions and might say things like they hope babies with medical conditions die quickly. That's why they have to stick to the mantra "Fluoride is safe and effective without harm to anyone." They are ignorant and heartless shills.

I once flew into a beautiful quaint town at the top of the Shenandoah Valley to debate continuing fluoridation. The water operator was concerned, because he could read and asked for a discussion regarding the efficacy. He showed me the bags of Chinese silicofluoride his department added to the pristine well water. He thought that it was a shame to pollute clean water.

The USPHS had tapped a recent dental school graduate to support the addition of fluoride at the open meeting. She was a diligent student and had done her homework, reading the 2006 National Research Council (NRC) review of fluoride in drinking water and memorizing the 'safe and effective' mantra, a mantra that she repeated so often that I had to ask if she'd actually read the NRC review. Indignantly, she replied that she had read every page, so I asked if I could borrow her copy to show her an example of why no one should be drinking fluoride, especially not bottle-fed babies. She agreed.

I opened the book, and it flopped open to Table 8-2 at the end of Chapter 8 that Dr. Kathleen Thiessen had prepared, showing what dose caused what damage to the endocrine system, especially the thyroid. She'd even bookmarked it. Northern Virginia is part of the goiter belt, a problem of low iodine. The thyroid glands grow so large that the afflicted look like Mark Twain's Calaveras Frog.

I pointed out the minute amount of fluoride (0.03 mg/kg/day) in someone with an iodine deficiency would harm a thyroid while an average bottle-fed baby would be dosed at 0.25 mg/kg, a gross overdose.

Then I explained that babies with low thyroid function because of low iodine at birth (congenital iodine deficiency syndrome) are stunted in their physical and mental development. The condition was called cretinism until cretinism became a politically incorrect term—it is now called an IQ deficit.

I was not allowed to comment further that day, because they said I was being argumentative. Wasn't that the point of the debate? Apparently not. The safe and effective mantra is not debatable. Sadly, that community continues to fluoridate using Chinese products contaminated with arsenic, barium, cadmium, and God only knows what else because each batch of fluoridation chemicals is different. This stuff isn't quality-controlled. Just like it was in the 1940s, fluoridation water additives are the toxic waste products of industry.

My good friend and colleague, the late Jeff Green, had the right idea. His approach was to focus on the substance. He persistently reminded water workers and legislatures that first, nothing should be prescribed to people for ingestion that is not approved by the Food and Drug Administration (FDA) as safe as well as 99% pure, and second, nothing should be added to water that contains any known contaminant above the public health goal—the typical fluoride additive is 17% fluoride and 83% contaminants.

Regardless of the recommendations delivered by well-paid industry shills, the FDA has never approved fluoride for human consumption in order to prevent or treat cavities or any other disease that I know of. Not only is fluoride itself identified as a toxin, but each batch of fluoridation chemicals is invariably contaminated with a witch's brew of poisons such as arsenic, aluminum, lead, barium, etc. (Mullenix, 2014). Some batches also include radionuclides (radioactive contamination).

In the End

When a judge examined the testimony and science submitted in court in a lawsuit brought under the Toxic Substances Control Act (TSCA), he arrived at the conclusion of "unreasonable risk," just like I and so many others had decades ago (Chen, 2024). This historic court case (Case No. 17-CV-02162-EMC) was the first time fluoridation was on trial in a federal court with an appropriate jurisdiction and with verifiable plaintiff standing. Subsequent to the verdict, Health and Human Services (HHS) Secretary Robert F. Kennedy, Jr. advised that HHS no longer promotes fluoridation practice and curtailed the funding to the chief Centers for Disease Control and Prevention (CDC) fluoridation promoters.

The criminal waste-disposal program envisioned by the immoral dentist and toxicologist, Harold Hodge, as an expedient way to dispose of a toxic byproduct from nuclear weapon production soon will become a relic of the past. But this chapter should serve as a lesson to the military and our representatives that their task is to serve and protect the people, not weapon production and not corporate interests. If you don't protect the children of your nation, you inevitably will lose your nation.

As I write this in 2025, San Diego remains fluoridated, even though the citizens have voted it out three times since 1954. The city has spent more than $200 million to truck hydrofluorosilicic acid (HFSA) from Florida and add it to the public drinking water for the last 13 years. Not surprisingly, every city council member's office has non-fluoridated bottled water delivered, just like the state legislature and governor. They are debating whether to close restrooms and institute cuts to city services because their retirement funds have drained the public coffers, requiring over half a billion yearly to keep the golden parachutes, with thirteen monthly payments a year and retirement benefits greater than their working salaries. I've suggested they stop fluoridation, but they aren't listening to me. They keep on repeating the magic-potion mantra that has mesmerized them for years.

I have a plethora of references, but I will simply recommend you check out the bibliography of *Fluoride Harm* and watch some of the documentaries I've uploaded to my YouTube channel (@davidkennedydds). A good place to start is the acclaimed documentary, *Fluoridegate: An American Tragedy*, which was attacked by the censors. It has been seen by well over a million viewers—350,000 viewed it in just the first ninety days after its release.

I wasn't part of the early battles against fluoridation, but I'm grateful I have been a front-line participant in two significant campaigns to protect oral health during my lifetime, one against mercury amalgam fillings and the other against fluoride. Amalgam fillings were recently banned in Europe, have been non-existent in Japan and Norway for over a decade, and have been "not recommended" in the US since 2020 for young children, fertile women, pregnant or nursing mothers, those with neurological diseases such as multiple sclerosis, Alzheimer's disease, or Parkinson's disease, and anyone with impaired kidney function or a heightened sensitivity (allergy) to mercury.

For all of its rhetoric, the United States lags behind the rest of the world when it comes to protecting patients, consumers, and children. The American life span has dropped since the implementation of fluoridation 80 years ago, so now we live six years less than our non-fluoridated European cousins.

Like mercury amalgam, fluoridation has begun to be phased out in America thanks to the efforts of a concerned public and enlightened legislatures. I am optimistic that I will see the end of this criminal act, this American tragedy, in my lifetime.

AUTHOR'S NOTE: The contents of this piece include my opinions and my memories. Additional references are provided at the end of this book. I will share other references upon request.

Fluoride as a Hidden Cause of Acne

By: Melissa Gallico

ABOUT: *Melissa Gallico is a former FBI intelligence analyst, naval intelligence officer, and Fulbright scholar to the United Kingdom. She graduated with honors from Georgetown University with a degree in Science, Technology, and International Affairs and holds a master's degree in International Studies from the University of St. Andrews. She is the author of "The Hidden Cause of Acne: How Toxic Water Is Affecting Your Health What You Can Do About It," published in 2018 (second edition) with a foreword by Stephen Harrod Buhner.*

CHAPTER 2

"One percent out of 1100 cases presented evidence or undesirable side. effects from the fluoride therapy. Skin rashes, headaches, epigastric distress, varying from slight discomfort to bloody vomiting were among the symptoms. The lowered threshold of allergic patients to allergens or intoxicants such as fluoride is discussed. It is pointed out that if fluoride is the allergen or intoxicant, by the tablet method of administration, the source is readily removed by the discontinuance of the therapy. This cannot be readily accomplished when communal water supplies are the source."

—Reuben Feltman, DDS (1956)

WHEN I JOINED the Federal Bureau of Investigation, fresh off five years of active duty as a naval intelligence officer, I never imagined the subject of fluoride would consume my energy more than any case I'd encounter on the job. The turning point came a couple of years later when I returned to the United States from a year in Scotland as a Fulbright scholar at the University of St. Andrews. Immediately upon settling into my new home in South Florida, the familiar symptoms reappeared: difficulty sleeping, a vague mental haze, and—most impossible to ignore—painful, chronic cystic acne.

I consulted multiple dermatologists and other doctors regarding my acne over the years and tried a variety of treatments, but no one was able to provide an answer for why my skin reacted so violently when I lived in certain locations. If acne is caused by genetics, hormones, or bacteria, why was my face effortlessly clear when I lived in places as diverse as Scotland, Senegal, Tunisia, Curaçao, and Puerto Rico? Why was I still dealing with acne well into my twenties and beyond while living in New England, Jacksonville, Washington D.C., Norfolk, and Delray Beach?

My first clue as to the cause should have come years earlier, when I started washing my face with bottled water. Something about washing my skin with tap water felt uncomfortable at times, almost a burning sensation, leaving a sheen that couldn't be rinsed away. But I never suspected that drinking tap water could cause a reaction on my skin—or that fluoride could be the culprit—until one day when I was standing in my sister-in-law's kitchen, talking to her about my acne, a glass of tap water in my hand. Maybe it's because she lives in Polk County, the heart of the phosphate fertilizer industry, the industry that supplies America with the bulk of its fluoride, but for whatever reason, the question popped into my mind: could my acne be caused by drinking fluoride in the water?

The hypothesis seemed easy enough to test. I started drinking distilled water, the only water I knew to be free from fluoride at the time. The relief was immediate and striking. But while my skin improved dramatically, I still experienced occasional flareups of acne. Each time, I analyzed what I ate or drank and then searched scientific articles on PubMed to see if I had consumed a significant source of fluoride.

The learning curve was steep. Some sources of exposure were obvious in hindsight, such as pasta or rice made with fluoridated water at a restaurant, or beer from a fluoridated brewery. But why would wine contain fluoride? It's made from grapes, not water.

What I discovered surprised me: grapes from California are commonly treated with fluoride as a pesticide, often leading to wine with fluoride levels several times higher than those in fluoridated tap water. European authorities were the first to notice this troubling trend in 1989, after measuring high amounts of fluoride in wine imported from California.

As a curious person and a dog lover, I wondered if raisins were also high in fluoride, and whether that had been investigated as a possible cause of raisin toxicity in canines. I was struck to see that 1989 was the same year the ASPCA's Animal Poison Control Center began noticing that dogs who consumed grapes or raisins were developing acute kidney failure (ASPCA Animal Poison Control Center, 2004). This was the same year California reached the height of its use of fluoride pesticides on their grape and raisin crops—over 1.3 million pounds per year. It was also the year, according to the online database of California's Department of Pesticide Regulation, the state that supplied half the world's raisin supply suddenly stopped inspecting them for pesticides.

This suspicious convergence of events prompted me to look into the veterinary research on raisin toxicity in canines (did they consider fluoride?—no), the complex web of government pesticide restrictions and inspections (did they test for fluoride?—no), and the bizarre history of America's Raisin Administrative Committee and its long-running National Raisin Reserve (did it play a role in all this?—possibly).

The full story of American raisins is too long to include here, but if you search online for "*How to Keep Your Dentist from Killing Your Labrador Retriever,*" you'll likely find a several thousand-word article I published on *Medium* with further details (Gallico, 2016).

Other sources of fluoride are even more insidious. For example, poultry products were among the most difficult to root out, even though they caused some of my worst flareups. The reason some poultry products contain high amounts of fluoride is due to fluoride pesticides in their feed. Just like with humans, fluoride bioaccumulates in their bones—bones that are then used to make soup or stock, or crushed into powdered fragments that end up in mechanically deboned meat products, like lunchmeat or chicken hot dogs. A study published in the *Journal of Agricultural and Food Chemistry* by researchers at Oregon State University found that a single serving of chicken sticks could provide half of a child's upper limit of safety for fluoride (Fein and Cerklewski, 2001).

After moving to a non-fluoridated neighborhood and experimenting over many months with my diet, I was able to clear my skin completely. I suspected I was not the only person experiencing this strange reaction to fluoride so I shared everything I learned in a free ebook I posted online. In addition to explaining how to eliminate fluoride from the diet for clear skin, I summarized the existing research on fluoride sensitivity, a phenomenon that has been documented in one percent of the population since the earliest days of fluoridation (Feltman and Kosel, 1961). The number of positive emails I received in response to the ebook made me wonder if fluoride-induced acne—sometimes referred to as fluoroderma—is more common than anyone realizes.

When I received an email with the words "your book saved my life," I knew I had to share this information with a wider audience. I expanded my 70-page ebook into a full-length book and self-published it on Amazon. I eventually published a second edition called *The Hidden Cause of Acne* with a foreword by Stephen Harrod Buhner through Healing Arts Press, an imprint of Simon & Schuster (Gallico, 2018). While writing the book, I delved into the existing research on acne and found very little related to diet. A team at Johns Hopkins University conducted a comprehensive review of the scientific literature published on acne during the second half of the twentieth century and concluded that 99.6 percent of all acne studies failed to mention diet at all. The main exception was a series of studies that provided evidence acne is "a disease of Western civilization" and nonexistent amongst certain people groups who consume a traditional diet (Cordain et al., 2002). These findings later played a key role in the founding of the popular paleo diet.

Another subject I explored in the book was the genesis of public water fluoridation in the United States. Surely, there must have been comprehensive studies on its safety. Surely, trials were held to the highest standards attainable at the time. Unfortunately, as those of us who have already been down this rabbit hole can attest, this is not what happened. *The Case Against Fluoride* by Drs Paul Connett, James

Beck, and H. Spedding Micklem, details the inadequacy of the safety studies conducted on fluoridation (Connett, Beck, & Micklem, 2010). Christopher Bryson's book, *The Fluoride Deception,* painstakingly dissects the outside influence on the science at the time (Bryson, 2004).

This last point captured my attention. Underneath government platitudes about fluoride being *"safe and effective"* and *"one of the greatest health achievements of the twentieth century,"* lies a tragic but fascinating story about the biggest pollution scandal in American history.

Most opponents of fluoridation are aware that the fluoride added to water is a hazardous waste product of phosphate fertilizer mining. However, it's less commonly known that fluoride was the most litigated air pollutant of the twentieth century. According to the USDA, it caused more harm to domestic animals than any other air pollutant (U.S. Department of Agriculture, 1972, p. 41).

Until the 1950s, lawsuits over fluoride air pollution focused on damage to agriculture—cattle, peach trees, fish hatcheries, gladiolus crops. But in 1955, when industry lost the first personal injury lawsuit, every major fluoride polluter in the country joined the appeal. These were some of the biggest companies in the world—U.S. Steel, Reynolds Metals, the Aluminum Company of America—and they lost to a lone farmer and his wife who sued over a variety of health conditions caused by fluoride.

As corporate lawyers stated in their appeal of the 1955 ruling, acknowledging the negative health effects of fluoride would set a precedent that threatened industry's very existence. If they were vulnerable to litigation from anyone living near a smokestack, what about their own employees? Internal documents show that some of these companies had been concealing the harmful effects of fluoride on their factory workers for decades. The biased research they funded to shield themselves from future personal injury lawsuits ensured that the health risks of fluoridation would go widely unrecognized for generations to come. Meanwhile, dentists' claims about its supposed benefits (also heavily influenced by industry) were presented in court as proof of its safety.

Bryson's book about the pollution story behind fluoridation is compelling, but I wanted to see the primary source evidence myself. My efforts eventually led to Dr. Michael Dolan, who helps maintain a special collection of material on fluoridation at the University of Massachusetts Amherst Libraries (Appendix A). There—in stark black and white—reside thousands of pages of official documentation detailing the forgotten history of fluoride air pollution in America.

After sifting through nearly a century of research and correspondence, I created a limited series podcast called *#FPollution:*

The Pollution Story Behind Fluoridation. Whenever possible, I included interviews with key players—such as Dr. William Hirzy, former President of EPA Headquarters Professionals' Union—as well as other contributors to this anthology who witnessed the pollution story behind fluoridation firsthand.

As I write this chapter from my little corner of South Florida, my county is presently fluoride-free for the first time in years. The remaining holdout fell without much fanfare a few months ago. A local dentist quoted in the news said he didn't mind seeing it go. The studies are relatively old, he said, and more information should be gathered to determine if it's really safe.

This was a strong contrast from the last city council meeting I attended when a large group from the dental lobby loudly demanded fluoride's continued inclusion in the public water supply. They accused me of being an opportunist selling a book, a clear attempt to discredit my reputation. They did not see the irony in the fact that they sell fluoride treatments for a living, and that their primary spokesperson was a professional advocate who travels the country trying to stomp out local efforts to end fluoridation—the same lobbyist who later mocked me as "pimple lady" in a tweet about his victory at the meeting.

Florida is on the verge of banning fluoridation altogether. The Farm Bill recently passed by the Florida Senate would restrict the use of any water additive not classified as a "water quality additive." [Update: On July 1, 2025, Governor Ron DeSantis signed Senate Bill 700, also known as the Florida Farm Bill, into law, effectively banning fluoridation throughout the state.] I wonder how many people will suddenly notice improvements in their acne or other health issues, and never realize why.

Dogs rarely die from raisin toxicity anymore. The fluoride pesticide once commonly used on raisins has been largely replaced with other methods of pest control. Veterinarians never determined the cause of this odd turn in the experience of man's best friend.

Not every mystery is solved, but the pursuit often tells us more than we expect.

EDITORS' NOTE: We found a cancellation order for registered in the United States, which forbids the distribution, sale or use of those specific products (cryolite), published in the U.S. Federal Register with a June 8, 2021 effective date.

Doctor, Nurse, and Thyroid Power

By: Dr Richard Shames, MD

and

Dr Karilee H. Shames, RN, PhD

ABOUT: *Richard L Shames, MD is a graduate of Harvard and the University of Pennsylvania Medical School. After doing research at the NIH lab of Nobel prize winner Marshall Nuremberg, he became a founding member of the American Holistic Medical Association. Over the years he has also served as adjunct faculty at UCSF Medical Center and Florida Atlantic University. Currently, he is a telemedicine thyroid practitioner and coach at* www.ThyroidPower.com.

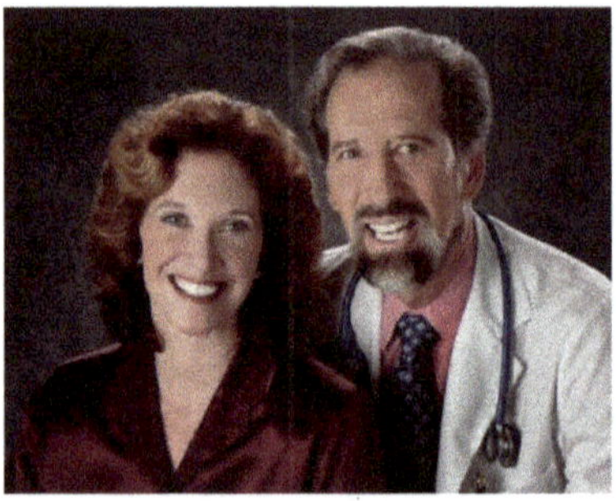

ABOUT: *Karilee H. Shames, RN, PhD is a clinical specialist in psychiatric nursing, and a certified holistic nurse. She served at Walter Reed Hospital and as assistant professor of nursing at Florida Atlantic University. A low thyroid person herself, Karilee has for many years led thyroid recovery support groups and now works with Dr Richard Shames providing telemedicine thyroid consults and speaking at Thyroid Power conferences.*

CHAPTER 3

"There are numerous mechanisms by which uncontrolled dosing of fluorides through water fluoridation can potentially harm thyroid function, the body and the brain."

—Dr Mark Hyman, MD (2016)

AS A DOCTOR-NURSE team with substantial health care training, we had always accepted water fluoridation as a safe and beneficial public health measure. We believed the official doctrine that fluoridation played a major role in large scale reduction of cavities in the general population. Plus, we understood that it easily provided this major benefit with no downside.

We grew up in the 1950s and 1960s. We always used fluoride toothpaste. We had fluoride treatment at the dentist. All throughout grade school and high school we were taught in order to fight dental decay, fluoride was added to water supplies and that fluoridation was one of the crowning achievements of the 20th century. We believed that these benefits were crucial to low-income communities where access to dental care was limited.

Later in college, and then professional school, we drew comfort from the endorsements of fluoridation by well-respected groups like the American Dental Association (ADA), the Communicable Disease Center (CDC), the Public Health Service (PHS), and the World Health Organization (WHO). It seemed like an irrefutable phalanx of agreement.

In fact, after we received our MD and RN degrees, we each considered ourselves to be emissaries of health education, revealing to those uninformed that fluoridation was silently 'strengthening' tooth enamel and thus lowering decay rates in the entire population, regardless of differences in socioeconomic status or individual dental hygiene habits.

After we completed our separate doctor and nurse training, we independently sought jobs at the same preventive medicine clinic. There we met, fell in love, and started a family. We raised our three kids with fluoride toothpaste. We gave them fluoride treatments at the dentist, we even once considered a doctor's advice for Karilee to take a 1 mg fluoride tablet each day during the latter part of her pregnancy, so as to strengthen the teeth of our unborn child. We ended up not following that advice, partly because Karilee had recently been diagnosed with Hashimoto's thyroiditis, the low thyroid condition common to her side of the family.

We worked together at the preventive medicine center, each getting more comfortable with our respective health care roles. At this time, we were firmly in the pro-fluoride camp. It seems to be such a widely accepted and successful practice, so ingrained in our understanding, that we never thought to question it.

That is, until many years went by and the clinic was seeing a significant percentage of low thyroid patients. This happened gradually as we became increasingly adept at treating low thyroid with an integrative approach, rather than simply one pill daily of prescription hormone.

Our center's huge success with these multifaceted thyroid programs gradually became well known. After a couple of magazine articles about what came to be called "better thyroid care" a major publishing house offered us a contract to write up some of our case histories for a new book on thyroid optimization.

The editors were especially interested in what was causing the surprisingly increasing incidence of thyroid problems all over the country. Our initial research to try answering this question led us to a startling revelation. To our astonishment, we uncovered good scientific evidence suggesting that fluoride could significantly disrupt thyroid function.

The deeper we dug, the more disbelief set in. Had we, along with so many others in the medical field, blindly accepted fluoridation, a widely used health practice that might actually have the significant side effect of diminishing thyroid function?

It seemed unbelievable. We had long assumed that if there were any harmful side effects, the various regulatory agencies would have intervened. We had never heard of anything to suggest that fluoridation could pose health risks. If there had been any sign of danger, surely this would have been thoroughly investigated. In fact, we had long ago dismissed the skeptics of fluoridation as being misinformed, untrained in health matters, or irrational with conspiracy theories.

We simply wanted to write a thyroid book, not go out on a limb of controversy about fluoride. There were plenty of other environmental chemicals coming under scrutiny. And yet, the fluoride factor seemed too huge to ignore. What we once considered an unquestionably useful and benign health maneuver was now demanding a closer look.

Karilee wanted to put these findings into the thyroid book's chapter on "Foods and Chemicals to Avoid." Richard was hesitant to do this, even though the research we were now reading was medically sound and from reliable sources.

He was concerned that including this material in our thyroid book would cast us as flaky and our book unreliable. We had heard about the 'fluorophobes' on the Internet and in town halls who used conspiracy theories to blame fluoride for every illness imaginable. Instead, we both wanted our thyroid book to be based entirely on the best new science.

But the more of the best new science we investigated, the more reasonable it seemed to indeed include fluoride in a list of foods and substances that thyroid glands don't like.

To be fair, we decided to also include studies that showed fluoridation to be both safe and effective for the general public.

That proved to be harder than we first thought. When we looked for fluoridation safety studies, we were amazed to find that there were none. How could the government have green-lighted and promoted a widespread health practice without the usual safety studies?

That was merely the first of many surprising eye-opening revelations. We began to dig deeper. Maybe the safety studies were done but under another name. Maybe approval came after a large clinical trial.

We decided to read up on the initial fluoridation debate in the late 40s and early 50s, and how it was originally decided that fluoride should be put into city water systems. We found that there was substantial controversy on this topic before it became approved. After all, fluoride had been used for years in Europe as an effective rodent poison. Also, the people that worked in the mining and refining of fluoride had long known it to be a grim workplace poison, capable of making factory workers very sick.

To help settle this post war controversy, it was decided to test for safety and efficacy on large numbers of real people. Two similar cities in Michigan were chosen for the clinical trial. Grand Rapids would have its municipal water supply fluoridated and nearby Muskegon would serve as a non-fluoridated control group.

At the end of 10 years, the incidence of tooth decay in both cities would be compared. It was thought that this large-scale study would settle the question once and for all.

At the end of five years (half the time allotted to the study) both cities had seen a substantial reduction in cavities. Something was having a real benefit, but it wasn't fluoride, because both cities saw the same reduction in childhood cavities, though only one city had been fluoridated.

Nevertheless, the study was ended at that half way point and fluoride was declared a winner, even though the process was not shown to reduce cavities in the test city above that of the control city. The benefit that both cities enjoyed was most likely due to improved hygiene and healthier eating all across the country in the post war economic boom. But that seemed not to matter. What people were told was that the fluoridated city had seen a definite decrease in cavities. Therefore, the process met with wide approval.

Shortly after the study of the two Michigan cities was stopped early, the Public Health Service, and the American Dental Association endorsed fluoridation. Then it was decided to fluoridate eight other cities in Michigan, even though the original study had ended early. Soon more and more cities all over the country followed suit.

Non-government scientists, however, were also on the job. A series of 1950s studies conducted by Pierre-M. Galetti, with other scientists, demonstrated that fluoride was toxic to thyroid function at concentrations as low as just a few parts per million. This meant that even the low concentrations of fluoride in city water were sufficient to slow down thyroid function. None of this research was mentioned in our medical training.

We kept digging, still hopeful that we would find a study, supporting the use of fluoride in municipal water supplies. No such luck, although there were plenty of studies about the definite effectiveness of fluoride when applied to teeth in a dentist office or when applied to the teeth at home via fluoride toothpaste. But it was hardly beneficial when applied to the teeth via fluoridated drinking water.

Plus, there was a distinct downside to the drinking water maneuver. When you drink fluoridated water, fluoride can build up inside your body and might adversely affect other tissues like the thyroid. Also, it is impossible to know how much fluoride any one person is getting. Some people drink much more tap-water than others, such as athletes on hot days. What about the amount of fluoride that's in the water used for bottled coffee or tea drinks, plus soda and juices? How much gets inside the body when we shower or bathe in fluoridated water? Basically, there's no way to tell how much some people might be ingesting.

What if the big tap water drinker also is one of the millions of people who already have a tendency for low thyroid? At this point in our questioning, Rich remembered something from his medical school pharmacology class. The professor had stated forcefully that, "Human body chemistry is extremely complex. There is no active substance that when added to the body has just one effect. Instead, there are always multiple effects, some good, some bad." Basically, it was magical thinking that fluoridation could have a wonderful beneficial effect on teeth and be totally free of side effects elsewhere in the body.

Now that we had dug more deeply into high-quality peer-reviewed fluoride research, it became clear to us that fluoridation of drinking water was only MINIMALLY effective in regards to children's teeth, and

NOT effective at all in preventing cavities in adult teeth. Moreover, it now seemed to be capable of having an important thyroid side effect.

Despite all of this, more and more cities joined the increasingly loud drum beat for fluoridation. Looking over the government fluoride literature from that time, all one found there were endorsements and opinion reviews, not true studies of safety and effectiveness. Fluoride in tooth paste and at the dentist's office appeared safe and effective. Fluoridated drinking water was neither.

Also, we now found that part of this drumbeat was the deliberate minimizing of anti-fluoride research. Here is but one of many such instances. Studies had summed up fluoridation's effectiveness on teeth by describing it as amounting to about 40% reduction in cavity formation (CDC, 1999). This was a relative reduction. The absolute saving was about a ½ of a tooth surface out of 128 tooth surfaces.

That is a very poor showing for any medicine or medical maneuver. Nevertheless, the pro-fluoridation forces touted this research project all around the country as showing that water fluoridation yielded a 40% reduction in cavities. That is not at all true, but it is what millions of people heard.

Even though the initial and follow up impetus for fluoridation was, shall we say, a bit questionable, more cities began to utilize the process. There should have been numerous safety studies, but none could be found.

Such studies were needed even more, now that the substance being put into the water supply was usually not actual sodium fluoride, but instead was hydrofluorosilicic acid. This is a toxic byproduct of the phosphate fertilizer and aluminum industries that reacts with water to yield fluoride. But not only fluoride. It yields a number of other chemicals and heavy metals as well. That's because it is obtained by scrubbing the inside of the smokestacks at fertilizer plants.

Surely someone would have performed safety studies on this byproduct that was now being substituted for fluoride in everyone's drinking water. Once again, amazement. No, such studies have ever been done on hydrofluorosilicic acid. One would think that the mayors, city councils, and water departments of communities considering fluoridation would want that information.

Nevertheless, in the early 50s, the Public Health Service gave its blessing to the use of this alternate source of fluoride, without having researched it adequately. At that time no one had any data on the long-term detrimental health effects of the silico-fluorides. Even now, neither the EPA or the CDC have data on the safety of this product that a great many of us are still drinking today.

According to researcher Myron J. Coplan, co-author of the famous Dartmouth study, about 90% of all fluoride-adjusted water today is treated with a silico-fluoride chemical (Coplan et al., 2007). Whereas laboratory research was initially performed using pure sodium fluoride, this is not what's being added today to municipal water supplies as they fluoridate. And when communities do use sodium fluoride, it is also a contaminated by-product of industry.

In fact, Dr. Mike Coplan together with Dr. Roger Masters and other scientists found an association between the presence of silico-fluorides in drinking water and the harmful uptake of lead in young children in several studies (Maas et al., 2007; Masters et al., 1999; Masters et al., 2000). This is in addition to possible fluoride poisoning. According to the national library of medicine's tox-net database, hydrofluorosilicic acid is easily capable of accidental poisonings in the people who must work with it.

As for the rest of us, the concentration of silicofluoride put into our water supply may not be toxic initially, but who is monitoring the long-term accumulation and total intake from multiple sources such as dental treatments, fluoride toothpaste at home, plus the amount in various foods and drinks?

The Department of Transportation guidelines for hydrofluorosilicic acid say "TOXIC: inhalation, ingestion, or skin contact may cause, severe injury, or death." Workers handling such a dangerous product are advised to utilize eye and face protection, respiratory protective equipment, and protective clothing especially for the feet and legs. This toxic waste product might cost the fertilizer company thousands of dollars per truckload to dispose of it properly, but instead they get paid to unload it full strength into city reservoirs.

If we as health professionals had not heard of such hazards, then it was most likely the general public had not heard about them either. We began to wonder what was the experience in other countries. We were surprised to learn that only 2% of Europe fluoridates their water, and overall, water fluoridation reaches less than 5% of the world population. A number of countries, including India, Japan, Finland, Denmark, Sweden, and Holland, have either rejected or banned the addition of this industrial waste product into community drinking water supplies.

Then we found out that large studies in New Zealand showed little or no difference in the teeth of children living in fluoridated and non-fluoridated communities. That is, except for one thing. Fluoridated communities had way more cases of dental fluorosis—the visible defect in teeth enamel from too much fluoride early in life. In its mildest forms, dental fluorosis appears as white mottling or striation on teeth. Moderate to severe dental fluorosis is unsightly and damages dental function (Colquhoun, 1984; Colquhoun, 1987; Colquhoun, 1994).

Meanwhile, our thyroid research had revealed that the thyroid problems were increasing steadily in the general population. Many doctors and epidemiologists were beginning to refer to the situation as the "thyroid epidemic". Only it was still unclear why the number of cases was increasing at such an alarming rate.

We had earlier become acquainted with the widespread health hazards of insecticide pollution from the 1980's book *Silent Spring* by Rachel Carson. More focus on danger to the thyroid and adrenal glands was the 1990s environmental volume called *Our Stolen Future*. We began to wonder if one of the chemicals causing such a high incidence of thyroid imbalance might be all that fluoride in our drinking water.

To understand the scale of the problem, consider this. At one point in our book writing, we learned that Synthroid, one of many thyroid medicines, was the second largest selling drug in the country. Checking with pharmacists, we heard that drugstores were filling more prescriptions for thyroid pills than almost any other category of medication.

It began to look as if the thyroid epidemic might be due in part to the bombardment of our collective thyroid glands by chemicals polluting the environment, some of which were once considered to be helpful and without any harmful side effects. (The now banned insecticide DDT is but one example.)

Our medical office was near that of John Lee MD, a long-time practicing physician, lecturer, and author of the national bestseller, *What Your Doctor May Not Tell You about Menopause*. He reported to us that in his many years of observations, vulnerable people in his practice were either low thyroid or normal thyroid, depending on whether or not they lived in a fluoridated community. In fact, he has seen patients who had gone in and out of hypothyroidism solely related to their moving into and away from cities with fluoride added to the water.

This crucial observation was confirmed later by a large study in England. The researchers analyzed data from nearly 8000 medical clinics. They found that areas with higher fluoride levels in the drinking water had about double the prevalence of hypothyroidism, compared to areas with lower fluoride levels (Peckham et al., 2015).

Of major interest to us in the late 1990s was a statement released from the National Treasury Employees Union, chapter 280. This union represented 1500 scientists, engineers, lawyers, and other professionals at the Environmental Protection Agency headquarters in Washington, DC.

Their statement reads "Our epidemiology studies suggest a causal link between fluoridation and medical problems such as cancer, genetic damage, neurological impairment and bone pathology." These union members were not "fluorophobes" from the Internet, but were instead scientists and other solid, concerned professionals employed by a major health guarding agency of the US government. If these scientists and professionals strongly felt that fluoride could be implicated as a causal link to various diseases, then linking it to thyroid was now a distinct possibility (Hirzy, 1999).

Now came the last straw. Our investigation into the history of thyroid treatment turned up something startling. Fluoride had once been used by the medical profession to deliberately slow down overactive thyroids. In the early twentieth century doctors in the United States, and especially Great Britain used fluoride, not in the water supply, and not directly applied to the teeth, but instead as a prescribed drug to be taken internally in order to slow down thyroid hormone production as a way of treating hyperthyroidism (high thyroid).

Because of the development of newer anti-thyroid medicines, including propylthiouracil (PTU) and methimazole (Tapazole), fluoride has not been used to treat hyperthyroidism for many decades. Only now, it seems that fluoride is still being used, although unknowingly, to slow down thyroid function in large numbers of previously normal people.

At this point we were no longer hesitant to discuss the fluoride topic in our upcoming Thyroid Power book. In fact, we were now seeing it as a "duty to warn." We were hoping to reach people in government and private agencies, who were still in thrall of fluoride's supposed benefit without side effects.

Even as more and more deleterious fluoride side effects became known to scientists, some of those in power refused to believe it. This is not hard to understand. The Public Health Service and various other agencies promoting fluoridation are unlikely to ever take responsibility for committing the most colossal mistake in the history of government science.

Here's a brief example of what the government might call damage control. In 1990 the environmental protection agency fired the office of drinking water's chief toxicologist, Dr. William Marcus. He was dismissed for refusing to remain silent on new research showing multiple fluoride risk issues. Dr. Marcus sued for reinstatement and won his case when the facts came out in open court. Events like these remind us that we cannot always rely on the wisdom of long-standing government policy.

We began to realize that this was not just a scientific question. There are also ethical issues. People opposed to water fluoridation expressed concern about the government's power to put any substance in the community drinking water without the expressed consent of the individuals affected. This power could set a dangerous precedent, and it contradicts an individual's right to choose what he or she ingests. Some people feel very strongly that the public is being mass medicated—without its consent.

At each new revelation, we became more and more interested in sharing what we had learned with future readers. During such a chaotic time in the history of medicine, it is up to each health consumer to vigorously guard his or her own wellbeing. We wanted to help people keep an open mind, review the science, listen to the concerns of others, and consider becoming involved in health issues.

We were especially hoping that our book would help people find their own voice, and make sure that all decisions are guided by the ethical principle to which physicians, nurses, and other healthcare professionals have pledged to adhere: "Above all, do no harm."

What would this mean for thyroid sufferers reading our book? It would mean trying to decrease exposure to fluoride. If living in a fluoridated area, try drinking only bottled water with known low fluoride content, or purified water such as distilled or reverse osmosis. (Simple filtration, even with the best of filters, does not remove fluoride.)

It also means using toothpaste without fluoride if you or a close family member has a tendency to low thyroid. Such fluoride free products are indeed available, but one might have to do some careful shopping. Even many of the "natural" toothpaste products at health food stores contain fluoride.

When our Thyroid Power book eventually was published, we advised our readers with a thyroid issue to discuss their personal concerns and needs with their dentist. Hopefully, they could find a practitioner respectful of their wishes and beliefs. We urged them to explore non-fluoride options, to encourage their children to eat less sweets, and to brush and floss regularly.

On the other hand, if they or their genetically related family members do not have thyroid issues, then by all means they could use fluoride toothpaste, but definitely not drink fluoridated water. For those who wanted to use fluoride toothpaste, we reminded them to spit it all out instead of swallowing any. We made sure to mention that this advice is especially important advice for children.

During our book tour we were shocked to find that good researchers all over the world in many different fields were tackling the same problem. As more scientists wrote up their studies, a very troubling trend was emerging. Just as fluoride had been strong enough to kill rats, it now appeared strong enough to affect a wide variety of human body tissues, even at the low concentrations of fluoride-adjusted city water. It is our hope that people of good conscience will heed the warnings implicit in all this new research, especially if they or anyone in their family has a thyroid problem. We now firmly believe that fluoridation is a bad idea whose time has passed.

Please accept our fondest wishes for your ongoing good health.
Richard and Karilee Shames

AUTHORS' NOTE: We are grateful to the editors for gathering such a diverse group of contributors to speak in one voice opposing fluoridation, and while we appreciate Dr. Ladapo's foreword and his ending water fluoridation in Florida, we do not necessarily agree with his other positions.

How a Single Mom Threatened an Empire

By: Brenda Staudenmaier

ABOUT: *Brenda Staudenmaier, a named plaintiff in the historic TSCA*

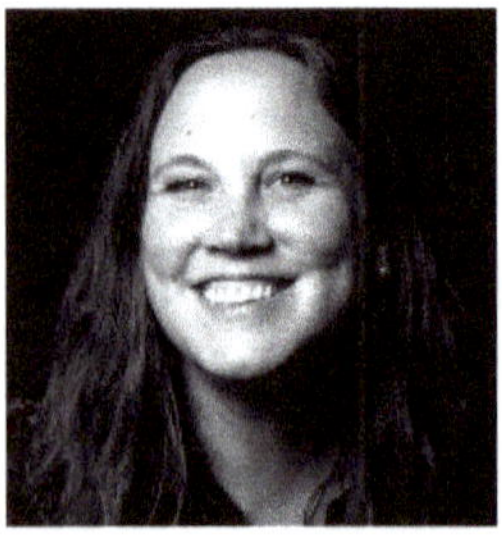

lawsuit against the EPA and former low-income single mom, turned her experience with fluoridation and health into motivation to pursue an associate degree in Environmental Engineering Technology–Waste and Water Technician. In 2016, she authored a proposal for a zero-carbon emission energy device for a National Science Foundation (NSF) College Challenge, which the White House recognized on World Water Day as one of the top ten innovation projects addressing air and water pollution. During COVID, she completed an online course at Harvard University, where her final project focused on wastewater contaminants of emerging concern and strategies to reduce them at the source. After several years working in wastewater, Brenda now serves as a technical trainer for water and wastewater operators, well drillers, plumbers, and engineers on operation, compliance, and safety in the water industry. Despite pushback from the Wisconsin Department of Health Services and fluoride promoters, she continues to build on her personal and professional successes.

Visit FluorideLawsuit.com for more about the lawsuit and the science.

CHAPTER 4

"Plaintiffs have proven, by a preponderance of the evidence, that water fluoridation at the level of 0.7 mg/L —the prescribed optimal level in the United States— presents an unreasonable risk of injury to health."

—Judge Edward M. Chen (September 24, 2024)

THAT SOUNDS LIKE it should be an ending, doesn't it? The death knell of fluoridation. Apparently, it isn't. Not yet, because the foot soldiers in the fluoridation army continue their assault on the people with gaslighting, name-calling, disinformation, and falsified data. But perhaps I should begin at the beginning.

The First Stand

On April 8, 2013, I stood trembling before the Green Bay Water Commission. It was the first time I had even attended a city or commission meeting. I didn't know what to expect. I didn't have a polished speech. I didn't know anything about the meeting procedure. I was just a single mom on food stamps, juggling waitressing shifts at Caffe Espresso. Since my water filters had expired, and I couldn't afford new ones, I was hauling a five-gallon glass jug of water up and down stairs in order to keep my kids safe from the poison my community added to our city water.

Public speaking terrified me, but something bigger than fear drove me that day. Protecting my two sons was more important than my fear. I had just lost my friend Frankie. He had osteosarcoma—bone cancer. Hospitals, surgeries, chemo, radiation, pain, poison. During his final year, we had talked about fluoride. A small epidemiological study by New Jersey authorities documented an association between osteosarcoma and community fluoridation (Cohn, 1992). A Harvard study linked fluoridated water to osteosarcoma in boys during a critical age range (Bassin et al., 2006). My son Hayden was in that window. I couldn't unsee the science, and I couldn't ignore my gut. So, I did what scared me most: I stood up and spoke.

I asked the commission to stop adding hydrofluosilicic acid to city water. Hydrofluosilicic acid is a corrosive byproduct of the fertilizer industry. It's a slurry—a cocktail of hazardous waste containing lead, arsenic, aluminum, and mercury along with some fluoride ions. The EPA MCLG (maximum concentration level goal) is zero for lead and arsenic. Yet, we are adding this junk to Green Bay & Madison's drinking water. I thought the science would speak for itself: fluoride wasn't FDA-approved for ingestion, and public water supplies shouldn't be a delivery system for medication.

Naïvely, I believed they'd listen. I believed that once people saw the science, they would agree that fluoridating the public water supply was wrong. I thought it was a simple misunderstanding. Instead, I faced a wall of resistance: Judy Friederichs from the Brown County Health Department, Carrie Stempski of the Oral Health Partnership, and Matt Crespin from the Children's Health Alliance of Wisconsin. They wielded logos, titles, and polished talking points, claiming fluoride was safe and essential, dismissing my concerns with lies about studies showing harm only at "400 times" our levels. Green Bay was fluoridated in the same range used in the Harvard bone cancer study! Crespin also downplayed dental fluorosis, calling it cosmetic and visible only to a dentist. But not only do many pay for cosmetic dentistry to repair stained and brittle fluorosed teeth, fluorosis was widespread enough that the recommended fluoride levels were lowered just two years later from a range of 1.2 - 0.7 mg/L to a single target of 0.7 mg/L. Most American communities, including the entirety of Wisconsin, had been fluoridating for decades at 1.0 ppm, so this represented a 30% reduction.

Crespin, brandishing his association with hospitals, dental associations, and nonprofits, was either dangerously misinformed or deliberately misleading the public. He deftly used talking points, logical fallacies, emotional manipulation, and outright lies to protect the policy instead of the people. He was a member of the government-backed fluoride response team. I was just a mother who wanted to talk about science, my lived experience, and about carrying jugs of water. He had institutional backing. The commission sided with him.

I was stunned. I realized I was a low-income mom going up against a team that included a woman with a designer handbag that cost more than my rent. I was drowned out by an empire committed to protecting a policy that worshiped a toxic chemical. Back in 2013, I never could have imagined that a dozen years later, I'd be the one telling this story.

Standing on the Shoulders of Giants

"If I have seen further, it is by standing on the shoulders of giants."
—Sir Isaac Newton

I stood on the shoulders of those who came before me who were ignored, defunded, censored, and discredited for daring to tell the truth about fluoride. They were silenced for being scientifically inconvenient. Their data was buried, credibility attacked, careers quietly dismantled, and voices muted, but their courage was the bedrock of my future.

Fluoride wasn't just in the water. It was in the culture—in assumptions, in institutions, in policies that protect industry over people. I wasn't just up against misinformation. I was up against an empire. They didn't follow the science—they followed the script.

I didn't just battle misinformation—I battled a well-oiled machine of public health officials, grant-funded operatives, school nurses-turned-propagandists, and a dental industry more concerned with appearances than with accountability. Many of the very dentists I was up against—who claimed to champion fluoride "for the poor"—would not even accept low-income patients in their practices. Their concern for poor families was a performance, not a practice. To truly protect children from harmful chemicals in municipal drinking water with life-altering effects, I had to speak out—and speak with authority.

That fall, I went back to school and studied environmental engineering, focusing on drinking water and wastewater. I learned more science. While I earned my degree, my life felt like a multi-ring circus: my boys, bills, books—and my brother Brent.

Brent, my bright, kind, and fun-loving brother, ended his girlfriend's life just weeks after that 2013 meeting. She was the director of the battered women's shelter. He was prescribed Adderall for attention issues and the two had been drinking—a dangerous combination which was a fact not allowed into evidence at trial. Multiple studies indicate that fluoride exposure increases attention deficits (Malin 2024; Fiore 2023; Geier 2025; Riddell 2019; Bashash 2018; Malin 2015).

If reducing fluoride exposure can reduce the number of people with ADHD, then less people need to be on medication like Adderall.

Living through this nightmare, I often felt as if my soul had detached from my body. I was watching my family's pain from a distance I couldn't bridge. I needed more than a distraction—I needed purpose. I needed to fight for something that could protect families like mine, and friends like Frankie.

TSCA Petition and Round Two

The next time I brought the fluoride issue forward in Green Bay was in 2017, shortly after I joined a group that filed the 2016 petition under TSCA Section 21 with the EPA—an unprecedented move to demand accountability through federal environmental law.

Many of the key players in Green Bay were the same as before, but a few new names had entered the mix. The tension on the City Council was also more obvious this time around. The fluoride-related mudslinging between alderpersons in 2017 became so outrageous it was turned into parody videos on the now-defunct "Green Bay Sausage" YouTube channel. The YouTuber—a woman battling MS—later disappeared from the platform. She seems to have deleted everything from YouTube, but both that video and the meeting are seared into my memory.

One unforgettable moment was Councilwoman Barbara Dorff yelling at Aldermen Scannell and Zima, accusing them of embarrassing the Council and warning them that their bad behavior was being recorded on video.

Another member of the fluoride response team who stood out was Michael Schwartz, the new Executive Director of Oral Health Partnership. He was one of those "nice guy with a smile"-types known by many in the community. He had polished talking points but no apparent interest in nuance. My heart sank when he gave his address at a public meeting. He lived in the giant house on the edge of the park, just a block away from the one-bedroom apartment I rented for myself and kids. He drove an electric car and kept a muscle gas-guzzling car in the garage. I was working, attending college full-time, and doing everything I could to make ends meet. Meanwhile, Michael stood in his front yard with a Roundup jug in hand, misting his lawn with the carcinogenic pesticide while families and children passed by en route to the park.

Michael Schwartz leaned hard on the CDC's dental myths and marketing materials. He presented "I Like My Teeth" talking points and the Wisconsin Dental Association's marketing one-liners as though they were peer-reviewed science. And sadly, many on council fell for it.

But the empire had to work for their wins. I made sure of that.

The Fluoride Rapid Response Team

I realized how threatening I'd become to the fluoride lobby—when I walked into the Green Bay City Council meeting before the final vote and spotted Johnny Johnson, Delta Dental's favorite frequent flyer, in the front row (CDHP, 2015). Johnny Johnson is the fluoride front man who preached the gospel of fluoride with the religious fervor of a snake-handling minister. In my opinion, Johnny serves the role as Sock-puppet-in-Chief for other more circumspect groups. If fluoride is on an agenda almost anywhere in the country, his small group, the American Fluoridation Society (AFS), dispatches him like a first responder. He flew all the way from Florida in order to discredit me. He told the Council that I was "spreading misinformation" and that he would be "the first to alert them if there were any red flags." He was already sitting on a mountain of red flags but chose to bury them under rehearsed lines, fear mongering, and industry spin.

The Green Bay City Council voted to keep fluoride after Johnny Johnson and associates convinced them that my 2016 petition had "no merit." Classic deflection: dismiss the messenger to protect the chemical.

It turns out the truth has more staying power than fluoride spin.

The Federal Lawsuit

Two months later, that petition became a civil lawsuit and I became a named plaintiff in Food & Water Watch, Inc. et al. v. Environmental Protection Agency et al. in the United States District Court Northern District of California in San Francisco. We sued the EPA to force them to protect the public and susceptible sub-populations from the neurotoxic risks of fluoride by banning the addition of fluoridation chemicals to water, pursuant to section 21 of the Toxic Substance Control Act (TSCA), 15 U.S.C. § 2620. Obama-appointed Judge Edward M. Chen was assigned to our case.

The American Fluoridation Society had another tactic up their sleeve. Knowing I wouldn't back down from fighting for safe water in Wisconsin, they held their annual retreat in Green Bay, where they cozied up to Nancy Quirk of the Green Bay Water Utility and Mayor Jim Schmidt. Their goal was clear: build relationships with local allies who could serve as foot soldiers, aka useful idiots, and keep the national players informed of events in my neighborhood.

A New Chapter

In 2018, I graduated with highest honors from Northeast Wisconsin Technical College in Green Bay. At the time, I had been simultaneously enrolled at the University of Wisconsin–Green Bay, pursuing a degree in Cellular and Molecular Biology, but I made the decision to drop out and take a summer position as a wastewater operator assistant. That opportunity led me to Madison, where I accepted a full-time role as a wastewater operator at the Madison Metropolitan Sewerage District later that fall.

In 2019, I bought a small home in downtown Green Bay for $50,000. I called it my "fuck you" home—a symbol of independence and long-term security. With a mortgage with taxes and insurance under $400 a month, it cost less than a storage unit in New York City. It was my backup plan, my screw-the-system sanctuary. Living without a car payment, with a mortgage that any minimum wage job could cover, and maintaining a cushion in my savings account is my version of success and security.

Nothing is ever easy and 2020 turned out to be a difficult year for me, like it was for most of us who didn't belong to the laptop class. As a single mother working an essential on-site job, I had no option to work from home when the pandemic hit. In Madison, Wisconsin, the schools shut down and were converted into paid daycare programs. The cost was high, and my son Ko struggled in that environment—he didn't get along with the sassy, sometimes aggressive, kids who made it hard for him to focus or feel safe. To give him a better experience, I often made the three-hour drive north to drop him off at my parents' farm outside Peshtigo. It was a good arrangement for Ko and my parents, but the separation took a toll on my emotional health. Weekends became sacred—my only real time with my youngest son. The little house I had bought in Green Bay became our weekend hub, a place where we could reset and be together, even in the midst of the chaos.

Our case was one of the first trials to be held over Zoom in 2020 because of the COVID lockdowns.

In a courtroom where truth had to rise above industry spin, the world's leading environmental health scientists stepped forward. They weren't fringe figures. These were career-long public health experts, respected globally, with hundreds of peer-reviewed publications between them. Their testimony would reshape the fluoride debate forever and expose the serious neurodevelopmental risks of early-life fluoride exposure.

The landmark TSCA fluoride lawsuit launched into federal court with extraordinary momentum. For the first time in history, world-renowned experts in environmental health—including Dr. Howard Hu, Dr. Bruce Lanphear, Dr. Philippe Grandjean, and Dr. Kathleen Thiessen—testified under oath that fluoride poses a significant neurodevelopmental risk, especially during pregnancy and infancy. Their testimonies were grounded in peer-reviewed science, including NIH- and EPA-funded studies, and clearly demonstrated that fluoride exposure at levels found in fluoridated drinking water is unsafe for the developing brain.

We won that lawsuit in 2020, in theory. But because the EPA begged the Judge to delay his verdict until after the National Toxicology Program (NTP) published its research on the effect of fluoride exposure on cognition and developmental neurotoxicity, we waited. There isn't enough space in this chapter for me to relate either the courtroom testimony or the behind-the-scenes duplicity of the fluoride empire that tried to derail our lawsuit and the NTP publication. (Connett 2025; Ross 2023)

Ultimately, we prevailed in 2024 with a second courtroom drama and an unequivocal verdict in our favor. And still the evil empire of fluoridationists work to protect their false god (Baletti, 2025a; Baletti, 2025c).

International Response

Between the first and second trials, I continued to engage with the appropriate Wisconsin authorities. In response to my contacts with the Green Bay City Council and Madison's Water Board, Johnny Johnson activated his international network of fluoride defenders from the U.K.,

Australia, and Canada, pulling dental directors from across the country to swamp local proceedings with industry-aligned propaganda.

One of the more absurd examples came from Dr. John N. Dane, Dental Director for the Missouri Department of Health and Senior Services. In an ADA article, he bragged, "I was alerted to this and that anti-fluoridationists were planning on stacking the speakers list. While I wasn't able to get on the speakers list, I could write a letter. I encouraged my staff to do the same and they all wrote letters. So, we sent six." His letter appeared highly official, complete with the emblem of Missouri Governor Michael L. Parson and a header naming Randall W. Williams, MD, FACOG as Director. In it, he falsely claimed, "Even those groups that are against water fluoridation will admit that removing the fluoride will result in at least one additional filling per person per year." Really? According to him, if Green Bay stopped fluoridating, every single person would end up with 10 extra cavities after a decade. How could any rational person take this seriously?

But the disinformation campaign swamping our Wisconsin communities didn't stop there. At the July 13, 2020 Protection & Policy Committee meeting, Florida dentist Johnny Johnson again showed up over Zoom. I was one of the first to speak. My attorneys, Michael Connett and Chris Nidel, followed with details about our lawsuit. Johnny, as usual, waited until the very end—his go-to strategy to get the last word in. And when he did, he delivered a blatant lie, telling the Council that my fluoride lawsuit wasn't really about the fluoridation of drinking water but about the "Toxic Substances Act" (sic), as if the two were unrelated. I nearly choked. The lawsuit was specifically about the developmental neurotoxicity of fluoridation chemicals added to drinking water. Yet, he twisted it again, right in front of elected officials, and nobody challenged him.

Democracy Silenced

During the committee level meetings in Green Bay, we were repeatedly told that the issue would move to the full council where our voices really mattered. If someone didn't get their chance to speak, they would have their opportunity in front of the full council.

On December 1, 2020, the Green Bay City Council made an unprecedented and deeply undemocratic move. Councilmember Chris Wery motioned to open the floor for public comment, and Councilmember Veronica Corpus-Dax seconded. Yet, despite the motion and a meeting full of concerned citizens, Mayor Eric Genrich shut it down. The moment was captured in full on the City's official YouTube channel—video proof of a democratic process deliberately derailed. Residents, some of whom had waited nearly an hour to speak on the fluoride issue, were denied their right to be heard. This was the first known instance in Green Bay's history where the public was completely silenced despite showing up and signaling their intent to participate.

Mayor Genrich interrupted the process and overrode our efforts, blocking citizens like Elliot Christenson, Guy Zima, and David Bartikofky from speaking.

This brazen disregard for the public led to an official ethics complaint against Councilmembers Barbara Dorff, Bill Galvin, Randy Scannell, Craig Stevens, Jesse Brunette, Lynn Gerlach, and Mayor Genrich. Their actions violated Section 4 of the City of Green Bay's Code of Conduct for Elected Officials, which explicitly requires members to encourage public participation, maintain fairness, and respect community voices. I also requested William Vande Castle, legal counsel for the Green Bay Water Utility, excuse himself from evaluating this complaint for his conflict of interest and prior attempt to intimidate me. He had tried to pressure me into removing a legally protected video from my YouTube page, in which a Green Bay Water Utility employee had confessed: "I'm pretty health conscious, like I mean, I don't use any fluoride in my toothpaste, any of that stuff. I mean, I know how bad it is for you. I don't drink our water." My complaint was thrown out by city employees who were on the ethics committee.

Marquette Connection

Nancy Quirk's support for fluoridation was unwavering, driven not by science but by family pride. Her nephews had attended Marquette University Dental School, and that was enough for her. WI DHS Dental Director Dunkel was closely tied to Marquette too—he seemed to care more about protecting its reputation than protecting public health.

Ironically, my own dentist, also a Marquette graduate, chose not to use fluoride. That dental office looked at the actual research and found it wanting. They were among the few with the humility to admit the science had shifted.

Nancy Quirk was well-connected—she sat on the EPA Drinking Water Advisory Committee, had worked at Wisconsin's largest fluoridating utilities, and was an influential voice within the American Water Works Association. Her blind support delayed protective actions not only for Wisconsin but across the nation. Worse, her name appeared as a member of the American Fluoridation Society, used on letters pressuring other communities to keep fluoride in their water.

When I contacted Andrea Hay of the Green Bay Water Utility to confirm this, she clarified: "Nancy never granted permission nor willingness to serve on this group. She saw her name on it, cleared up the misunderstanding, and they deleted her from anything that had indicated she was."

And that's the kind of operation we're up against. Deception by default. Membership by assumption. And a campaign powered not by truth, but by repetition and intimidation.

Wisconsin & World

In Wisconsin, like elsewhere, decision-makers fall prey to the bystander effect and to normalcy bias. The Department of Health Services (DHS)—filled with MDs, RNs, and PhDs like Jeffrey S. Lafferty, PhD, Environmental Epidemiologist, and Sarah Yang, PhD, Manager of the Hazard Assessment Section—has the expertise to sound the alarm about fluoride's risks but, instead, it defers to dental dogma. Responsibility is diffused and coworkers feel pressure to support one another and not "step on toes"—especially when careers are tied to promoting fluoridation. No one wants to offend a colleague or risk their own position.

It is safer to be the bystander who assumes someone else will follow the science, who justifies misery as normal, and who just copies and pastes talking points that originated eighty years ago than it is to take affirmative action.

Wisconsin played a critical role in launching fluoridation, driven by overzealous dentists determined to fluoridate 50 communities by 1950. I discuss this dental history in an article published by my college newspaper, "I am Suing the US EPA Over Fluoride Added to Our Drinking Water" (Staudenmaier, 2021).

Fluoride Harm provides a more modern context, which includes the corruption of public health players, politicians, and polarized media outlets that parrot marketing misinformation. Thank goodness for small independent media because the major platforms are in service of their sponsors, and what should be public service broadcasting manufactures consent by promoting propaganda and compliance—like Madison, WI, WORT Radio, which features AFS spokesman Johnny Johnson and DHS staffer Paula Tran.

But cracks are forming in the narrative. HHS has already signaled reform: Removing fluoride from water supplies is listed as a key public health priority by MAHA—a stunning shift after decades of knee-jerk defense. At the EPA, Administrator Zeldin has declared fluoride will finally be regulated under the Safe Drinking Water Act. Yet, paradoxically, the Department of Justice has appealed Judge Chen's landmark 2024 ruling on behalf of the EPA. So, we wait: will justice for our children's brains prevail, or will politics stall the inevitable?

The Road Ahead

Since 2022, Karen Spencer and I have written a series of protest letters to the CDC Oral Health Division, which long served as the mouthpiece for outdated fluoridation policy and the distributor of participation trophies to utilities dumping a toxic industrial slurry into public drinking water. Their response was essentially: go pound sand.

The CDC Oral Health Division was largely dismantled in early 2025. In September 2025, Health and Human Services (HHS), under the direction of Robert F. Kennedy, Jr., released the interagency MAHA strategy report to Make America Healthy Again (MAHA). Several of the leaders of the U.S. agencies engaged in that initiative mentioned investigating fluoride exposure as an environmental threat to health in a joint meeting.

Consequently, I can see a light at the end of this long road—I am impatient to reach it. The days of rubber-stamping, funding, and rewarding fluoridation practice are ending. Science has evolved. The public is watching.

Those of us who have fought the empire of deceit for more than a decade—and those who have carried this fight for over half a century—who have championed clean, safe water against all odds, are no longer asking politely. We are demanding accountability. We are demanding the truth. And we are demanding safe water for every community—now, and for generations to come.

To Fight or Not to Fight.

That was the question!

By: Dr Robert C. Dickson, MD, CCFP, FCFP

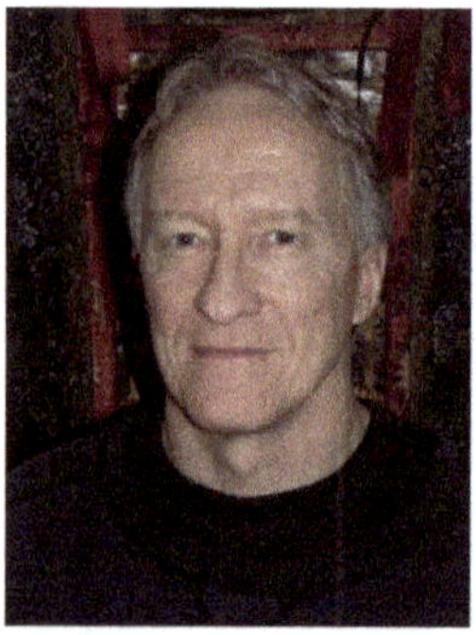

ABOUT: *Dr Robert C. Dickson is a newly retired Family Physician in Calgary, Alberta. He is the Founder and President of Safe Water Calgary (safewatercalgary.com), the Chair of Fluoride Free Canada (fluoridefreecanada.ca), and an active member of FAN, the Fluoride Action Network (fluoridealert.org). He is currently taking the City of Calgary to Court for adding a known neurotoxin to public water.*

Dr Bob has volunteered in several countries around the world, including with Medical Mercy Canada in Thailand/Myanmar, and in rural Guatemala assisting communities with medical, dental and humanitarian programs with Project Ixcanaan. He has served as the Chair of: Tools for Peace, the Arusha Cross-Cultural Centre; and Four Worlds Centre for International Development Learning. He was also the President of Change for Children and a Senior Volunteer with RESULTS Canada and the Calgary Distress and Drug Centre.

Dr Bob's pre-medical careers include unionized labour; truck driver; air traffic control; child care counsellor; Emergency Medical Technician; and paramedic. His current afflictions are biking, hiking, travelling, golf, dancing, spiritual journeys, and winning pickleball medals.

CHAPTER 5

"Truth is treason in an empire of lies."

—George Orwell

AS A FRONTLINE medical doctor, I supported water fluoridation. Glitzy and persuasive brochures and advertisements crossed my busy medical desk and frequently hit the airwaves and press.

I voted YES for fluoridation in the 1998 plebiscite, the sixth in four decades, in my home city Calgary, Alberta, Canada! Activist friends, who had been fighting against the pro-fluoridation juggernaut for years, challenged me to look at the science and to not rely on the so-called experts.

Stunned and surprised by the plethora of good anti-fluoridation science, I consulted my PhD/MD friend and mentor from the University of Calgary, Dr James Beck. Raised and trained in the USA, Jim admitted he knew little about water fluoridation, thinking it to be safe and effective. He surveyed the literature and within weeks, Jim was adamant that fluoridation was indeed a mistake, and that we should do something about it. His infamous words in 1999 were, *"Bob, with all this science behind us, we should have this harmful practice stopped in months!"*

Flash forward 12 years, we were lobbying and educating City Councillors and staff, Deans of Medical Schools, Medical and Dental Officers of Health, and Public Health policy makers, and writing numerous articles, letters to the editor, and op-eds alongside several tenacious grassroots activists. Our efforts finally paid off—our Calgary City Council passed an excellent motion! In 2011, Council put fluoridation to rest after 20 years, and they have been attacked tenaciously and relentlessly ever since by the insidious and aggressive pro-fluoride lobby.

One of the attacks on City Council and professionals opposing fluoridation had to do with the fact that in 2011, there was no public vote to end fluoridation. But one need only apply common sense—nobody should be voting on what medication their family, friends, colleagues, and strangers take. Public plebiscites should not replace good science and debate.

Common sense, unfortunately, is not so common anymore. But it worked in 2011, along with the steadfast resolve of several champions for the cause on the City Council whose courage and persistence prevailed. They were adamant that they were not scientists and were, for the most part, untrained in that field. However, what they were competent and confident in was that they could make decisions based on the ethics and morality of medicating all their citizens with, at the very least, a highly controversial and polarizing substance. It also helped that the industrial waste product hydrofluosilicic acid added to our public water had essentially destroyed the injection and metering systems, and the rebuild was to be several millions of dollars, along with almost $1 million yearly for the toxic waste and ongoing training, HAZMAT suits, maintenance and supplies.

It is said that if a lie or mistruth is repeated often enough, it will eventually be accepted as true. Such is the case with the oft-stated mantra of the pro-fluoridationists, persisting for decades—water fluoridation is "safe and effective". Sadly, we hear that mantra repeated recklessly and often, across many forums, for entities and treatments that are neither.

Is water fluoridation safe and effective? The short answer is a resounding NO. The long answer—well, excellent books have tackled and dealt with this contentious and polarizing subject over several decades. One of the earliest which delved into the bad politics and poor science behind fluoridation was *The American Fluoridation Experiment* by the esteemed Dr George Waldbott, penned in 1957. Another, by a leader in the anti-fluoride charge in Europe, was the 1987 book *Fluoride: The Freedom Fight* by Dr Hans Moolenburgh, which was instrumental in keeping Europe 97% fluoridation-free to this date.

Want to read a spy thriller that is based on 10 solid years of research and investigative journalism? Christopher Bryson's brilliant exposé *The Fluoride Deception* takes one down a journalistic ride through the underbellies of dark science, government corruption, malfeasance, and the manufacturing of consent. Hard to put this one down!

Unabashedly, one of my all-time favourites is *The Case Against Fluoride,* meticulously researched, written and published in 2010 by mentor and my dear friend stricken now with dementia, Dr James Beck, PhD, MD. Co-authored by arguably the most knowledgeable man on the planet in the fluoridation arena, Dr Paul Connett, PhD, from the USA, and by the late Dr Spedding Micklem, PhD, from the UK, this highly-referenced book is still a major tome in the fight for clean and safe water.

The Case Against Fluoride was instrumental in our education of City Councillors in 2010. Dr Beck and I hand-delivered free copies to all Councillors and Mayor Nenshi, the latter who most likely never opened it because of his staunch pro-fluoride biases—"we must help the poor kids", which has remained a pro-fluoride mantra and anthem for decades. Paradoxically, I have been accused by several pro-fluoridation leaders of deliberately harming poor children. Quite the opposite is true, as attested by my participation and leadership in projects locally and in the developing world with RESULTS Canada, Medical Mercy Canada, the Arusha Cross-Cultural Centre, Change for Children, and financial support for many organizations such as Doctors Without Borders and Amnesty International.

Turning off the fluoridation taps in 2011 in Calgary was monumental! We were the largest city in the fluoridated world to say no to this failing public health program. But the pro-fluoride lobby, led by the relentless and poorly informed Juliet Guichon, a history major and lawyer from the University of Calgary, and aided and abetted by the grandfatherly Johnny Johnson, a retired dentist from Florida, relentlessly attacked City Council overtly in the press and covertly with every means at their disposal. Pressures mounted and time took its toll. Dr Beck retired from the 18-year struggle in 2017. Left without my co-leader and mentor, and with several of the supportive City Councillors tiring of the battle or moving on, I took action that was a profound adventure for me, founding Safe Water Calgary and launching the website that endures to this day (safewatercalgary.com).

And then the bombshell, the nemesis of conscientious medical professionals everywhere—there was a major complaint against me to the CPSA (College of Physicians and Surgeon of Alberta), our licensing body and guardians of the medical universe.

I was travelling through the hinterlands of eastern Australia and got a data signal on a hilltop. Stopped roadside, I quickly perused my long list of emails and spotted a Private and Confidential message from the CPSA—Complaint Dismissed! What complaint? This was February 2019, and the first I'd heard of anything awry on the College front. Delving into it later, Juliet Guichon, along with former Head of Pediatrics Dr Ian Mitchell and others, had registered a very long and detailed complaint against me in January, a month earlier. My first knowledge of said complaint was this dismissal letter from the Chief Complaints Doctor at the CPSA in which the body of the letter stated tersely that I was walking on a tightrope and that I should watch my back! Strange wording from the College but, hey, the complaint was dismissed!

However, not one to rest or take defeat lightly, Juliet, along with her cabal, launched an appeal to the CPSA, stating that they had grave concerns that Dr Dickson would convince Calgary City Council to keep this lifesaving, safe and effective program away from the poor kids—their major talking points—pulling on the heartstrings of the public and decision-makers alike.

The Complaint was reinstated, with the sway and influence of College insiders. Time to lawyer up! Most cases in Canada brought against MD's are covered by the CMPA (Canadian Medical Protection Association), and I was fortunate to qualify. My expensive lawyers at Bennett Jones immediately got to work, and we drafted an excellent 75-page document to the College with realms of science and defences of free speech.

Whew, that should be the end of it! But no, the CRC (Claims Review Committee), likely with "safe and effective" biases, deemed that Dr Dickson required further investigation! We took the matter to Provincial Court, claiming that the initial dismissal should stand. However, after almost two years of wait and see during the tumultuous times of the little virus, the court ruled against us. Onward with the CRC.

While being 'investigated' by the CPSA, I continued to try to educate Calgarians about fluoride harm, all along being careful to state, as I had been warned, to repeat that it was 'my opinion' every time I spoke against fluoridation. I had written an OpEd with Dr Hardy Limeback which was initially promised to be published by the editor in chief of the Calgary Harold. Inexplicably, it was pulled and no one at that news outlet would respond to our concerns and tell us why. That letter is in Appendix H, along with the letter I wrote to Naheed Nenshi, the Mayor of Calgary at the time. There were many other examples of the media ignoring our Safe Water Calgary team. Being ignored is one thing, but the organized attempt to take my medical licence away from me over my opposition to fluoridation was obviously just plain nasty and playing dirty. Lawyers really do play dirty.

Back to the CPSA 'witch-hunt.' Several investigators independent of the College were assigned, yet none ever contacted me personally, and very seldom did *my* lawyers either. In the meantime, the College in 2023 obtained 2 expensive "expert" opinions against me and my views—one from an Edmonton family physician who was obviously very poorly informed on fluoride, and another by an Albertan public health MD, who spouted the tired and traditional "safe and effective, trust the experts and the science" talking points.

A year passed, and the College did not divulge that the CRC was meeting in September of 2024 to decide if I should go to Tribunal Trial or not. That resulted in them deciding that a Tribunal Trial was needed for this rogue doctor in January 2025 before they had the opportunity to read the incredibly detailed and supportive report from one of Canada's most imminent and leading MDs, scientists, and researchers, Dr Bruce Lanphear. This report tracked not only the major studies and talking points leading up to the 2019 charges, but also the plethora of new science, data and evidence up to his October 2024 report. It supported and exonerated my stance and positions completely!

Next up, negotiations around charges and Tribunal Trial set for five full days, January 27-31, 2025. Much angst and bartering with College lawyers, insistence from my Bennett Jones lawyers that I couldn't fight them on everything, and a deal was struck.

On January 27, it took only half a day in the Tribunal Trial for the College to drop 3 of the 4 charges against me. In essence, I won on the science of fluoridation, as they knew better than to attempt to fight us on that battle ground. I also won on the major issues of free speech, and of practicing outside the scope of my medical training.

The accepted penalties were first, admission of guilt for calling public health and medical/dental officers of health liars when I had proof that they were lying to the public and to decision and policy makers; second, the requirement to take a 2-day psychological boot camp course (like that imposed on the infamous Ontario psychologist Jordan Peterson) at my own expense of approximately $2,000; and finally, to pay fines and Tribunal costs of over $6,000.

Heavy sigh! But also, a huge breath of relief at this six-year marathon finally attaining a modicum of finality, and that the CPSA's ability to take down truth-telling physicians was battered and wavering. They were out of their lane for way too long, as many of my colleagues will attest.

Before battle with College of Physicians and Surgeons of Alberta—meditate, chop wood, carry water, travel, play pickleball, golf, commune with dear friends, fight the Evil Captain Fluoride.

After battle with College of Physicians and Surgeons—meditate, chop wood, carry water, travel, play pickleball, golf, commune with dear friends, fight the Evil Captain Fluoride—and trust that I will never have to deal with those Orwellian bullies ever again as I am now retired!

At the time of writing this chapter there is an attempt by Safe Water Calgary to launch a legal challenge to try to end fluoridation within weeks of it being reinstated after a 14-year pause. As of June 30, 2025, pregnant moms, infants and toddlers were once again being exposed to inappropriate levels of fluoride ingestion. Fluoride Free Calgary is dedicated to protecting susceptible Calgarians and will not stop until fluoridation ends once again in Calgary.

Unsafe, ineffective, unethical, costly, devoid of common sense—water fluoridation should be put where it belongs; in the **Museum of Failed Medical and Public Health Practices**.

Fluoride out. Dr Bob.

> **AUTHOR'S NOTE**: The content of this chapter are my views and not necessarily those of my colleagues or the College of Physicians and Surgeons of Alberta.

Clean Teeth or Dirty Little Secret

Fluoride is mining's dirty little secret

By: Erik E. Crown

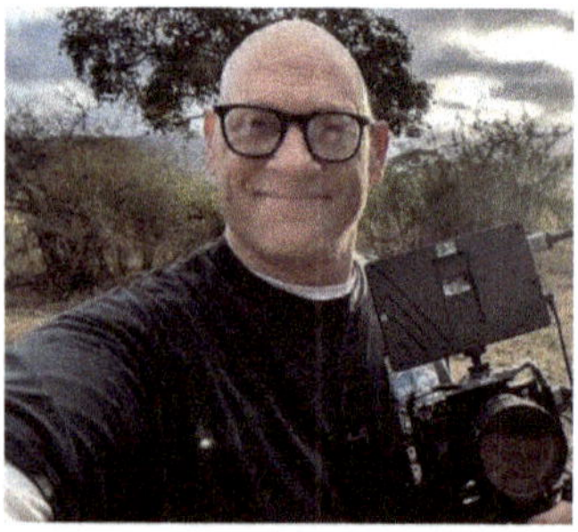

ABOUT: *Erik Crown is an award-winning filmmaker who has worked in the industry for over 30 years, creating unique investigative documentaries. He started out in Hollywood on productions like Scrubs, Enemy of the State, and TMZ, but after finding out his environmental cancer was incurable, he decided to give up his place in Los Angeles to travel the world, trying to fight for a better ecological future. He left for the Amazon jungle in 2017 with Earthrace Conservation to help save animals through direct action campaigns, continuing his work in the South China Sea, the Philippines, Vietnam, Colombia, Tanzania, and many other locations. His documentary PHOSFATE focuses on the health effects a small town feels after being poisoned for years by a Fortune 500 mining company. Another documentary, Cancer Alley, explores a deadly 85-mile stretch of road between Baton Rouge and New Orleans. Erik recently started a production company called Humanimal Pictures with his partner in life and partner in movies, Sierra Williams. Together they continue to advocate for a cleaner, free, and a healthier future for all through investigative projects and direct-action work.*

CHAPTER 6

"The greatest enemy of knowledge is not ignorance;
it is the illusion of knowledge."

—Daniel J. Boorstin, SJD

BATTLING ENVIRONMENTAL CANCER since 2005 and investigating the toxic world that made me sick since 2018 has one repetitive element, we are poisoned because it's legal.

The doctors don't know how to help me, so we try everything. I have had 13 surgeries, radiation in multiple places, immunotherapy, oral experimental chemo, and regular chemo, and I have yet to ever be in remission. But sadly, I am not alone. According to the National Cancer Institute, men have a one in two chance of being diagnosed with cancer in their lifetime, and women have a one in three chance. Childhood cancer has skyrocketed. This diseases affects us all; whether you have cancer now, or are forced to watch your child or loved one battle cancer now or in the future, or you may get cancer yourself in the future.

Fertilizers and pesticides are two examples of how we are being legally and routinely poisoned. Mining companies make them from phosphate, and the industrial waste from that process is sold out of the front door as a legal additive for local drinking water systems. If it sounds crazy, that's because it is. It is a cancer of the body-politic.

Fluoride had always been a side fringe conspiracy theory where I grew up, and anytime someone mentioned fluoride, it was summarily dismissed. I was always quick to dismiss it until I learned not only were the claims of fluoride harming consumers true, it was worse than imagined, because this poisoning was not only legal, but encouraged by government agencies. My documentary that took me deep into the heart of phosphate mining provided me with an education that changed me forever.

Poison and Profit

But first, please stop calling it "fluoride." That conjures the quaint picture in our minds to cover the harsh reality that what's in our water is not naturally-occurring calcium fluoride—it is hydrofluorosilicic acid (HFSA), a toxic industrial waste from phosphate mining. Implying that fluoridation water additives are a natural mineral is a deceptive narrative that lulls the public into comfortable compliance.

These are the stories that allow companies to poison us for their profit; these are the stories that public relations departments and ad companies spin. What I love about documentaries is that they allow us to tell the rest of the story—the truthful residents' stories which return the power of story back to the people who are fighting for a cleaner future and often for their very lives.

What I love about the process of creating documentaries about activism and conservation is every story has a protagonist and antagonist, but the roles are not always clearly defined; these are complicated stories. In the story of fluoridation, who is the good guy and who is really the bad guy? Is fluoridated water a magic potion that is promoted in order to prevent dental decay? Or is there another agenda?

After hearing about high radiation levels in public parks and playgrounds in Florida, I headed there in 2018 to begin a documentary called *PHOSFATE* about a small town that stood up against Mosaic, a Fortune 500 company that mines phosphate in central Florida, taking the phosphate and leaving a legacy of cancer and chronic illness.

The residents drove me to various areas where we used Geiger counters and water testing to check the health of the area. With high radiation readings in the water and the ground, people living in the area are heavily impacted, according to an EPA study from the 1980s. But you don't need to live near the mines or work in them to experience higher cancer risks. Mosaic Mining treats and self-tests, then releases the water they borrow from the surface water (they are permitted to take up to 70 million gallons a day), because it all flows to a few larger tributaries where towns along that river pull drinking water from, and in so doing expands the risk area to whomever uses that water

Wait—the drinking water? Water is the building block of all life, but has it become a wrecking ball for genes after decades of careless chemical management? Why would they put this in our water supply intentionally? It was part of a toxic puzzle I needed to put together in my mind to understand my toxic exposure.

After my initial expeditions with local activists, I tried to interview Mosaic officials, but they refused to talk with me. But in short order, we noticed we were being followed by white Mosaic pickup trucks and vans wherever we went.

The story that unfolded was terrifying: communities being poisoned, legally, by these companies. In the middle of filming and facing harassment in many ways, I met the most amazing activist named Gary O. Pittman. Gary was a former mining worker who sued the industry for better safety conditions—and won. He paid a steep price for his job by getting cancer and dying early, but he made sure he made his industry pay a price, too.

Gary changed the world when he published *Phosphate Fluorides: Toxic Torts* in 2011 (Pittman, 2011). He detailed his experience and explained the process that creates HFSA. So, I reached out to him in order to hear more about this firsthand. Gary explained that hydrofluorosilicic acid is a byproduct of evaporating phosphoric acid during the beneficiation process of mining phosphate.

In Florida, the phosphate industry uses Best Management Practices, which means the polluters regulate themselves, and they are not cleaning it up. This is an industry tasked with a critical job of mining phosphate, but even more critical than digging it out of the ground is to do it safely in order to protect all animals and people nearby—during the process and after—by ensuring a safe product and environment. Unfortunately, they are not held accountable for harming people with their products and the regulators have made it even easier to dispose of radioactive waste in "byproducts" distributed throughout Florida and beyond (Appendix I).

> "*The economic benefit of recovering uranium from WPA* (Wet Process Phosphoric Acid) *phosphoric acid streams will be both in the value of the uranium and in* ***reduced regulatory demands*** [Editors' emphasis added] *on disposal of low-level radioactive wastes arising from the WPA process."* (World Nuclear Association, 2025)

It was hard to imagine that toxic waste mining by-products were being used in towns without anyone even knowing, from radioactive rocks for playgrounds and roadways in public parks, to arsenic-laced fluoridation chemicals in drinking water. This is mining's dirty little secret: the waste they create that is too toxic to throw away into the environment or re-introduce to the environment, so they legally sell it to an unknowing public as a product.

Naturally-occurring calcium fluoride is safe to hold in your hands whereas the man-made industrial waste is not. Why and how are we willingly placing highly corrosive and dangerous chemicals into our own water supply? Sadly, the fluoridation chemicals from industry are a cheaper alternative, but "cheaper" has a high hidden cost—human health.

The nostalgia and heartfelt embracing of fluoride originated in an interesting intersection of Commerce and Art. Norman Rockwell used his famous style and a mythology cooked up by the ad agencies to create a series of advertisements for Crest featuring fluoride. Today, we see the simplistic ideas of the 1950s being challenged by modern studies, and more people want to know– what's in their water?

Residents around the world are learning more about their water, and learning more about elements like the cancer-causing arsenic that hydrofluorosilicic acid introduces into the water supply.

Ever wonder how fluoridation chemicals are made from phosphate rock? It's a pretty simple process, but it can only be done in phosphate facilities. During the mining process, phosphate rock is treated with sulfuric acid to create phosphoric acid, and the leftover condensation is treated and collected so it can be sold as hydrofluorosilicic acid (HFSA), a legally-approved fluoridation water additive.

Studies suggest that HFSA may lead to higher levels of arsenic, lead, and radionuclides in drinking water. Additionally, HFSA has been linked to increased lead leaching from plumbing materials, potentially affecting children's brains and bodies (Masters & Coplan, 1999; Masters et al., 2000; Coplan et al., 2007, Mullenix, 2014).

Arsenic contamination from HFSA can increase the risk of lung and bladder cancer (Kurttio et al., 1999). Studies on radionuclides suggest that using HFSA as a fluoridation agent could result in significantly more cancer cases compared to using pharmaceutical-grade sodium fluoride (Alimam & Auvinen, 2025) even if it's only a trace amount of radioactive uranium that ends up in the HFSA. Industrial grade Sodium Fluoride that is used as a fluoridation additive is also contaminated with arsenic and other toxins.

According to the National Cancer Institute, arsenic is a known carcinogen that can cause bladder, skin, and other cancers after prolonged exposure, even at very low chronic exposures (Kurttio et al, 1999). Studies also suggest that even pharmaceutical grade fluoride is probably carcinogenic (Doull et al., 2006). Why add any known or suspected carcinogen to our water supply, at any level?

This has always been kept a closely guarded secret, but thanks to Gary Owen Pittman, a former phosphate mining supervisor with Occidental Chemical Corporation in northern Florida, the information finally saw the light of day (Pittman, 2011; Fluoride Action Network, 2022). Hydrofluorosilicic acid is a toxic waste byproduct from the phosphate mining process, and it's also the "fluoride" that is used for our water systems. Everyone really must watch the interview of Gary O. Pittman who was an experienced phosphate fertilizer plant manager where HFSA was made. It is shocking. Phosphate plants use a tar-like defoamer that is vaporized along with HFSA. Smokestacks build up a fluoride rich deposit (containing all the contaminants) which is then recovered in the water scrubbers with "fresh water" from plant wells that are already contaminated by the gypsum ponds leaching into the ground water (Fluoride Action Network, 2022).

It should come as no surprise that the Fortune 500 mining giant Mosaic based in Florida sells most of the fluoride in the US and Canada.

The radionuclide contamination in HFSA is particularly worrisome. Phosphate rock is a good source of uranium, which is being extracted from hundreds of phosphate fertilizer plants all over the world, with the US extracting the most uranium (World Nuclear Association, 2025).

Without reverse osmosis, these minute amounts of contaminants are not removed from drinking water and are consumed day after day from your communal (city) tap water. The heavy metals and radionuclides accumulate over the years in the skeletal system.

It appears very obvious that mined toxic waste should not be added to the public water supply, so why does it continue? We all grew up with the concept of fluoride as something that prevented cavities. No one wants cavities. They are literally holes in our heads. But I have to wonder what other holes must exist in the heads and souls of those who continue to champion the legal poisoning of phosphate workers, consumers and the millions of people who drink unpurified tap water.

Marketing v. Education

Fluoridation began in the 1950s and many people were lulled into a false security by Norman Rockwell's "Look Ma, No Cavities" Crest campaign in 1958. Our country truly believed that water fluoridation would help save our teeth, but it's key to remember that even this was not natural. Artificial fluoridation of public drinking water supplies in the United States began on an experimental basis in 1945 using sodium fluoride, largely derived from by-products of the aluminum smelting industry.

Presently, about 90 percent of drinking water systems adding fluoride use HFSA including its derivative sodium salt (known together as "silicofluorides") as the fluoridating agent. Well over 150,000,000 people in the United States consume silicofluorides in their drinking water. They are not pharmaceutical-grade substances. Collectively, the public water supply systems of the United States are a hazardous waste disposal system for these products.

People are demanding better from the government, and making changes across the country as many communities no longer want HFSA in their water, and it's being removed through legal and political challenges. Gary not only stood up to the giants that poison us, he mentored and inspired many of us, helping us navigate the complex road of intimidation we all face when working on investigating pollution. The job doesn't sound very dangerous, and it shouldn't be, but you would be amazed at how crazy the other side gets when you expose the truth.

The awakening of the "fluoride deception" is leading us to a new revolution in thinking. People now understand protests against fluoridation is not evidence of susceptibility to a conspiracy theory, it's demanding accountability from polluters and politicians. Objecting to fluoridation is refusing to allow our bodies to be used as dumps for the mining industry's toxic waste.

Looking Ahead

Tonight, teeth all clean and fluoride-free, I am ready to head out to a screening of *PHOSFATE* with Sierra. We can't believe the movie is going strong since its release in 2020! Mosaic never stops working their toxic byproducts into everyday life, from toothpaste to the newest innovative way to turn toxic waste into profit—roads.

Soon it won't matter where you live, you'll be exposed to radiation without even knowing it as they add gypsum to building materials. Gypsum is so toxic they are not allowed to dispose of it. There are 25 immense phosphogypsum stacks in Florida, which is about a third of the 70 'gypstacks' nationwide.

When I tell people about radioactive playgrounds and roads, or that the fluoridation chemicals added to their drinking water are mining waste products, many of them look at me like I am crazy and brush it off as conspiracy nonsense. I wish it were nonsense, then people would have less cancer.

However, many people around the nation are paying attention. Florida looks for answers from politicians. Conspiracy theory dismissals fade as information comes to light. More people who walked into the fluoride discussion hoping to disprove that there is harm end up switching to fluoride-free toothpaste. I know I did, and I will never buy fluoridated toothpaste again. No one should hide behind deceptive slogans or stories, but instead stand proud next to facts.

Although many of the politicians who have sold the residents out continue to ignore their calls and emails, the fluoride discussion has done something really big and really important. It has opened a Pandora's box of a water revolution, and you can join this revolution of everyday residents around America just by asking: "What's in your water?"

EDITORS' NOTE:
We are appalled to learn of the presence of radioactivity in the fluoridation water additives and horrified to learn that there is no regular batch testing by NSF. Even a very small trace of radionuclides increases the risk of cancer (Alimam & Auvinen, 2025).

The NSF admits that their annual spot check finds detectable radionuclides in a minority of their samples (NSF.org, 2024). Interviews with Gary O. Pittman reveal that industry subterfuge and omissions make it impossible to believe any pretense of safety.

- Gypsum stacks become more concentrated with heavy metals and radionuclides as the water from these ponds is used over and over again.

- Pond water leaches into the groundwater that is the source of 'fresh water' for the wet scrubbers to isolate the HFSA.

- Tar-like defoaming agents and kerosine additives used in processing are likely recaptured with the HFSA collected by the water scrubbers, but no tests are done to verify those substances have not contributed to the contamination of HFSA.

- Annual NSF testing of a few hundred samples cannot detect the maximum contamination that occurs on a daily or weekly basis in specific HFSA batches, each of which is unique.

- When the (smoke) stack crew is asked to get a sample of HFSA, the workers might say *"Hey man, you ain't going to pass."* Gary explained, *"We just go open a blind way back down the line somewhere and let fresh water rush in and then they pass, you understand... but you don't understand, if you want to keep your damn job, yeah."* (FAN Interview, 2022)

Gary O. Pittman, author of *Phosphate Fluorides Toxic Torts* died on April 3, 2025, at the age of 71 years. He became disabled while in his forties. He suffered from many chronic illnesses due to hazardous workplace exposures at Occidental Chemical Corporation, a North Florida phosphate ore mining operation. He settled his lawsuit with the company after seven years of litigation. They just wanted him to go away (Pittman, 2011; Pittman, 2017).

Dirty Water

Medicated water is criminal

By: Erin Brockovich

with

Bob Bowcock

ABOUT: *Erin Brockovich is an internationally known environmental health activist whose origin story centered on a water pollution cover-up by PG&E in Hinkley, California which resulted in the largest settlement ever paid in a direct-action lawsuit. Her story was made into an Academy Award winning 2000 biographical legal drama starring Julia Roberts in the title role. Erin's subsequent work has earned her many awards as a consumer advocate. She is the author of several books including "Superman is Not Coming: Our National Water Crisis and What WE THE PEOPLE Can Do About It."*

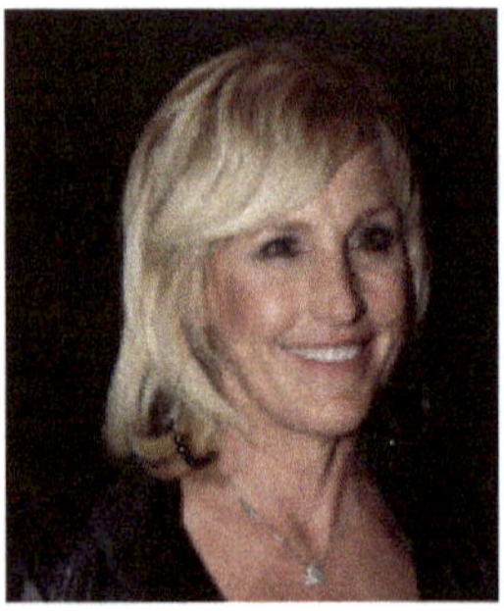

ABOUT: *Bob Bowcock is the founder and Managing Director of Integrated Resource Management (IRM). He has extensive leadership experience in water operations, nationally and abroad. He routinely provides expert witness testimony to both state and federal courts, conducts research, and writes reports for law firms in the specific area of water resource management. He is also a Superior Court Appointed Watermaster. Bob, with and without Erin, has testified before many legislatures concerning water resource management issues.*

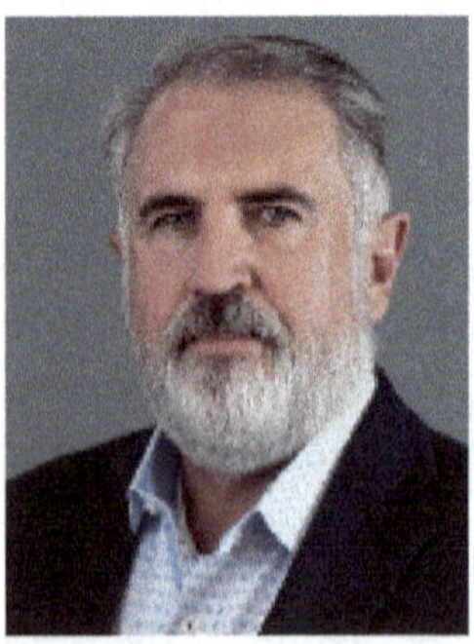

CHAPTER 7

"A nation that destroys its soils destroys itself.
Forests are the lungs of our land, purifying the air
and giving fresh strength to our people."

—U.S. President Franklin D. Roosevelt (1885-1945)

SEVERAL YEARS HAVE PASSED since I got my kick start into the world of environmental advocacy. Since then, my name has sort of become more of an adjective than a noun.

As the requests for help investigating environmental matters became increasingly unmanageable, I vacillated between feeling utter disbelief and being as mad as hell. Frankly, it was overwhelming. I had been blessed with the opportunity to be engaged as a motivational speaker, which I'd turned to as a newfound career—it paid the bills. I was still a single mother of three trying to make it all work, and I was inundated with pleas for help from moms and communities across the globe seeking to understand why their children were sick, covered in rashes and had their hair falling out, thousands of pleas a month. Many of the requests came from moms who had formed groups, and they had no understanding of the word "No." From Kettleman City, California, to Newton Creek, New York... all across our nation, these serious cases requiring real investigation poured in.

And then there's Bob. Not really a part of my coming out story in Hinkley, but always right there by my side, whether I wanted him there or not. Bob sort of just appeared one day, mysteriously quiet, always standing in the back of the room, annoying really. Bob always heads out in front, gets dirty, and helps the community leaders better understand just how they can best help themselves.

While I sort the continuous stream of messages from desperate moms and try my best to reply, Bob heads out on the more critical cases, digging in and swiftly finding the responsible polluter. I have always maintained my sixth sense about these things, while Bob pursues science. It's not pretty. We fight constantly, but we always get to the bottom of the situation. We have scores of road stories, fighting in a car driving down the road in a Michigan Lake driven blizzard to running out of gas, my fault, in a hundred-degree lightning storm somewhere in the south. We've shared the podium at a thousand community meetings for over three decades.

After our first few years working together, we both realized what we were doing just wasn't sustainable. We were burning out, and the requests just kept pouring in. Bob and I sat down one day after a long road trip to try to figure out if we could continue. While we were able to work on cases that led to litigation, which enabled us to cover our costs, more than ninety-nine percent of the cases really didn't have a responsible party. Bob, being an old water utility manager, would never litigate against a water utility, and most requests somehow involved failing drinking water systems.

It was then that Bob explained to me the basic problems many community drinking water systems face. It's simple to understand when you break it down to this simple concept: clean the drinking water. Bob was often criticized by his peers for oversimplifying the science when he said, "take the dirt out of the drinking water." It wasn't oversimplification, it was brilliance.

Based on this simple point, we decided to focus on the foundational concept of clean, healthy community drinking water and sharing this message with moms across the nation in order to better help them to help themselves.

Long before the passage of the Safe Drinking Water Act in 1974, it was universally recognized that the cleaner the water is, the fewer chemical reactions that form toxic compounds would occur. But by now, you are probably asking, "What does this have to do with the practice of dosing fluoride into our community drinking water systems?" The answer is "Plenty."

The idea behind the federal regulation of community drinking water began with the railroads. The goal was everyone should be able to rely on the drinking water being consistently safe as you traveled across the United States. Then things began to go wrong.

Starting in 1962, the United States Public Health Service recommended that public water supplies contain between 0.7 and 1.2 mg/L of fluoride to help prevent tooth decay. Simultaneously, communities across the country began to fall in line with those recommendations.

It seems that almost everything that begins with good intentions creates webs of myopic and self-centered plots intended to manipulate people in order to protect policy. That's when Bob and I see the unintended consequences of regulatory compliance spin out of the bureaucratic silos like the destructive winds of a Kansas tornado.

For example, when the Safe Drinking Water Act was just taking hold in the early 1980s, the Surface Water Treatment Rule required minimum disinfection to rid drinking water of bacteria and other disease-causing organisms. Increases in chlorine levels, rich in organic precursors (dirt), cause the formation of regulated toxic disinfection byproducts. As a result, many drinking water systems elected to add ammonia to dirty drinking water to sequester the chemical reactions that form these disinfection byproducts. Simultaneously, adding ammonia to form *chloramine* increased the water's corrosivity, which leaches lead from pipes and brass fixtures. Since lead does not have a maximum contaminant level, only an action level, utilities pinky swear they will "take action" to reduce lead in drinking water. This so-called action resulted in the addition of phosphates to reduce corrosion effects.

Bottomline, rather than cleaning out the dirt using proven, cost effective, age-old water treatment techniques like activated carbon, making the water safer to drink, thousands of utilities opted to haphazardly add ammonia, still forming toxins (just at reduced levels), and then adding phosphates as a countermeasure. I just didn't get it, WHY? Why wouldn't a community opt for cleaner drinking water over adding more chemicals?

Many utilities use cost as a scare tactic to influence decision makers. They'd say that activated carbon just costs too much. Well, that just didn't make sense to me. Hundreds of drinking water utilities have been using activated carbon for decades with overall costs often less than those utilities that choose to destroy their own infrastructure as well as the plumbing, fixtures and appliances of their consumers. The City of Cincinnati, Ohio, was so committed to granular activated carbon treatment they constructed a carbon activation kiln at the water treatment plant on the Ohio River in 1974.

Here's the kicker. Many of the same utilities that claim *it just costs too much* to clean the water are the same utilities that will die on a battle hill in support of fluoridation programs. Why? Fluoride, although a toxic waste, isn't free. Storage and dosing systems aren't just handed out... or are they?

What I discovered is that there are more grants and government assistance programs to promote using our community drinking water systems as medical dispensaries than to make drinking water safe to consume. Why is the fluoride advocates' lobby so large and well-funded?

This was where we began to investigate what was going on. I knew some drinking water utilities dose fluoride into their drinking water but I didn't really understand the effect of fluoridation on infrastructure, environment or consumers.

As I began to dig into it, what I learned was most disturbing. It is what led me to repeat as often as I could, rallying community groups, "The use of the public drinking water system to dose any substance to achieve a medical result is criminal!" Followed by, "Water treatment professionals are not pharmacists—our drinking water is not their medical dispensary," and "Don't mess around with fluoride. It's dangerous... turn it off and never turn it on again. It's not the job of the city to dose any substance in the community drinking water system for the sole purpose of achieving a medical result. If you continue, you're morally corrupt!"

These are harsh words, but I mean them. The question of whether dosing fluoride in public water supplies is morally wrong is complex with arguments on both sides. It essentially boils down to a conflict between alleged public health benefits and individual rights.

Arguments against water fluoridation based on ethical concerns include the violation of Informed Consent because adding fluoride to public water is mass medication without individual consent. Informed consent is central to medical ethics. Individuals should have the right to choose whether to consume fluoride as a preventative dental treatment. Fluoridation programs remove that choice, forcing many to opt for expensive bottled water.

There is a complete lack of control over dosage, people consume varying amounts of water, leading to overexposure in many and possible under-exposure in others. And finally, fluoridation as a form of mass medication disregards individual differences in health and vulnerability to adverse effects.

Views on the most effective fluoride therapy for community prevention of tooth decay have always been mixed. Some believe water fluoridation is the most effective, whereas, others see no systemic advantage and prefer topical application strategies. Those opposed argue that water fluoridation has no or little cariostatic benefits, may cause serious health problems, is not effective enough to justify the costs, and is pharmacologically obsolete. Once again, Bob and I agree that the dosing of our community drinking water with any substance is just wrong.

After seventy years of U.S. fluoridation, the recommended concentration in drinking water was cut to single fluoride concentration of 0.7 mg/L in 2015. That's almost half of the previous upper limit. A claim was made that the reduction allowed for

the fact that people now get more fluoride from other sources (such as toothpaste) than in the past.

I call BS! Fluoridation policy causes dental fluorosis (white or brown spotting on teeth) whether at 1 ppm or 0.7 ppm and regardless of any other exposures. Fluoridation policy also causes a condition called skeletal fluorosis, when fluoride builds up in the bones as a result of years of consumption. This can eventually result in joint stiffness and pain as well as lead to fragile bones and more fractures in older adults.

Studies have shown an association between the use of fluorosilicic acid and its sodium salt to fluoridate water and increased uptake of lead into children's blood. Lead is acknowledged as a neurotoxin that damages the child's developing brain. Lead, as well as arsenic, aluminum, and other toxins, contaminate the fluoridation water additives used in American and Canadian communities. Lead toxicity is largely unaddressed in developing countries.

I, I mean we, Bob and I, have remained constant in the fight against dosing community drinking water with fluoride. We have, and will continue to, take on shameless criticism from those committed to the practice of forced medical treatments. Call us leaders of the tinfoil hat community all you want, we can sleep at night knowing we are on the right side of the issue.

I advocate for the truth and transparency—a person's right to know. I believe that in the absence of the truth, all of us are helpless to defend ourselves, our families and our health, which are our greatest gifts.

As with everything, some people always go too far, too far to the right, too far to the left, and this is true of environmentalism. In many instances, our protests fall on deaf ears because of preconceived notions and limited understanding. Often, we don't think about or worry about or understand what is happening to another person until it happens to us, and then it is too late.

Disease doesn't recognize the color of our skin or our political party's affiliation. Deceits have no boundaries. When it comes to cover-ups and the destruction of our environment, we and our drinking water are up for grabs.

One of the truths that Bob and I have consistently said that confirms human rights and defies deceitful rhetoric is; "Fluoride doesn't belong in drinking water. Period."

Paradigm Shifts in Science

Barriers to communicating new science with decision-makers

By: Dr C. Vyvyan Howard, MB, ChB, PhD, FRCPath

with

Dr Paul Connett, MA, PhD

ABOUT: *Vyvyan Howard is a medically qualified toxico-pathologist specialising in the problems associated with the action of toxic substances on the fetus and the infant. He is Emeritus Professor of Bioimaging at the University of Ulster and has written a number of papers and book chapters and spoken in a variety of forums to draw attention to the threat posed by environmental pollutants to the developing fetus. He has a scientific interest in the toxico-pathological mechanism responsible for IQ loss in the fetus and infant through fluoride exposure.*

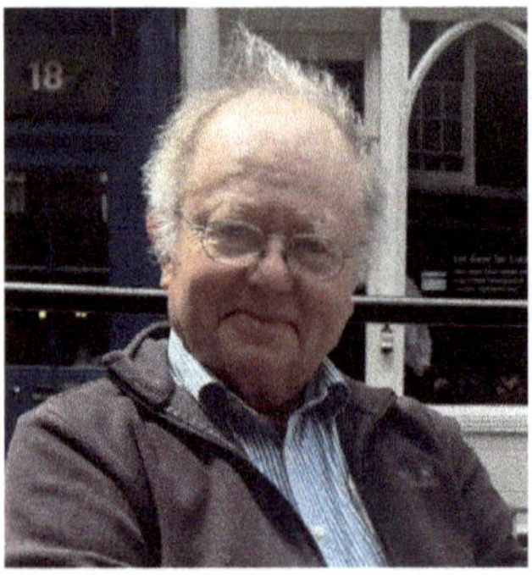

Dr Howard is a Fellow of the Royal College of Pathologists, Past President of the Royal Microscopical Society, Member of the British Society of Toxico-Pathologists, Past President of the International Society of Doctors for the Environment and Emeritus Fellow of the Collegium Ramazzini. He served for six years as a toxicologist on the UK Government DEFRA Advisory Committee on Pesticides.

See Paul Connett's chapter for his biography.

CHAPTER 8

"There are none so deaf as those who will not hear."

—John Heywood (1546)

WHEN THE BASHASH et al. (2017) paper was published, a number of scientists and clinicians knowledgeable of the scientific literature on fluoride toxicity embarked upon activity to bring the findings in the paper to the attention of regulators and governmental decision-makers. That paper, and those which followed, completely changed the nature of the prior debate. In the face of developmental neurotoxicology, leading to significant loss of IQ when fetuses and infants are exposed to fluoride, there should be little to debate. Developmental toxicological damage is permanent, while dental damage is repairable.

We do not know of any parent who would trade an iota of their child's intelligence for the questionable saving of a fraction of a filling over a lifetime. This is particularly so since the judgement of the California Federal Court under the Toxic Substances Control Act (TSCA), commanding the US EPA to take measures to deal with the 'unreasonable risk to public health' posed by fluoridated community water supplies. These aspects of the recent history of fluoride toxicity are dealt with extensively by other authors in this book and we will not restate them here.

However, we have included a compilation of letters we delivered to decision-makers in an attempt to bring the scientific evidence and ethics to the attention of the Government of the UK and of the astoundingly refractory response in Appendix B of this book.

Our initial series of letters were sent by Royal Mail recorded postal delivery, and we have a record that they were delivered to 10 Downing Street (the UK Prime Minister's office). There was no apparent way of sending the letters to 10 Downing Street electronically. We received no acknowledgement to these three letters. However, they were widely distributed to parliamentarians. When we attempted to send Letter 4 by Royal Mail recorded delivery, we were informed that the postcode was no longer available for direct posting.

Consequently, I asked my MP, Hon Gregory Campbell, to have the fourth letter delivered by him to the Prime Minister's Office with a request for a response. A response came as a letter from Hon Stephen Kinnock MP (see Appendix B). Mr. Kinnock's letter is not encouraging.

Firstly, it completely ignores the two UK Government funded studies, CATFISH and LOTUS, which both show that artificial water fluoridation is not efficacious in preventing caries and does not protect socially deprived groups, a major driver for implementing water fluoridation.

Secondly, it misstates science. The judgement made by Judge Chen, at the end of a seven-year court case which included consideration of the National Toxicology Program (NTP) systematic review, did NOT find that fluoride below 1.5 mg/L was not associated with neurological damage. In fact, 0.7 mg/L was considered to be associated with fetal neurological damage.

Thirdly, the tenor of Mr. Kinnock's letter on behalf of the UK Government seems to ignore the findings of the recent US studies showing loss of IQ in fluoridated populations. He seems to be prepared to risk reduction in the UK population's IQ because a review of the NTP stated that there was "*moderate confidence*" in the effect. This appears to be a bizarrely casual attitude to the use of precaution in public health.

World-Wide Prejudice

The difficulty in getting those in positions of authority to listen to scientists, doctors, and dentists with strong credible evidence of the harm caused by their fluoridation policy is not limited to the UK. We also see it in the Americas, Australia, and New Zealand.

When we spoke at Otago University in New Zealand in 2018 at the request of a Citizens' Group, there was a very small group in attendance, none of whom were professors or teaching staff. Our small audience was comprised mostly of students, and most of them wore fantastical hats fashioned from tinfoil—the obvious implication being that the learned Professors Howard and Connett, along with co-presenter Irish scientist Declan Waugh, were crazy conspiracy theorists deserving of ridicule (International Experts at Otago University, 2023).

We directly and respectfully addressed the adolescents in our presentations and to do them credit, they stayed and listened without causing any disruption. They did not, however, at any time apologize for their disdainful insult to us or ask any follow-up questions.

It does beg a larger question: if our educational institutions emphasize conformity with policy instead of critical evaluation of facts and those who rise to positions of power in government and other organizations prefer to respond to matters of fact with fictions and ridicule, is the world slipping deeper and deeper into a totalitarian mindset where scientific discipline, justice, and health are no longer valued?

Conclusions

There are clearly many obstacles in the way of concerned scientists (and citizens) making their views known to governments and other decision-makers. Initially we were surprised to discover that there was no obvious way to send information electronically. We found that you could post letters to the Office of the Prime Minister and obtain proof of receipt. We did not receive any sort of acknowledgement to our first three letters. Then this mode of communication was also blocked, and it became impossible to post directly to 10 Downing Street.

In another chapter in this book Paul Connett has described our similar efforts to get the BBC to live up to its standards of professionalism and objectivity in its reporting of the science pertaining to the fluoridation debate. Sadly, its coverage of the same scientific studies and events covered in this chapter has been lamentably poor and more consistent with the apparent opinions of the tin-hat student brigade in New Zealand. As with our efforts with three Prime Ministers, as of this time of writing, the response of the BBC has been equally disdainful. We would also draw the attention of readers to another chapter in this book written by a BBC reporter, Michele Paduano. He writes about the blatant censorship of his work on fluoridation by his superiors at the BBC, which led him to resign after nearly 30 years of service.

We close with one more question for our readers to ponder: is propaganda and protection of policy more important than public and personal health in the twenty-first century?

Why I Quit the BBC Over Fluoride

By: Michele Paduano

ABOUT: *Michele Paduano is a successful investigative journalist in the UK. He broke the story about Dupont's fungicide Benomyl causing lack of eyes in the fetus (Paduano et al., 1993). Dr Vyvyan Howard subsequently became the causation witness in Castillo vs Dupont—an American lawsuit that found for the plaintiffs against Dupont in 2003. This was one of a series of successful PFAS-related lawsuits against Dupont tried by environmental attorney Robert Bilott. Although primarily a Health Correspondent, Michele also covers Social Affairs, Environment and various other specialist subjects. Michele's approach to his craft is: "I always hope to stumble across that bit of information which could unearth the story that would make that fundamental difference."*

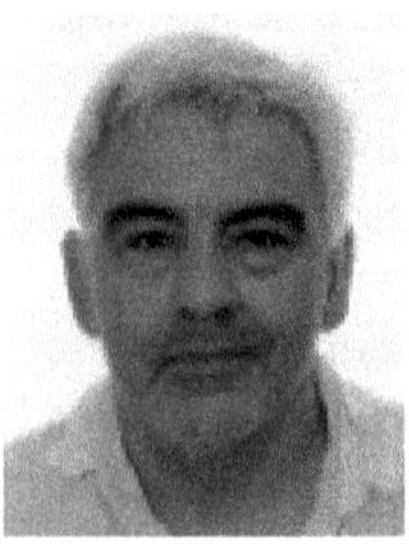

CHAPTER 9

"Our liberty depends on the freedom of the press, and that cannot be limited without being lost."

—U.S. President Thomas Jefferson (1786)

I FIRST MET Professor Vyvyan Howard whilst investigating a mysterious cluster of children without eyes—born in Lincolnshire. With his help and the support of *The Observer*—a British Sunday newspaper—the problem was linked to chemical usage and notably to a fungicide called benomyl. The product was eventually withdrawn and ten years after the investigation, 13-year-old John Castillo won $7m compensation in a landmark judgement in the United States. His empty eye sockets were linked by a court to exposure to benomyl (Reed, 2003).

I then began avidly reporting on environmental issues—linking childhood brain tumours to potential *in utero* exposure to pesticides and suggesting early links between landfill sites and cancer. But by 1993, I was poor and I joined the BBC—eventually becoming the West Midlands Regional Health Correspondent.

The West Midlands was the first place in the UK to adopt fluoridated water in 1964. I was aware of Professor Howard's concerns, but apart from a broadcast on dental fluorosis in the nineties and a report when documents were leaked to me to show that Severn Trent Water—the regional water company—had over fluoridated water, I stepped back from environmental health issues and began exposing the problems of day-to-day care in the NHS.

I didn't even report Professor Stephen Peckham's work which suggested a possible association between fluoride and hypothyroidism —even though the study was conducted in Birmingham in the heart of my region (Peckham et al., 2015).

However, when Professor Howard contacted me after decades in 2019 saying a number of scientific studies on fluoride were showing a neurotoxic effect, I began asking questions of the authorities, but I received such vehement rebuttals that I knew that the chance of getting the BBC to publish anything—whatever the quality of the science—was remote. I didn't even try.

It was only when, out of the blue, Professor Howard called me in September 2024 to inform me that Judge Edward Chen in a federal court in California had ruled that fluoride represented an unacceptable risk to the unborn child (Chen, 2024) that I looked again. I read the judgment in full and felt that I had a public duty to report on it.

After all, Chen was demanding an EPA response to his concerns regarding 0.7 mg/litre of fluoride added to water. In the UK West Midlands, water fluoridation has occurred at 1 mg/litre since 1964, and it is acceptable in law to fluoridate at 1.5 mg/litre which is right on the edge of the World Health Organisation's permitted limits.

I wrote up a preliminary online news version of the story. A TV interview with Joy Warren from West Midlands Against Fluoride was set up. There was a date pencilled in to run the story. Professor Howard provided a down the line interview where he stated:

> *"This judgement is a game stopper. The fact that it is neurotoxic to the foetus and causes an irreversible change in outcome in the child's brain, there are no other arguments."* he said.

Shortly before the Joy Warren television interview, I was contacted by my editor, Lucy Collins, asking who had commissioned the story. I replied that it hadn't been commissioned, but I am the Health Correspondent, and I regularly offer stories based on my expertise.

There was a degree of prevarication, but eventually, I was asked to pull the interview scheduled for October 17th and I contacted Ms Warren to explain.

She was naturally disappointed when I called her, but genuinely understanding. I explained that it wasn't my decision and that I was convinced that it was a minor hiccup and that I had a long history of pushing boulders uphill—most of which I did manage to finally push over the edge and send crashing down the other side.

During the conversation, she mentioned that she had heard that an anti-fluoride campaigner was being interviewed in Cumbria regarding the plans to expand fluoridation there. I was somewhat bewildered that an article was being prepared in another region—the North—and I was being stalled in the West Midlands.

The day that I was originally scheduled to film the interview with Ms Warren, I met, instead, with my editor, Ms Collins and the Regional head of online news, Tom Warren.

I tried to explain the science, the judgment, and the National Toxicology Program (NTP) findings in the United States, but everything that I put forward was parried by the concern that an article would cause unnecessary alarm among the population of the West Midlands and that the British authorities said fluoride was safe.

I countered by saying that history was littered with examples where the authorities had said a substance was safe: PCBs, 245T, Thalidomide, organophosphates, lead in petrol, diesel. In the case of diesel, it was promoted as environmentally beneficial for decades—even though I had attended a conference in the early 90s that already defined micro particulates as dangerous and a risk to health.

I was also challenged on a lack of a detailed rebuttal. My riposte: I can only ask the questions, but if the Department of Health and Social Care is only prepared to state that "The fluoride levels permitted in the UK are proven to be safe and are well below the levels quoted in this study and WHO safety guidelines (1.5 mg/litre). There is a duty to monitor effects of water fluoridation schemes on health. The next health monitoring report will be published in 2026," then I was somewhat limited.

I had also quoted the British Dental Association stating that it was safe and had always intended—and had stated—that I would interview Barry Cockcroft, the chair of the British Fluoridation Society.

I explained too that I had read the last fluoride health monitoring report for England in 2022, and it didn't address neurotoxicity as a specific issue. But I was happy to include whatever they wanted if it was relevant.

I reminded my management of my credentials as a reporter, a health correspondent, and my history as an environmental health reporter at national level. I also brandished my cuttings from my time working on newspapers. I asked on what basis they were challenging my expertise.

Ms Collins said that it was merely one court in the United States and one federal judge which could be overturned at a later date.

I pointed out that we didn't fail to report on court verdicts because they might be overturned in the future, but in whatever way I challenged the logic, I was countered by the accusation that it was scaremongering and that UK authorities said that adding fluoride to water was safe.

I was also told that Carol Rubra, senior health news editor, had been consulted and had concerns about the quality of the science being used.

When the conversation became more heated, Tom Warren accused me of being biased and presenting fluoride harm as fact.

I walked out of the meeting upset—stating that never in my 30 plus years as a BBC journalist had I ever been accused of bias or been found to have been biased. I went home and reread my proposed article—reflecting on what had been said.

I then prepared a detailed apologia which demonstrated that at no point had my article overstated the science or presented the evidence as fact. I quoted a study abstract:

> *The tendency to ignore new evidence that does not conform to widespread beliefs impedes the response to early warnings about fluoride as a potential developmental neurotoxin. Evolving evidence should inspire scientists and health authorities to re-evaluate claims about the safety of fluoride, especially for the fetus and infant for whom there is no benefit* (Till & Green, 2020).

At this point, I was still of the opinion that I would be able to get my article published and I asked what specifically needed to be done to get it over the line. I advised them that I was happy to undertake any further work required to ensure publication.

On October 28th, I received advice from BBC Editorial policy regarding BBC guidelines which stated that stories must be well-sourced, based on sound evidence and corroborated when reporting statistics and risk. I am directed to the editorial guidelines:

- ***3.3.8*** *We should reserve the same scepticism for statistics as we do for facts or quotes and not necessarily take numbers at face value. When our output includes statistics, we should explain the numbers clearly, put them into context, weigh, interpret and, where appropriate, challenge them, present them clearly and attribute them. The statistics must be accurate and verified where necessary, with important caveats and limitations explained. We should use a range of evidence to put statistical claims into context and help audiences to judge their magnitude and importance. Where claims are wrong or misleading, they should be challenged.*

- ***3.3.9*** *The reporting of risk can have an impact on the public's perception of that risk, particularly with health or crime stories. We should avoid worrying our audiences unduly and contextualise our reports to be clear about the likelihood of the risk occurring. This is particularly true in reporting health stories that may cause individuals to alter their behaviour in ways that could be harmful. We should consider the emotional impact pictures and personal testimony can have, particularly on perceptions of risk*

There are objections to the quality of a Canadian study (Green et al., 2019) which was published in *JAMA Pediatrics*, a suggestion that wider deprivations may impact on IQ in fluoridated areas, and a questioning of how much credence should be given to the US judgement in a country that is highly litigious and where lower court judgements are subject to challenge.

In the meantime, I had been working hard to provide further balance for the article. I had spoken to Barry Cockcroft, chair of the British Fluoridation Society who insisted on the safety of fluoride. Interestingly, he suggested that maybe there should be emphasis on fluoridation in the North of England not the South. The North is considered more deprived and has worse dental health. The latest research from the Universities of Manchester, Aberdeen, and Dundee which showed only "modest" benefit from fluoridation. Therefore, the inference was that fluoridation might not be required in the South where there was less dental decay.

And I had contacted Professor John Fawell, who wrote the book on fluoridation and who advises the World Health Organisation. He, of course, stressed that fluoridation is safe and pointed to Health Canada's 2024 conclusion on safety:

> *"...based on several considerations, the panel agrees that there is not a sufficient basis at this time to recommend a specific point of departure and health-based value for neurocognitive effects."*

But, and it struck me as a big but, when pushed further he said that he did think that Britain should review its dosing level in the light of new evidence—given that the USA and Canada medicate at 0.7 mg/litre.

I had it. This was a game changer. This had to be a story. The leading proponent for fluoridation suggests that we should consider reducing our fluoride levels by 30% in the UK based on the latest science and the precautionary principle.

It's worth pointing out that there had been no coverage anywhere on the BBC online pages of the US Federal Court Judgement or of the US National Toxicology Program findings at all.

I triumphantly take my Fawell response to Deborah Turness, the head of national news and to my senior managers locally.

A week later—complete silence—so I try again, this time approaching Tim Davie, the BBC Director General, Ms Turness again, and Samir Shah, the chairman of the BBC.

The following day I am told by Lucy Collins that we are not running the story and that it is her decision. I am again referring to the idea of causing unnecessary anxiety, the relative value of a US court judgement and specifically the previously mentioned: 3.3.9 of the editorial guidelines.

I try to point out that there must be a story of some sort in the Fawell comments and that we appear happy to report on the findings of a US Court when it relates to Prince Andrew—so why not in this case?

There is one further recourse within the BBC—Sir Nicholas Serota. He is the senior independent director on the BBC Board. His blurb says that he is "responsible for upholding and protecting the independence of the BBC by acting in the public interest and exercising independent judgement." It is his duty too to ensure that the BBC fulfils its mission to inform and educate.

I explained to him my concern that no BBC outlet had reported the Fluoride Judgement, the National Toxicology Program findings or the new position expressed by Professor John Fawell—despite the fact that the Government was about to make a decision following a consultation to expand fluoridation in the North East. I told him that this appeared nothing short of censorship.

I suggested that with the arrival of Robert F. Kennedy, Jr. as the Secretary of Health and Human Services in the United States (the equivalent of the UK Health Minister), the BBC could also end up with reputational damage.

Eleven days later, on 26 November 2024, an anonymous pro fluoridation article appeared on the England page of BBC Online regarding the fluoride debate in the North East. Its headline quotes the British Dental Association saying that fluoridation would be a great leveller. But, finally, halfway down the article, the following passage:

> *"A US Court recently concluded fluoridation posed an 'un-reasonable risk of reduced IQ in children', though the ruling did not 'conclude with certainty' that fluoridated water is injurious to public health".*

An anti-fluoride campaigner, Ms Standen, is quoted urging the UK government to be careful. "If you don't really know what the impact is going to be, you should be cautious about putting it in the water," she said. "In fact, you should not put it in the water until you've established 100% safety."

But Oliver Jones, a professor of chemistry at RMIT University in Australia, said the evidence was inconsistent and people should not be concerned by the US judgement. "If X causes Y, then we should see that consistently," he said. "We shouldn't be getting some results showing something and some of the results showing something else completely."

I later found out from Vyvyan Howard that he had been interviewed by BBC television in the North East regarding fluoride—but his contribution had never been used.

I was not told that article was going to be published, but when I became aware of it, I naturally asked why it was possible to do a story in the North, but not in the Midlands and why there was no mention of the need to review the concentration of fluoride that was being put into water in the UK?

Ms Collins' riposte was that there was no news line for the West Midlands.

I was exasperated. How can we ignore a leading proponent for fluoridation suggesting that we should look at reducing the levels of fluoride currently being put into our water? How can it not be a West Midlands story, as well as a national story, since the vast majority of people who receive fluoridated water in the UK live in the West Midlands?

I even suggested a much watered-down version of my article which emphasised merely that it is in the safety interests of babies in the West Midlands to consider reducing the amount of fluoride added to water to the levels used in the USA and Canada.

Four days later, a story appeared on the BBC Hereford and Worcester Web website. This is another part of my patch as West Midlands Health Correspondent, but the story was written by a non-specialist who reports on municipal and public meetings. It's headlined: "Calls for the whole country to have fluoride in water." The article extolls the virtue of adding fluoride to water and reassures the public that "it is a safe and effective strategy." (Wilkinson-Jones, 2025)

There had been no consultation with me—the region's health expert—ahead of its publication by the online team. Most telling, the online site is run and overseen by Tom Warren who had accused me of bias earlier.

After thirty-one years, I had by now made the decision to leave the BBC. I had been offered voluntary redundancy even though my job was not at risk. I articulated that growing censorship was a reason for wanting to go. Knowing I was leaving, management stopped engaging with my protests and played a waiting game.

At my farewell party, I cited the fact that the BBC's mantra of impartiality which was constantly rammed down our throats had begun to cudgel stick in my craw. I loved the BBC, but it was now anything but impartial. My fight was over, but it was time for others to take up the and fight for its soul.

Not a single member of the senior management team attended the event—dozens of those whom I had supported over the years in their personal fight for truth and justice did.

EDITORS' NOTE: As this book was going to press, Michele informed us that his article concerning fluoride exposure during pregnancy and lowered IQ in offspring was published elsewhere (Paduano, 2025).

Malpractice

Civil Service Labor Union's Opposition of Water Fluoridation

By: Dr J. William Hirzy, Jr., PhD

ABOUT: *Dr Hirzy went to university in 1954 with a U.S. Navy Regular ROTC scholarship, intending to have a career in the regular U.S. Marine Corps. He did his national service for 27 years in the Civil Service instead of the Naval Service. He was the Senior Scientist for Risk Assessment, Toxics Office at U.S. EPA for over 27 years, and former several-term President of the EPA Professionals Headquarters Union in Washington DC (NTEU 280), Chemist in Residence and Adjunct Professor, American University Department of Chemistry 1995–2013. The details of how and why the EPA professionals 'labor union fought the fluoride fight—and others—can be found at epaunionhistory.org.*

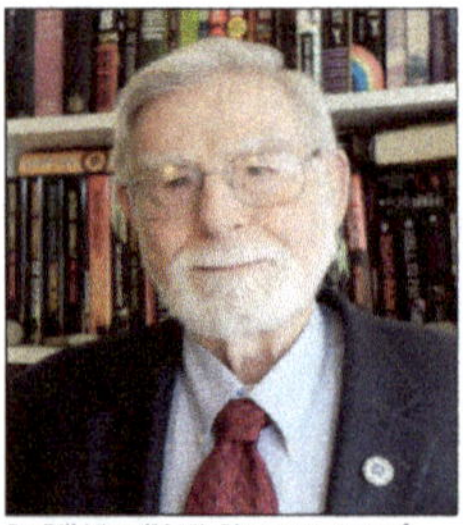

Dr. Bill Hirzy (2015). Photo courtesy of Ellen Hirzy.

CHAPTER 10

"It is my belief that nearly any invented quotation, played with confidence, stands a good chance to deceive."

—*Mark Twain*

WHILE THE U.S. Environmental Protection Agency (EPA) is rightly considered a science-based entity, there is another aspect of the EPA not generally recognized by the American public. There are actually two cultures there: the scientist culture and the lawyer culture. When they are in harmony, it is a beautiful thing; when they are not, it can get ugly. I was naïve about how differently scientists and lawyers see the world when I joined EPA.

Service vs Servant

When I arrived at EPA headquarters as a Senior Scientist in the Assessment Division of the Office of Pesticides and Toxic Substances in May 1981, EPA professionals—including prominently Dr. Robert J. Carton, who became the first EPA employee to pick up the cudgel against fluoridation—were anxious about the future. New President Ronald Reagan was known as anti-environment and anti-labor, and his EPA Administrator had virtually no management experience outside a 30-person telephone office in Denver. Organizing was in the air. Eight of us professional employees (as defined in the Civil Service Reform Act of 1978) began the task of organizing what became, after two years of hard work, the National Federation of Federal Employees Local 2050, which was chartered in 1983. In 1984, Local 2050 won an election to become the exclusive representative for the professional bargaining unit at EPA Headquarters. Our main focus during the election campaign was working to secure an ethical work environment for professionals, shielded from undue political influence. We campaigned on being able, as the legally authorized representative, to bargain with management over working conditions. An ethical work environment was one such critical working condition. Our first contract proposals included a "code of professional ethics." The exact term "scientific integrity" wasn't in wide use at the time, but it came to be—in actions by the Union.

The first action of Local 2050 along these lines made clear how differently the scientists (and those who think like scientists) and lawyers reacted to upper management's 1984 withdrawal of proposed asbestos regulations [under section 6 of the Toxic Substances Control Act (TSCA)] due to political pressure. We learned of that withdrawal during a press conference in the Administrator's office. I organized employees in the Office of Toxic Substances to protest what we learned was the President's Office of Personnel Management (OMB) being the source of that pressure. One hundred twenty-eight staff and management employees signed on to a letter to the Administrator I had drafted on that subject. I pointed out the scientific basis for the abandoned regulations. The letter said that neither he nor we had come to work at EPA just to draft options for OMB to select from for controlling health risks. Management's response to the 128 signatories of our letter was to call a mass meeting to explain the withdrawal from asbestos control via TSCA. I asked the Acting Administrator why the fiction of "We just discovered section 9 required us to withdraw" when staff knew that was not true. I next asked, "What is the ethical duty of an attorney in that situation?" ***The two-culture reality at EPA then became crystal clear. He replied, 'It is the duty of an attorney to get his/her client where they want to go without violating the law. And our client was the President of the United States."*** Scientists have no "clients." They ask questions of Mother Nature, try to make sense of her answers, and publish their understanding of the science so that other scientists can test those understandings. If they receive compensation for their work, they also deliver their understanding to their employer. Period! That union action was reported on by the *New York Times*, and people fighting fluoridation noticed.

Some of those folks contacted us and invited EPA professionals to a seminar on fluoride toxicity. The seminar was presented by Dr. John Yiamouyiannis and attended by a number of EPA professionals, including Local 2050 leaders. The seminar was an eye-opener for all of us in attendance. At the time, EPA had just proposed new drinking water standards for fluoride that included the health-based drinking water standard—now called the Maximum Contaminant Level Goal (MCLG) of 4 milligrams per liter (4 mg/L) for fluoride. The Agency did so even though it knew moderate to severe dental fluorosis would affect many people. First, a non-enforceable standard to protect against known or anticipated adverse effects on health, known as the Maximum Contaminant Level Goal (MCLG), is set. Then, an enforceable Maximum Contaminant Level (MCL) is set based on feasibility and economics. The Natural Resources Defense Council (NRDC), an environmental advocacy organization, had filed a lawsuit against the EPA for setting that MCLG, contending it did not protect public health as mandated by the Safe Drinking Water Act. (More on this also below.)

Also, around this time Paul Price—the employee assigned to write the Federal Register Notice of Proposed Rule Making for the new drinking water fluoride standards—came to Bob Carton with a complaint. Paul told Bob he had been ordered to change the MCLG from 2 to 4 milligrams per liter. Paul, incensed at that order, had then composed a bitterly satirical bulletin board announcement (before emails came to be the method of communication) because he was aware that severe dental fluorosis (DF) occurs in children with nephrogenic diabetes insipidus who drink water with 0.5 mg/L of fluoride. Severe DF results from fluoride exposure of the developing tooth during crucial stages of development. The severe category shows enamel mottling and brown stains. The announcement said that management had opted for that higher MCLG, which was already known by management to cause severe dental fluorosis because it was cheaper for people to keep their mouths shut than to remove fluoride in compliance with a lower standard.

Brick Walls

Duly alarmed, Bob and I went to the Director of the Office of Drinking Water (ODW), asking him to arrange a seminar from the contractors who had written the Technical Support Document on which the 4 mg/L MCLG was based. We expressed our concern that the public would think EPA scientists were responsible for that flawed document. No Dice. We were told that ODW had followed normal practice for its proposed standard, namely, publishing it on the Federal Register and asking for comments. Case closed.

We then went to the Agency Inspector General (I.G.), who is charged with ferreting out fraud, waste, and abuse and is responsible for doing something about any found. Bob laid out the scientific justification management used for the proposed MCLG and why it constituted fraud. The I.G. pleaded his inability to assess whether the MCLG's justification was fraudulent, and he declined to take action. So much for staying within the system.

Upon learning of the Union's concerns, NRDC asked Local 2050 to join their lawsuit in the DC Federal Court of Appeals against the EPA over that standard with an *amicus curiae* brief; NRDC would handle the legal wording, and we— principally Bob Carton—would handle the science section. We polled union members, got their approval for joining NRDC, and filed the *amicus* brief. Judges Bork and Ginsberg wrote for the Court that the brief would not be entered into the case because it would be like the EPA suing itself. We argued that Local 2050 was not a creature of the EPA, but that didn't change the Court's ruling.

Sensing that just folding our tent and retreating from the field would be an abandonment of our duty as health and environmental professionals to protect the public, as well as our oath to "...defend the

Constitution against all enemies, foreign and domestic," we consulted the National Federation of Federal Employees (NFFE) national office for advice. The General Counsel advised us that we could use our own time and resources to pursue this fight. And so we did. But first we paid a visit to Ralph Nader, a well-known and respected campaigner on consumer safety issues.

I also contacted Bob Eckhardt, the "Congressional Father" of TSCA, two other important environmental lawyers, and a family friend about the withdrawal of asbestos. Bob had triggered a Congressional investigation that revealed the extent of OMB's secret contacts with Canadian asbestos mining interests. The revelation prompted an EPA/OMB Memorandum of Understanding that forbade such future secret meetings.

Nader told us he always had bad feelings about the Federal Government's drive to fluoridate drinking water supplies as a way to lessen the incidence of dental caries. He suggested we consult with attorney Jim Turner, one of "Nader's Raiders," the famous cadre of attorneys and investigators Nader employed in exposing and addressing threats to consumer safety.

A New Direction

We met with Jim several times to discuss strategies for ending the threat fluoridation posed to the American public. I pointed out that section 21 of the Toxic Substances Control Act was a route to "drive a hemlock stake through the heart of fluoridation." Section 21 permits citizens to petition the EPA to take regulatory action on any chemical substance that constitutes an unreasonable risk to health or the environment. Turner pointed out that, assuming an EPA denial of a petition to ban fluoride addition to drinking water, a lawsuit would have to be filed to force the EPA to act. Such a lawsuit would be a costly affair, Jim declared, and we were at a loss in 1986 as to finding the necessary funding. After the Connett family joined the fight, using the Fluoride Action Network (FAN) to build alliances that were able to get the necessary funding, an outstanding science capability was built. It was "Game On!"

On November 14, 1985, EPA finalized the 4 mg/L MCLG in a *Federal Register Notice*, having made an official finding that severe dental fluorosis was not an adverse health effect. The next day Bob Carton **again** wrote to EPA Administrator Lee Thomas detailing the unethical—to say the least—behavior he had allowed in setting the MCLG by ignoring advice from health experts about severe dental fluorosis. He pointed out that the original Report of the Surgeon General's ad hoc panel on non-dental effects, which EPA had solicited, recommended an MCLG between 1.2 and 2.4 mg/L to prevent moderate to severe dental fluorosis, which the Committee described as an adverse effect on health. Input from the National Institute of Mental Health was that individuals with moderate to severe dental fluorosis were probably at risk for psychological and behavioral problems. Likewise, the National Drinking Water Advisory Council, an outside body that EPA uses, advised the Agency that moderate to severe dental fluorosis is an adverse health effect. EPA sidestepped language of the Safe Drinking Water Act that requires an MCLG to prevent "any known or anticipated adverse effect on health with an adequate margin of safety" by declaring severe dental fluorosis a "cosmetic" effect. Bob later testified under oath that he had never—in his twenty years at EPA—ever seen such a blatant disregard for expert advice. He went on to say, "...someone in the upper echelon was...basically telling their own scientists to go to hell."

After getting advice and the okay from NFFE National's General Counsel, the Union started responding to requests for our take on fluoride toxicity. Bob Carton was Local 2050's principal spokesman and I was his wingman. Bob went alone to several communities that were dealing with proposals to fluoridate their water supplies. I later accompanied him on some visits and went myself on others. Locations he and I visited during this period are not accessible to my memory bank, though I do recall some trips to New England. During these visits we explained to officials and citizens in attendance what our professional credentials were, that our opinions and beliefs were ours—and the union of which we were elected officers—alone, not the EPA's. We always made that clear during our presentations. We did not represent the agency for which we worked. Such was the advice we received from the NFFE General Counsel, and it kept us from crossing a forbidden line. Later, I write of Bill Marcus's struggles in the EPA concerning unspoken lines, where he was fired, sued the EPA for wrongful dismissal, and won reinstatement as well as a financial settlement.

In addition to this outreach work, Bob represented the Local in presentations on fluoride toxicity to several EPA consultant organizations and its Science Advisory Board. The SAB and consultants were to recommend ways to improve science used by the Agency, and the SAB's job is to keep EPA from making big, embarrassing mistakes on science. He emphasized the difference between the original version of the Surgeon General's report that recommended a 2 mg/L MCLG and the version cited as justification for the proposed 4 mg/L MCLG.

I'm convinced that these presentations were well received and believed by some in upper and middle management and outside consultants. Nevertheless, the EPA stuck to the 4 mg/L MCLG; it did so, we thought, because of its "junior" status in the Federal

Government (i.e., not a Cabinet Agency). EPA had to play the role of "taking a hit for the team" on fluoride toxicity. The Agency was bombarded from heavyweights, like John Small and Michael Easley, in the pro-fluoridation camp, to discipline and fire Bob and me and to quash our Union's efforts on the issue. But management didn't do any of that—yet, more later on that. After Bob Carton left EPA in 1992, I always replied to Easley's and similar slanderous comments about us, copying EPA management on my replies. More than once, I challenged Easley to come to EPA and debate me in front of employees on fluoridation. There never was a response from him.

The first heads-up to the professional community about fluoride was published in our November 1985 newsletter, *Inside the Fishbowl* (Carton & Hirzy, 1985). Here is a partial transcription of that "Heads Up" article written by Dr. Robert J. Carton, our Union's first and foremost advocate on fluoride, and me:

FLUORIDE IN DRINKING WATER—WHAT ABOUT THE SCIENCE?

> *"On October 31, Lee Thomas signed the Notice promulgating a new Recommended Maximum Contaminant Level (RMCL) for fluoride in drinking water of 4 mg/L, up from the old level of 1.8 to 2.4 mg/L .....Most Americans....were not aware...of the incidence of "Texas teeth" in our Southwest...nor of...premature aging related to high levels of fluoride in drinking water in other parts of the world...and that the Government would—always and only—act in our very best interest...(But)...with each increment of increased understanding of the effects of fluoride on human health, an all too predictable reaction has occurred (concern, opposition). Those whose professional reputations and commercial interests are tied to a one-dimensional public perception of fluoride - benefit, period - try to discredit any detrimental information. We in the public health and environmental protection profession are no strangers to such actions...We just need to be aware of them and to base our professional actions on the best scientific evidence.*
>
> *And that brings us to the new RMCL. Was the scientific analysis objective, or was it influenced by 'defenders of fluoride? Why in the world should a labor organization care, one way or the other?"*
>
> *This labor organization cares because it is an organization whose members' livelihoods depend exclusively on their reputations for professional objectivity and competence. The slightest hint that a scientific document for which EPA is responsible is tainted, does*

terrible damage not only to public confidence in EPA, but to our reputations as well, and we will not have it!"

Later, during the "toxic carpet crisis" of the late 1980s and early 1990s, management threatened to prosecute me under 18 U.S. Code section 205. They falsely alleged that I represented private interests on official time, a federal criminal statute with a $10,000 fine and 5 years in prison upon conviction. EPA management also brought in a "union buster" consultant trying to break our union and teach us a lesson in labor-management relations.

Making Waves

By the summer of 1989, Local 2050's fluoride activities were drawing media attention. Bob Carton participated live in an investigative report on the *Gary Null Show* on WMAC, New York, and that broadcast was then broadcast on 50 other stations the following week. Syndicated investigative correspondent Jack Anderson wrote a complimentary column on NFFE's work titled "EPA gnashes teeth over fluoride." The *Washington Post* refused to run the column, so we copied it for the EPA community's information into the July-August *Inside the Fishbowl*. *Science* magazine told Local 2050 that it intended to publish a piece on the issue. I was invited to present a seminar before the Institute for Policy Studies on Local 2050's activities inside EPA. My summary of that presentation is given in the September-October 1989 *Inside the Fishbowl*. The Environmental Law Institute invited me to write a piece for the February *Environmental Law Reporter*, which I titled "The Other Voice From EPA." The piece covered our fluoride fight, among other activities.

The February 1990 issue of *Fishbowl* had two articles on fluoride and cancer: 1) "*Fluoride and bone cancer – the heat is on Californians and so are the denials!*" and 2) a guest editorial by Dr. John Lee titled, "*Fluoride and Cancer*." The first one dealt with results of the National Toxicology Program that found osteosarcoma in exposed rodents, and the bobbing and weaving by EPA's Office of Drinking Water, the American Dental Association and the U.S. Department of Health and Human Services to downplay those results. Dr. Lee's piece was a findings summary of the committee he chaired, charted by the Marin County Medical Association in order to study fluoridation.

Thus, did Local 2050 inform the EPA Headquarters community, and this is when some heavy stuff starts hitting the proverbial fan.

The February 15, 1990, issue of "*Environment Week*" quoted Administrator Bill Reilly as complaining about the misuse of risk assessments in some circumstances. Bob Carton wrote to Reilly about that citation and commented that the union agreed with him of one such misuse of a risk assessment, namely the assessment that justified the fluoride 4 mg/L MCLG.

Bob wrote a scathing review in the May *Fishbowl* of the April 17, 1990 *Washington Post* coverage of the scientific review panel's assessment of the NTP cancer study on fluoride. The *Post* had parroted the U.S. Public Health Service's endorsement of fluoridation consistently—"No Significant Cancer Risk Seen in Fluoride"—even in the face of that panel's finding that fluoride "caused statistically significant cancer in male rats" (this was before Jeff Bezos acquired the paper. The *Washington Post* continues, in 2025, to be reluctant to publish anything adverse about fluoride).

In the November 1990 *Fishbowl,* Bob wrote, for its first publication, about the outrageous order Bill Marcus, Office of Water Senior Toxicologist, received from his immediate supervisory chain of command. In essence, "Don't provide us with any more information about fluoride toxicity. Or if you insist on doing so, you must do it on your own time, not as part of your professional duties here." That was followed by other actions in support of Bill Marcus, which resulted in more public awareness of the protected status of fluoride and the need for more public support to overcome that situation. More information on Bill Marcus' firing and his successful fight for reinstatement, with massive support from the people working to end fluoridation, can be found at the epaunionhistory.org website.

Bob Carton resigned from the EPA on May Day, 1992, after a career doing groundbreaking work on asbestos, arsenic, and other high-profile chemicals, which brought down wrath from the Nixon administration. That was manifested in management's refusal to honor his work by keeping him at a GS-13 position for 17 years. Bob also produced and distributed at his own expense and on his own time a periodic newsletter on fluoride toxicity that went to people he knew who were interested in the subject. His fingerprints and boot tracks are all over this subject and have been for years.

Bob took a job with the U.S. Army Medical Research Command at Ft. Detrick, Maryland, where he reported directly to the Commanding General. The general said to Bob, "I hear you got into some fights at EPA; that's good because we like fighters here!" One of the first jobs Bob took on was to prevent the resumption of fluoridation of Ft. Detrick's water supply. He won eventual approval of his work by the Commanding General, who agreed that the soldiers under his command drank more than the EPA standard of 2.0 liters/day, thus getting toxic doses of fluoride. The Secretary of the Army, however, after doing his political homework, turned his thumbs down. The "Protected Pollutant" remained untouchable in the U.S. military.

With Bob's departure it fell to me to assume the lead in Local 2050's efforts on fluoride toxicity. That involved a lot of travel, using my personal leave allotments from EPA. I spoke at the invitation of Crystal Harvey to the Arkansas State Legislature, at the invitation of Mike Ewall to the Pennsylvania State Legislature, and at the invitation of the Dean to a Grand Rounds session of the Oregon University Medical School, and to a variety of other city and state officials, and attended forums along with such notable scientists as Roger Masters and Mike Coplan (who tied increased blood-lead levels and crime to use of HFSA), Hardy Limeback (who once pushed fluoridation for the Canadian Dental Association), Chris Neurath (whose outstanding ability as a researcher and writer continues to this day), and the Connetts (founders of the Fluoride Action Network). I also made the acquaintance of the poltergeist, Olly, at Knox College in Dunedin, New Zealand, and made presentations there and in Australia and Canada.

In 1997, California Citizens for Safe Water asked for Local 2050's endorsement of their Initiative Legislation to prevent a statewide fluoridation mandate. I called a General Meeting of Local 2050 to consider that request and to ratify the recently concluded Collective Bargaining Agreement with EPA management. I invited Bob Carton and Professor Paul Connett to make presentations reviewing the latest information on fluoride. After their talks, we took votes on the contract and the Californians' request, both of which were approved unanimously. Thus began my affiliation with the new entity, the Fluoride Action Network (FAN).

I, as a union leader, kept my sisters and brothers in the other EPA labor unions across the country up to date on Local 2050's—and later NTEU Chapter 280's—efforts toward applying scientific integrity on the fluoride toxicity issue.

Fluoride and Cancer

The Union's reputation for truth-telling led to many requests for a summary of why we were doing this work on fluoride toxicity. I wrote a White Paper in 1999 that detailed with 24 literature citations and 15 endnote references why the Union chose to oppose fluoridation. It also was useful when preparing presentations. In 2000, I was invited to explain our Union's action before the U.S. Senate Committee on Environment and Public Works. (My testimony can be viewed via the FAN website and on YouTube).

I cited the judicial findings in three trials in Pennsylvania, Illinois, and Texas that all found, in essence, that fluoridation should be stopped. I called for a review of the NTP cancer bioassay slides of tumors that were downgraded based on political pressure that changed NTP's findings of "clear evidence of carcinogenicity" to "equivocal evidence of carcinogenicity," thus saving the U.S. Public Health Service from having to halt promotion of fluoridation. I called for a new comprehensive Congressional review of fluoridation; the last one being done in 1978. It never happened.

The only beneficial effect of my 2000 testimony was its continuing on-line availability for citizens' use in fighting the community fluoridation practice.

I engaged the EPA rank and file and authored a letter to EPA Administrator Johnson in 2005 saying:

"We, the undersigned representatives of a majority (eleven) of EPA's employee unions, are requesting that you direct the Office of Water to issue an Advanced Notice of Proposed Rulemaking setting the maximum contaminant level goal for fluoride at zero, in accordance with Agency policy for all likely or known human carcinogens. Our request is based on the overall weight of the evidence supporting the classification of fluoride as a human carcinogen, including new information from Harvard on the link between fluoride in drinking water and osteosarcoma in boys that was conveyed to you in a meeting with union officials on May 4, 2005....."

It is noteworthy that when industry becomes aware of important new scientific findings like this, it has (depending on the specific statute) a very brief time to notify EPA. The Agency is then expected to take timely and appropriate action based on the specifics of that notification. In the present case EPA is aware of important new, high-quality evidence of potentially serious danger to young boys drinking fluoridated water, and we believe EPA has an ethical duty to send an effective warning immediately about this hazard.

Edward Ohanian replied to the Union's letter saying the National Academy of Sciences' review—which EPA had asked for—was due soon, so no action would be taken on our "zero MCLG" recommendation now. And no action on the copious database on fluoride's carcinogenicity has ever been taken by EPA. Even now.

The biggest red flag during those days was raised by Elise Bassin, a PhD student of Chester Douglass who, while a professor at the dental school at Harvard, was also the editor of Colgate's *Oral Care Report*. Dr. Bassin's study on bone cancer and fluoridation had considerably alarming results (Bassin, 2001; Bassin et al., 2006). She wrote:

"Among males, exposure to fluoride at or above the target level (of non-fluoridated water—my insert) was associated with an increased risk of developing osteosarcoma. The association was most apparent between ages 5-10 with a peak at six to eight years of age. The odds

ratio for the high exposure group was 5.16 at 7 years of age with a 95 percent confidence interval of 1.64 to 16.20." (Bassin, 2001, page 75)

In a published letter Douglass, who was obviously not happy that Bassin was able to publish her results, warns:

"A parallel analysis of age-specific exposure to fluoride, especially during growth periods, is also being pursued by our study team in the second set of cases of our study. Accordingly, readers are cautioned not to generalize and over-interpret the results of the Bassin et al. paper and to await the publications from the full study, before making conclusions, and especially before influencing any related policy decisions." (Douglass & Josipura, 2006).

It took Douglass 19 years to publish the promised parallel study which turned out to be flawed. Because he was funded by NIH, the government agency wanted an investigation. It was done in house by Harvard and Douglass was cleared. The report was not made public. During the entire process, Douglass had donated $1 million to Harvard (epaunionhistory.org) which was no doubt a conflict of interest. Eliss Bassin did not do any further research.

Fluoride Neurotoxicity

Having co-authored with Paul Connett, David Kennedy, Bruce Spittle, and Quanyong Xiang an article titled "*Developmental Neurotoxicity of Fluoride: A Quantitative Risk Analysis Towards Establishing A Safe Daily Dose for Children*" (Hirzy et al., 2016), I presented its results to EPA Office of Water Officials and to the EPA Drinking Water Advisory Committee, in two successive years, and to FDA's Over-The-Counter Drug Monograph System.

I also gave a deposition covering all the above in the *Food & Water Watch v. U.S. Environmental Protection Agency* lawsuit so expertly and cogently prosecuted by Michael Connett and supported so generously by Movement Friends. My comment so long ago to Jim Turner finally sees its glorious fulfillment.

Setting the Record Straight

Hearing people claim that they trust fluoride in water is safe up to 4 ppm because the EPA says so is like listening to nails dragged across a chalkboard. Bill Marcus, Bob Carton, and I, along with the scientists and technicians in eleven EPA unions, have been steadfast since the 1980s and '90s in our condemnation of politically determined fluoride contaminant levels and of the intentional pollution of drinking water with fluoridation water additives.

This is my epistle to my countrymen and to the world on scientific integrity in organized federal labor. My final message is: Don't let the bastards get you down.

Fluoridation Fallacy

Death of the Precautionary Principle

By: Dr E. Griffin Cole, DDS, NMD, IBDM, MIAOMT

ABOUT: *Dr Cole practiced biological dentistry for 28 years in Austin, TX. He is ozone certified and received both his Board Certification in Naturopathic Medicine and his degree in Integrative Biological Dental Medicine from the School of Integrative Biological Dental Medicine (ACIMD). Dr Cole holds a Mastership in the International Academy of Oral Medicine and Toxicology and drafted the Academy's Fluoridation Brochure and the official Scientific Review on Ozone use in root canal therapy. He is a past President of the IAOMT and serves on the Board of Directors, the Mentor Committee, the Fluoride Committee, the Conference Committee (as Chairman) and is the Fundamentals Course Director.*

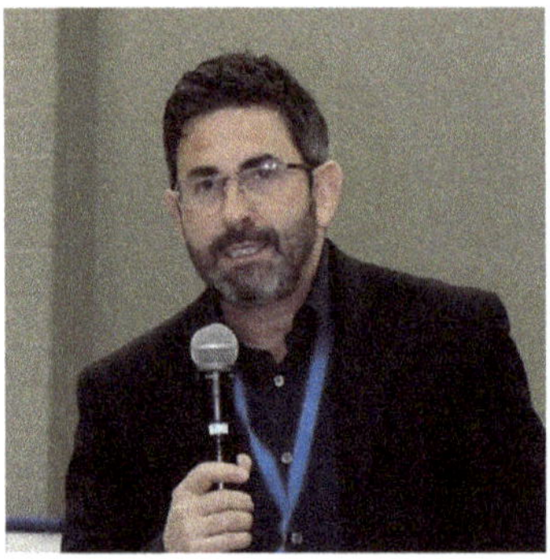

He has been featured on many radio and television programs including World News Tonight with Diane Sawyer. He has been published in numerous national peer-reviewed publications for his restorative and cosmetic dentistry.

One of the current fluoride experts in the country, he has published on the true costs of fluoridation. Dr Cole has lectured and testified before US councils and legislatures as well as internationally for over two decades on practice management and biological dentistry. He currently consults and is a featured expert for health summits and podcasts. A former clinical instructor at the University of Texas Dental School, Dr Cole is the co-founder and President of the Center for Advanced Dental Disciplines.

CHAPTER 11

"If the masses cannot be commanded, they have to be manipulated.
That's where modern indoctrination and propaganda was born,
as it is described in the works of people such as
Lippman, Trotter, and Bernays."

—*Professor Mattias Desmet (2022)*

"I'M SO SURPRISED you haven't been contacted by the ADA, Joe."

I was on the phone with Joe Conger, an excellent journalist and reporter for the TV station KENS 5 in San Antonio. He was working on a story about recent news from Health and Human Services (HHS), which had announced a plan to lower fluoride levels in drinking water due to the growing number of fluorosis cases in children. It was February 2011, and I was excited—and honored—to be the featured "expert" dentist in his piece.

This was groundbreaking: for the first time in the 66 years since fluoridation began, one of its staunchest endorsers was finally acknowledging a flaw in the policy.

"What are you talking about? Why would the ADA care about my little San Antonio story?" Joe asked with a laugh. "Hey, Griffin, I'm getting another call—can you hold?"

Ten seconds later, he returned, stunned.

"You're not going to believe this—it's the ADA!"

When I graduated from dental school in 1993, I believed everything I'd been taught: that mercury amalgam was safe, and fluoride was the miracle cure for tooth decay. Why wouldn't I? I had attended the University of Texas Health Science Center in San Antonio, which had just been named the top dental school in the country by *U.S. News and World Report*. I left school feeling fully equipped and confident in my training.

But it wasn't long before I began questioning some of the sacred doctrines of organized dentistry. I came to realize that my education had focused more on technical proficiency and less on critical thinking. The mercury amalgam issue was easy to unravel. The fluoride lie took a bit longer.

Fortunately, I started my career working alongside a holistic dentist—at a time when that label still drew accusations of quackery and ostracism. I quickly became a target of jokes and judgment from colleagues who had once respected me. But the ridicule only strengthened my resolve. I had to know the truth.

Books like *A Struggle with Titans* by George Waldbott and *Fluoride: The Aging Factor* by John Yiamouyiannis opened my eyes further. I eventually decided I could no longer support or promote water fluoridation. In 2000, I had my first opportunity to speak publicly on the issue in my hometown of San Antonio, one of the few remaining large cities not yet fluoridating.

I prepared obsessively for a public debate with Dr. Maria Lopez Howell, a respected dental professor of mine, in front of a packed room of concerned citizens. A popular radio personality would emcee the event, and I was introduced as an "expert," though I felt far from it. But I was ready.

Then came the announcement: Dr. Howell wouldn't be attending. She was a no-show. I wasn't surprised—deep down, I doubted she could publicly defend a policy that puts an entire community at risk just to prevent a cavity or two. While disappointed, I took the opportunity to speak anyway. What should have been a debate became a lecture, and I realized that day this was a cause I would champion for years to come.

Unlike many colleagues in this book, I've been lucky. I've endured little more than the occasional sneer or sideways comment. I've never feared speaking out, even when writing anti-fluoride pieces in periodicals and dental newsletters. But I know others haven't been so fortunate. Many of my co-author friends have suffered far worse, losing credibility, income, and even their careers for simply speaking the truth. It is shameful and criminal what happened to researchers like Phyllis Mullenix, Bill Marcus, and Hardy Limeback. I honor their sacrifices.

In 2009, I delivered my first lecture on fluoride to the International Academy of Oral Medicine and Toxicology, an organization I've been actively involved with for 25 years. While preparing for the presentation, I reached out to Phyllis Mullenix, a brilliant researcher from the prestigious Forsyth Dental Institute in Boston. Fourteen years earlier, she had published groundbreaking research on the neurotoxic effects of fluoride in rats. Despite the significance of her findings, she lost her position and funding for refusing to suppress the study. During our conversation, she recounted a visit from Harold Hodge in the late 1980s—the lead scientist of the Manhattan Project and a prominent advocate for fluoridation. Hodge reviewed her work and admitted that her results mirrored findings he had discovered decades earlier. Hearing this gave me chills. The very man who championed fluoridation as public health policy had known about fluoride's neurotoxicity for years—yet he not only remained silent but also misled the American public.

Fluoridation has become one of the most hotly debated topics in health, and I'm encouraged to see momentum shifting in our favor. It's astonishing to think that it all began with one curious Colorado dentist—Dr. Frederick McKay—investigating brown stains on his patients' teeth. His simple inquiries ultimately led to one of the greatest public health frauds ever committed. *

To be fair, I believe the original intentions were sincere. McKay spent 30 years investigating the cause of mottled enamel in children, and epidemiologist Dr. Trendley Dean followed suit. Dean's 1938 research suggested that 1.0 mg/L of fluoride might reduce decay with minimal fluorosis—but he also warned that more research was needed. In his 1938 paper he says:

> *"Inasmuch as it appears that the mineral composition of the drinking water may have an important bearing on the incidence of dental caries in a community, the possibility of partially controlling dental caries through the domestic water supply warrants thorough epidemiological-chemical study."*

Yet, once industry got wind of fluoride's potential, everything changed. The aluminum and phosphate fertilizer industries, desperate for a fluoride disposal solution, jumped at the opportunity. Public relations master Edward Bernays, along with a few scientists in white coats, was all that was needed to force this unproven and dangerous operation upon unsuspecting Americans. Bernay's use of propaganda and manipulation, no doubt a product of his uncle Sigmund Freud's teachings, helped spin the narrative. His chilling words still echo:

> *"In almost every act of our daily lives, whether in the sphere of politics or business, in our social conduct or our ethical thinking, we are dominated by a relatively small number of persons...It is they who pull the wires which control the public mind."*

And so, fluoridation began—not based on solid science, but on machinations and industrial convenience.

Initially, the American Dental Association and American Medical Association opposed fluoridation, rightly calling it reckless and unproven. In 1938, AMA President Charles Heyd declared, "I am appalled at the prospect of using water as a vehicle for drugs. Fluoride is a corrosive poison that will produce serious effects on a long-range basis. Any attempt to use water this way is deplorable."

His colleague, Dr. Flanagan, the Assistant Director or Environmental Health for the AMA, echoed that concern: "The AMA is not prepared to state that no harm will be done to any person by water fluoridation."

Today, decades later, their warnings seem prophetic. More than 80 studies now link fluoride exposure to neurological harm in infants. A federal court recently ruled against the EPA, and the new HHS Secretary has prioritized removing toxins from our food and water. The tide is turning.

The Precautionary Principle tells us: First, do no harm. If there's even a possibility of danger, especially without clear benefit, we must pause. Yet the U.S. continues to fluoridate more water than any other country —despite having no better cavity rates than those that do not.

One patient forever shaped my convictions. She was a teenager from West Texas, exposed to high levels of naturally occurring fluoride. Her teeth were severely mottled. She rarely smiled, ashamed of her appearance and was teased relentlessly. I still remember the moment she saw her restored smile in the mirror—her joy was indescribable. Her happiness paid me more than any amount of money could. A couple months later, her father called to say she'd made the cheerleading squad and was thriving in school. That moment reminded me: fluoride, whether natural or artificial, can profoundly affect lives.

I've made it my mission to speak the truth: fluoride was never the panacea we were promised. For many, it has been a harmful toxin. I will continue to speak out and fight against this injustice until fluoridation is fully banned—or until my last breath.

***EDITORS' NOTE**: There is considerable evidence that Dr McKay was not the initiator of the fluoride fraud, but only a useful tool for power players intent on evaporating the pollution lawsuits plaguing corporate fluoride polluters in the early and mid-20th century.

The Water System that Refuses to Comply with a State Mandate

By: Andy Anderson

ABOUT: *The Ozark Mountain Regional Public Water Authority provides*

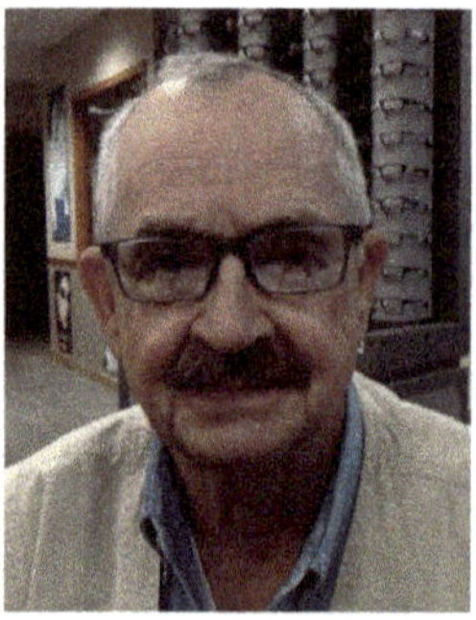

wholesale treated water to 18 cities, towns, and rural water systems in the Ozark Mountain region of Arkansas. At the heart of this operation is a 4.5 million gallon per day treatment facility located on the south shore of Bull Shoals Lake. This lake is a US Army Corps of Engineers Lake whose primary mission is flood control. Andy Anderson has been Chairman of the Board for this system since 2006.

CHAPTER 12

"A man dies when he refuses to stand up for that which is right.
A man dies when he refuses to stand up for justice.
A man dies when he refuses to take a stand for that which is true."

—Dr Martin Luther King, Jr.

OUR STORY BEGINS before the implementation of the Arkansas Statewide fluoridation mandate known as Arkansas ACT 197 of 2011.

Lay of the Land

Nestled in the rural expanse of north-central Arkansas, several water systems struggled with insufficient quantity of water during dry conditions and poor water quality. Those waters contain contaminants, such as radon, radium, and naturally-occurring calcium fluoride.

In 2004, twenty-two water systems joined together to form an alliance seeking a solution for our common water challenges. An engineering firm, Engineering Services, Inc. of Springdale, Arkansas, was chosen as the firm to carry this project forward. The Alliance looked at several ideas, finally deciding to pursue one which would take water from Lake Bull Shoals, treat it, then furnish it to the member associations through approximately 120 miles of transmission main lines. This was to be done over a period of many years.

The Alliance began seeking funds for the project, working through State and Federal agencies and our State and Federal congressional representatives, as well as applying for grants from area businesses. In 2006 the Alliance converted to Ozark Mountain Regional Public Water Authority (OMRPWA) giving it the ability to finance projects with construction bonds and to take land by eminent domain. The Authority is governed by a nine-member Board of Directors, with three directors from each county in the primary service area. Work continued toward getting started on engineering, obtaining funding, getting required cultural and environmental surveys, etc. In October 2008, word came down that there could be a federal stimulus fund. If the Authority received adequate stimulus funding, the entire project could be completed in the next few years. Everyone involved began working diligently so that all would be ready if the funds became available.

Final decisions on the location of the intake and treatment plant had to be made, and surveys of the properties were necessary before any construction could begin. Many meetings were held with the U.S. Army Corps of Engineers, the USDA, the State Health Department, the Arkansas Natural Resources Commission (ANRC), and other key agencies to ensure that every regulatory and logistical hurdle was carefully considered and addressed.

The Authority also needed to obtain appraisals of the properties involved, including the land where easements would be required. Once these appraisals were completed, the land purchases and easement acquisitions had to be negotiated and finalized—a process that took time, effort, and persistent communication.

One of the biggest hurdles we faced was the Corps of Engineers 'water allocation study. Under normal circumstances, these studies could take up to five years to complete. However, the Corps recognized the urgency and committed to expediting the process for our project—a crucial concession that kept us moving forward.

In 2009, we reached a significant milestone: we received signed water purchase contracts from 18 of the original 22 water systems. These contracts committed each system to a minimum monthly purchase amount, which was essential for demonstrating to the USDA that we would have the revenue needed to repay the construction loans.

It's important to note that all of this occurred before the state fluoridation mandate legislation was even introduced. At the time, many of the systems were using well water, some drawn from considerable depths. That water often contained radon, radium, fluoride, and other naturally-occurring contaminants—some at levels that threatened both the health and confidence of residents. These systems looked to the Authority's project as a solution: water that would be safe, reliable, and free from those undesirable contaminants.

Funding and Fluoride

We obtained letters of support from local cities, towns, and state and federal legislators, as well as from the Arkansas Department of Health (ADH). On May 1, 2009, the ADH sent a detailed seven-page letter to the USDA, strongly endorsing the need for our project to be funded. The letter emphasized the problems that the project would address if funded and, significantly, it listed **fluoride as a problem** no fewer than 14 times.

This date—May 1, 2009—is important because it clearly shows that at that time, the ADH itself regarded fluoride as an undesirable contaminant. Yet, just two years later, when the Arkansas legislature considered the proposed statewide fluoridation mandate under Act 197 of 2011, the ADH did nothing to oppose it.

In fact, a Director within the ADH actively promoted the mandate. He provided Arkansas legislators with information from a so-called "screening study" that he had conducted in 2002, which he claimed compared the dental health of school students in a fluoridated community versus an unfluoridated one in Arkansas. According to his testimony, the study showed a 50% reduction in cavities in the fluoridated area—a dramatic result that likely swayed the legislators. Within just 11 days of the bill's introduction, it was signed into law.

However, when a request was later made under the Arkansas Freedom of Information Act to obtain the data from this study, the ADH claimed that the study data had not been retained. For a study of such significance—one that influenced statewide policy on drinking water—it's highly unusual, if not suspect, that no data would be preserved. Typically, if a study truly showed such a dramatic benefit, the pro-fluoridation community would be broadcasting it from the rooftops.

Adding to the concern, representatives from the schools supposedly involved in the study were later questioned, and none of them had any recollection of any such study ever being conducted. Taken together, the missing data and the lack of local knowledge raise serious doubts about the legitimacy of the study. By a preponderance of the evidence, I believe that the ADH Director provided false and misleading information to the Arkansas legislature to get the fluoridation bill passed.

Following his successful advocacy for Act 197, this same Director was rewarded with a high-profile job in Washington, D.C., as the Chief Dental Officer for Medicaid and Medicare.

This brings us to the point in time when we at the Ozark Mountain Regional Public Water Authority (OMRPWA) had secured the necessary funding and were actively constructing the treatment plant and installing the transmission mains—well before Act 197 was signed into law. When the fluoridation mandate was enacted, we requested and received authorization from the Arkansas Department of Health (ADH) to delay the installation of fluoridation equipment until our system was fully operational.

Several of our customer entities expressed concern right away. They had signed water purchase contracts with OMRPWA specifically to obtain water **without** the fluoride contaminant—one of the key reasons they wanted to leave their existing, problematic wells behind. These customers made it clear they were opposed to purchasing water that contained fluoride.

When our system became fully operational, ADH began pressuring us to submit plans for adding fluoride to the water supply. However, our Board of Directors—representing the counties and water systems we serve—began voicing strong opposition to implementing fluoridation by feeding it into the water.

It is important to note that Act 197 requires water systems serving 5,000 or more people to add fluoride to their water. Not one of the systems we supply on its own has 5,000 people; individually, none of them would have been subject to this mandate had they not joined OMRPWA. Ironically, by seeking a reliable, safe water source free of contaminants, they now found themselves caught in the crossfire of a state mandate that would have otherwise left them alone.

Defiance and Fines

The wholesale water systems on either side of us initially also opposed the addition of fluoride to their water supplies. However, under increasing pressure from the Arkansas Department of Health (ADH), they eventually agreed to implement community water fluoridation, leaving OMRPWA as the **only** water system in the state still refusing to comply. This position of defiance only increased the pressure on us. On November 12, 2015, I, the Board chair of OMRPWA, was visited by staff members from two of our legislators who informed me that I could be personally sued for everything I owned if we did not comply.

My stance then—and now—was that OMRPWA is governed by a Board of Directors representing the customers in each of their counties. These customers never agreed to fluoridated water. They actively opposed it when they signed their water purchase contracts, and they were not willing to accept it now.

On June 18, 2015, the Arkansas Department of Health sent three representatives to our monthly Board of Directors meeting. They came to address our concerns and persuade us to comply with the mandate. Every one of our 18 customers had a representative in attendance, and each was given three minutes to speak directly to the ADH officials.

They arrived expecting to find "dumb Ozark hillbillies," but quickly discovered that our community members were far more knowledgeable about the risks of fluoride than the supposed experts from the big city.

Our part of Arkansas attracts many retirees who are drawn to its unspoiled environment—mountains, clear streams, rivers, and lakes. Many of these new residents come from polluted urban areas and deliberately seek clean, contaminant-free water. They are well-informed about the potential harms of fluoride—to humans, animals, and the environment.

But the ADH representatives refused to acknowledge any of these harms. One even claimed that the only harm fluoride might cause was some staining of teeth. None of them admitted knowing that powdered infant formula should not be mixed with fluoridated water, or that fluoridated water should not be used in kidney dialysis.

After the ADH representatives left, the Board held a vote, and **all 18 customers** unanimously agreed that we should continue to refuse to comply with the mandate. Some even declared that they would refuse to pay their monthly bills if fluoride was ever added. I explained that continuing to resist could mean needing an attorney and covering court costs, but the members readily agreed to be assessed extra to fund the legal fight.

After careful consideration, I requested and received a cost estimate from an attorney regarding the expenses we might incur in fighting the fluoridation mandate in court. This attorney was not only knowledgeable about the harms of fluoride, but had also worked with us previously and fully understood the stakes. He provided a clear estimate and verbally agreed to represent us all the way to the Arkansas Supreme Court for a fee of $12,500.

To cover this cost, letters were sent to each of our 18 customer systems requesting a contribution of $695 each. This would allow us to raise the necessary funds to proceed with the legal challenge and stand firm in our refusal to fluoridate the water.

The legal process began when we received a notice to appear before the ADH Administrative Board at 10 a.m. on March 29, 2016. That hearing unfolded exactly as we expected: the ADH acted as the prosecutor, judge, and jury all in one. They showed no interest in hearing our side of the story. Their verdict was straightforward: Act 197 is law, and "you must comply." If we failed to comply, they warned, we would be fined $500 per week.

Following the Administrative Board's decision, the case advanced to the full Arkansas Department of Health Board for a hearing on July 28, 2016. Unfortunately, that hearing was nothing more than a carbon copy of the first. Again, there was no genuine interest in considering our evidence or concerns. The ruling remained the same: Act 197 is the law, and you must comply.

Faced with no other choice, we appealed the ADH ruling to Circuit Court, filing the appeal on September 7, 2016.

The Arkansas Legislature meets only in odd-numbered years. In every legislative session since Act 197 was passed, we have introduced bills in an attempt to overturn the statewide fluoridation mandate. I, along with others from our community, have consistently tried to provide testimony before the committees where these bills were heard. So far, however, we have been unsuccessful. Arkansas politicians seem to be heavily influenced by lobbying groups with deep pockets and the ability to contribute generously to their campaigns.

During this time, we initially had an attorney who was both knowledgeable and deeply committed to working with us on this issue. Unfortunately, that changed when he left his law firm and we were assigned to another attorney—one who seemed more interested in serving the system than representing our interests. He refused to honor the verbal cost estimate we had arranged with his predecessor. Instead, he began billing us in quarter-hour increments for every email he sent or received, as well as every phone call. Our small legal defense reserve was rapidly depleted.

Over the next two years, we filed multiple motions to stay the legal action against us until the Fluoride Action Network's lawsuit against the EPA was resolved, along with other motions aimed at delaying our case. Unfortunately, we were unsuccessful.

Our hearing in Circuit Court was held on March 7, 2019. Despite our efforts, we were not given an opportunity to testify. The Court simply reviewed the Arkansas Department of Health Board's ruling that we were appealing and upheld it.

At that point, our only remaining recourse was to appeal the Circuit Court's decision to the Arkansas State Supreme Court. I firmly believed that I would get a chance to testify before the Arkansas Supreme Court.

There are three fundamental beliefs I hold regarding Arkansas's mandatory fluoridation law, and these are the very points I have been anxiously waiting to present—yet I have not been given the opportunity.

Number 1: Mandatory fluoridation is an **unjust law** because the people directly affected by it never had the opportunity to vote on it—neither to approve nor to reject it. Instead, a small group of ill-informed legislators made this critical decision on behalf of everyone, bypassing the will of the people.

Number 2: Mandatory fluoridation is an **unethical law** because it constitutes forced medication without informed consent. Legislators have no authority to mandate what medications are appropriate for the citizens they represent. This law removes individual choice and violates the ethical principle of consent that is foundational to medical practice.

Number 3: Mandatory fluoridation **violates the Federal Safe Drinking Water Act (SDWA).** The SDWA applies to all water systems in the United States and prohibits the addition of any substance to drinking water for the purpose of preventive health care. The sole reason fluoride is added is to prevent tooth decay but there is not one function in the human body that requires fluoride. While the SDWA does grant states "Primacy" to regulate their own water supplies, that Primacy is conditional: state regulations cannot be **less stringent** than federal regulations. If the federal SDWA prohibits preventatives but a state mandates a preventative, then the state's regulation is, by definition, less stringent. In that case, the state cannot legally mandate fluoridation and still maintain its Primacy.

Appeal

These three points form the backbone of my case, and I remain determined to present them before a court.

The appeal to the Arkansas Supreme Court was not at all what I had expected. Instead of reconsidering the validity of the Circuit Judge's decision, the Supreme Court only reviewed whether the lower court had followed the proper legal process. I did not get to testify, and the Court ultimately affirmed the Circuit Court's ruling.

One critical issue that emerged was that our attorney had failed to challenge the **constitutionality** of the fluoride mandate in the lower court proceedings. That misstep left us with no avenue to argue this important point during the Supreme Court appeal. As a result, the only remaining legal option is for us to file a **new court case** that specifically challenges the constitutionality of Act 197. Unfortunately, for a small, non-profit entity like ours, the cost of starting a brand-new legal fight is prohibitive. If, by some miracle, we do secure the funds, we will challenge this state law.

At every monthly Board of Directors meeting, fluoridation remains a standing agenda item. The Board has consistently and unanimously decided that we will **not** add fluoride to our water supply. It is not my decision alone; OMRPWA is governed by a Board of Directors, and they are resolute in their position to keep fluoride out of the system.

This journey has taught me a lot about how the government and the legal system work—and, often, how they don't.

- I have learned that our elected legislators are heavily influenced by lobbyists. A retired lobbyist once told me, "If you will give me enough money, I can get any legislation passed—good or bad." Those words have proven truer than I could have imagined.

- I've also learned that the legal system is, in many ways, a money machine. Lawyers often seem to churn paperwork more to bill the customer than to actually resolve the issue. If a lawyer refuses to listen to the client, they should be fired and replaced with someone who will. This is especially critical when the lawyer does not share the client's perspective or commitment to the cause.

- We made a fatal mistake early in our case—one that left us in a legal tangle with no straightforward way out except to file a new case from scratch.

Meanwhile, we are being fined **$500 per week** for refusing to comply with this unjust mandate. Yet if we were to comply, we would face an even bigger problem: many of our wholesale customers have already vowed to refuse to pay for water containing fluoride.

As a Board, we feel more than justified in our position, and we are committed to fighting this battle until we prevail.

Do Not Swallow

Liberty for all

By: Dr Bill Osmunson, DDS, MPH

ABOUT: *Bill Osmunson, DDS, MPH, is a retired cosmetic, comprehensive, neuromuscular, and general dentist with 45 years of practice in fluoridated and non-fluoridated communities, low socioeconomic communities, rural communities, tribal health centers, and very wealthy cities. Dr Osmunson has provided a wide range of dentistry from preventive routine dentistry, treating cosmetic and functional dental fluorosis, to complex stomatognathic disorders. Dr Osmunson is a past Director of Research, Director of Occlusion One and Clinical Instructor at the Las Vegas Institute for Advanced Dental Studies. He mentored his two sons in dentistry. He is a published author and gained Food and Drug Approval for a dental device. For the first 25 years of practice, Dr Osmunson promoted fluoride ingestion with either supplements or the addition of fluoride to public water. Reading both sides of the literature, he realized millions are being seriously harmed because they are ingesting too much fluoride. Dr Osmunson's mission is to turn off the fluoridation pumps. Questioning authorities has taken a toll on his health, family, and practices.*

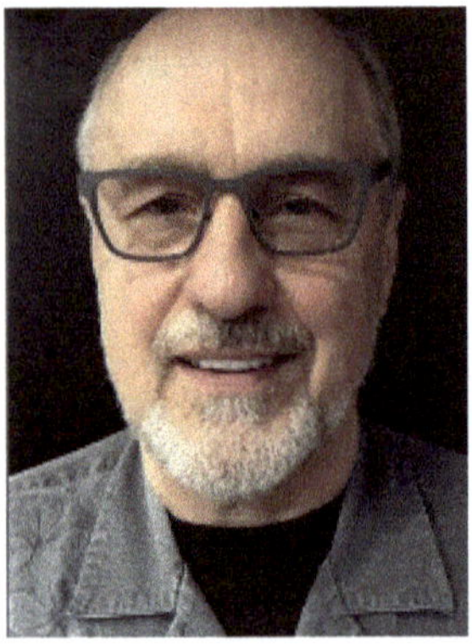

CHAPTER 13

"Is the glass half full or half empty?"

—Aphorism

ALL PROFESSIONALS WORK within the professional community of their peers. In dentistry, dentists frequently see patients from other dentists. Patients may be referred for specialized treatment, due to insurance coverage, or for any number of reasons. Patients who are moving to a new home may ask for a referral from their existing dentist for a dentist in their new community. And patients who have had bad experiences with a dentist or who feel they need a second opinion, will actively seek out new dentists. Moreover, dentists network with their peers and other dental associates at professional events. Consequently, maintaining a good image among your peers is important to maintaining a successful business— and make no mistake about it, a dental practice is a business.

I am retired now, but if I were asked if I lost business because of my opposition to fluoridation, I'd have to say, probably. Although there are more dentists than most people imagine who do not believe fluoridation does teeth any good, they know that it would be heretical to say otherwise. They know they not only risk being regarded as "odd" by their peers but also that some of their patients might question their professionalism for not sticking to the American Dental Association (ADA) dogma—and that might motivate patients to find another dentist.

One story I heard was from an out-of-state dentist who was having lunch with the head of the ADA affiliate for that state. The director was trying to convince her to sign onto a fluoridation promotion campaign, and she kept trying to get him to talk about the evidence that fluoridation caused or worsened thyroid disease and affected fertility and fetuses. In a fit of exasperation, she finally said, "You have daughters who are getting married. You know what the science says about thyroids and hormone disruption. Would you really want them to be drinking this stuff?"

The director held up his menu in front of his face so no one could observe him and whispered, "of course not! But we have to promote it for the good of our profession."

Profitability

Just like most people don't realize that fluoride is actually a poison, most people don't realize that the "safe and effective" image of fluoride as a panacea for cavities is very profitable to the dental profession. In-office dental treatments pump hundreds of thousands of dollars into the business. Repairing stained and brittle (cracked, split, broken) fluorosed teeth caused by poisoning while the tooth was forming under the gum line contributes to the bottom-line of the multi-billion-dollar U.S. cosmetic dentistry industry requiring crowns, root canals, extractions, bridges and/or implants (Osmunson & Cole, 2024).

Dental fluorosis is actual harm. As a cosmetic dentist, I treated dental fluorosis, both cosmetic and functional harm. Claims that fluoridation is cost-effective omit the costs of treating the harm and minimize costs of operations. Omitting harm is like trying to balance your check book without deducting the checks.

Dentists placing black and gold fillings tend to overlook the cosmetic damage of dental fluorosis, which in one study 95% of children wished to have removed. Damage is the cost, not the repairs. For example, a scratch on a car is damage for which the owner may desire compensation, even if they don't get the scratch repaired.

An EPA study reported that functional damage repair costs exceed cosmetic repair costs. My profession has failed to accept or measure the costs of treating the damage caused by fluoride, resulting in bones and teeth with lower tensile strength, increasing risks of fracture.

At least dental damage caused by fluorosis is visible, even if most people don't understand what caused it. Most people don't realize that kidney disease, arthritis, and other health complaints, like learning disabilities and brittle bones, have been exacerbated or caused by fluoride exposure from the low concentrations in the water.

Most people don't know how to judge their dentist recommendations any more than they know how to judge fluoridation policy.

Judgment

Should we judge fluoridation safety like the tobacco companies demanding absolute certainty of harm before issuing a warning or, from the ethical side, demanding certainty of safety before dispensing?

A Washington State law answers that question and orders the Board of Health to "Adopt rules necessary to **assure safe** . . . drinking water" (RCW 43.20.050 (2)(a)).* The word assure is defined as "to positively," "to confidently dispel any doubts," the water is safe. The only issue for fluoridation authorities to consider is safety.

Determining benefit, the job of the *Food and Drug Administration Center for Drug Evaluation and Research* (FDA CDER) and conducting cost-benefit analysis—or benefit-risk evaluation—are not the jobs of the Boards of Health, the Environmental Protection Agency (EPA), water purveyors, voters, Centers for Disease Control (CDC), or fluoridation lobbyists. Without FDA CDER approval of benefit, fluoridating authorities must be laser-focused on safety, confidently dispelling any doubt the water is safe to drink.

For over 15 years, the *Washington Action for Safe Water* members and I, made 22 rule change petitions to the Washington State Board of Health to protect the public health. We supported petitions with thousands of pages of peer-reviewed scientific studies reporting risks, harm, and lack of significant benefit.

The Board consistently denied any rules to protect the public, such as a warning label for infant formula made with fluoridated water addressing excessive fluoride exposure, dental fluorosis, and other risks. Most denials were appealed to the Governors as provided by law, and also denied. Early on, the Board gathered like-minded believers and sang the praises of fluoridation's benefits.

I petitioned the Washington State Board of Pharmacy, a different Board, to designate fluoride as a poison as provided by law or exempt when regulated as a drug. The Board of Pharmacy responded that fluoride is a legend drug requiring a doctor's prescription (RCW69.38.010)*. The Board of Pharmacy was soon eliminated, and responsibilities were placed under their bosses.

The FDA confirmed that fluoride is an unapproved drug, and their newsletter explained, "Manufacturers of unapproved drugs are usually fully aware that their drugs are marketed illegally, yet they continue to circumvent the law and put consumers 'health at risk'." (Boyer, 2009)

Authorities do not gain respect when they are the biggest pushers of an illegal drug. One could argue that the state legislature approved the use of fluoridation however, authorizing the use does not remove FDA approval requirements. The legislature may approve a road or building, but approval does not exempt building inspectors or building engineering laws, product quality, regulations and oversight.

One of our petitions requested the Board of Health to gain FDA CDER approval. I had previously gained FDA approval for a dental device and found the FDA scientists to be top-quality. I then tried to gain approval for fluoridation, expecting to be denied, and it was denied, confident the FDA would deny other petitions for drug approval based on their past denials, such as its 2016 Warning Letter to Kirkman Labs about marketing "fluoride drops" and 1975 Regulatory Letter to 35 manufactures about "fluoride lozenges" (Enziflur) regarding withdrawn approval.

Our persuasive carrot for the Board to talk to the FDA was the potential of an exclusive patent where the Board could then charge all the other fluoridating water purveyors, perhaps $1 a year per person. A tidy income of perhaps $200,000,000 a year was too hard for the

Board to pass up. The Board took the bait and contacted the FDA. The FDA responded that if the Board tried to gain fluoridation approval, fluoridation would be "banned." Exactly the response I expected.

Did the Board then stop promoting fluoridation and obey the law? No. The Board redoubled their promotion with essentially a cut-and-paste assurance of "safe and effective" from the fluoridation lobby.

Confident that hundreds of millions of people were being harmed by ingesting too much fluoride, my frustration ripped my guts up with stress, loss of sleep, time, money, and arguments in my mind. Seriously, if I saw a child swimming and in distress or a child running into a busy highway to get their runaway ball, I could not stand by and watch, much less millions of children being harmed by both my professions and my governments. All the while, I was making money treating both cosmetic and functional dental fluorosis caused by too much fluoride. Guilt pushed me to be an activist against fluoridation.

The National Research Council (NRC) in 2006, reported about 18 health risks, each raising serious doubts of fluoridation's safety, certainly for subpopulations such as infants. The NRC report screams risks and should have stopped fluoridation. The Board of Health rejected the scientific facts and put full faith in the fluoridation lobby endorsements.

I requested meetings with every federal and state agency and professional organization promoting fluoridation I could think of, and all denied or had me speak with their lawyers. Hitting my head against stone walls of tradition and endorsements, I (and others) petitioned the *National Toxicology Program* (NTP) in 2015 to review fluoride for thyroid harm, cancer, and developmental neurotoxicity, i.e. brain damage. The *NTP Board of Scientific Councillors and as* accepted the petition on developmental neurotoxicity, and the NTP expected two or maybe three years for a final report. The draft was politically blocked until the court ordered its release, and publication took 10 years after our nomination. There are thousands of toxins, and at this speed, just reviewing the risks of fluoride would take over a hundred years. One public health dentist told me: I will promote fluoridation until I receive a court order to stop or I see people dead on the street with "died from fluoridation" on their death certificate.

Presenting the 2024 NTP report with a determination of fluoride exposure being a moderate risk and the Federal Court's decision (Chen 2024) of fluoridation being an unreasonable risk to the new Washington State Board of Health members appears to have pushed the Board to finally consider science. At the end of 2024, the Board set up a panel of Department of Health employees and public observers to evaluate the science. As of May 2025, the panel has had 6 meetings and received a great deal of scientific evidence. No factual evidence presented by the Department's experts dispelled doubt in the risk of harm to any cell, system, organ, or tissue of the human body. The final Panel and Board decisions were expected by the summer of 2025.

The Panel members are mostly public health state employees who have promoted fluoridation and lack research education. The paradigm shifts for members trained to remain compliant with policy may prove impossible.

In a malpractice civil case, the confidence of harm needs to be greater than 51%. In a criminal case, confidence needs to increase beyond a reasonable doubt of harm. However, authorities by law must have an even higher level of confidence and dispel any doubt that the water is safe to drink. To assure safe water, the focus shifts from proving harm to dispelling any doubt of harm, which includes applying a margin of safety.

During the fluoridation trial in the U.S. Ninth District, an EPA expert was asked by Judge Chen what it would take to change his mind on fluoride's lowering of human IQ. The EPA expert responded to Judge Chen, "one or two more studies."

Fortunately, I was not in the courtroom when I yelled at my computer screen, "that's exactly word for word what the tobacco lobby said for decades." We now have over 70 human studies reporting harm from fluoride ingestion to the developing brain, some at very low fluoride concentrations in water. One or two more will not change the preponderance of the evidence, regardless of their outcomes.

Liberty, freedom from government oppression, is violated with the mass medication without patient consent, without a doctor's prescription, of an unapproved FDA drug and thus illegal drug. Moreover, despite any claims to the contrary, authorities are unable to assure the public that fluoridated water is safe to drink because we have the evidence that it isn't.

Finish Line

Did opposing dental dogma from the ADA harm me personally, professionally, and psychically? Yes, it did; and the time I spent fighting it took a toll on my family relationships. But fluoridation policy harmed millions of unsuspecting consumers, beginning in the womb. The references in this book, as well as the chapters of other authors, go into that detail.

In summer 2025, I was invited to present evidence to the FDA CDER and NIH under the organization of the Reagan-Udall Foundation on lack of benefit and the risk for pediatric patients from fluoride tablet supplements. I was also honored with an invitation to sit on a National Fluoridation Commission of experts to review the science on water fluoridation. The Commission includes both opponents and proponents, respectfully acknowledging those of us who were ostracized for many years.

I am happily retired from dentistry, but I will not rest easy until we retire fluoridation from government policy.

***Footnote**: Revised Code of Washington State (RCW 57.08.012)

Personal Perspective on the Grand Rapids Trial

By: Aliss Terpstra, CNP

ABOUT: *I am a Certified Nutritional Practitioner (CNP) and someone who suffers fluoride hypersensitivity and illness because of the chronic fluoride overdose I received from conception onward in a government public health experiment. I have been a fluoridation activist for the past 25 years because of where I was conceived and raised. My holy grail is to see the end of water fluoridation where it first began, in my hometown of Grand Rapids, Michigan.*

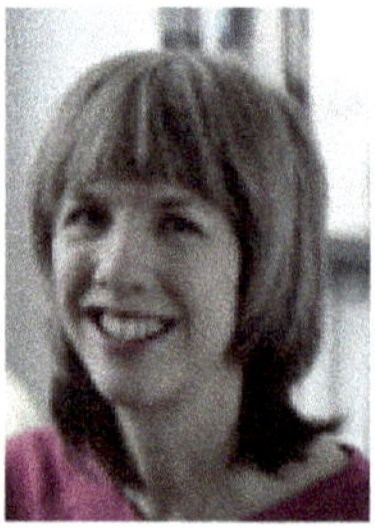

CHAPTER 14

"The plain fact that fluorine is an insidious poison, harmful, toxic and cumulative in its effects, even when ingested in minimal amounts, will remain unchanged no matter how many times it will be repeated in print that fluoridation of the water supply is 'safe'."

—Ludwik Gross, MD (1957)

FOR DECADES I have made eloquent deputations to Toronto Board of Health, written magazine articles, op-eds, and letters galore, and delivered white papers full of science, logic, and passionate truth to the unelected, unaccountable public health authorities who continue to recommend a harmful practice they refuse to re-examine critically despite ominous published, peer-reviewed research confirming neurotoxicity to fetus and child from consumption of Health-Canada-recommended fluoridated water. I have connected with NGOs, Council of Canadians, UNIFOR, the federal Green Party, local politicians and related advocacy groups and convinced them to issue public statements condemning fluoridation. I sat on boards, founded organizations and drove to meetings all over Ontario. But Toronto is still fluoridating its water at 0.7 ppm, and I still cannot drink the water.

Grand Rapids during WW2 did not have an apparent crisis of tooth decay, or a shortage of fluoride, since tea was in every kitchen. It was an orderly middle-class city in central Michigan, astride the Grand River that meanders across a fertile plain on its way northwest to Lake Michigan. Surrounding farms were, and still are, productive and prosperous. The sugar-rationing years of the war, in force until 1947, probably did everyone's teeth (and overall health) a service. Nevertheless, the city leaders were approached in early 1944—during the height of the Manhattan Project—to be the flagship city carrying forward the false banner for water fluoridation as an effective, safe public health measure for cavity prevention to the rest of America and the world. In some regards, it was overwhelmingly successful, except for the cavity prevention part.

The Nuremberg Code was several years away. Medical experimentation on uninformed patients, without placebo controls, was all too common. Eugenics was a popular theory even though Hitler's associated actions should have made it extremely distasteful to

Americans by then. The fluoridation trial as presented to Grand Rapids in 1944 should have been rejected as illogical, laughably unscientific, methodologically unsound, and unethical, and its proponents kicked to the curb. But the military-industrial complex had seduced Americans into a misplaced faith in paternalistic authoritarianism; their love child was Propaganda Inc.'s Edward Bernays, and almost everyone was dazzled by the media blitz and blinded to what really happened.

As detailed in Christopher Bryson's book *The Fluoride Deception,* fluoridation was not an experiment *per se*; it was a done deal from the get-go, cooked up during the war years by industries whose lawyers worried about getting sued for fluoride pollution damage. Fluoridation was dressed up to be a modern scientific health improvement exercise with no risk in order to fool the good-hearted but scientifically naïve councillors governing Grand Rapids, Newburgh and Brantford into signing up their populations, present and future, for a gamble that would result in uncontrolled irreversible effects on their health. I believe the proponents knew it would never be scientifically monitored or recorded once fluoridation was in place because the goal was never health, dental or otherwise.

In Grand Rapids, the groups of kids who were followed for only four years were carefully selected. They were only boys over age six who already had permanent incisors, and the children who got more cavities or who got sick during that time were dropped from the trial. The follow-up was supposed to be 15 years but was very sporadic and superficial. Those of us born after 1947 were ignored as a group except for a few individuals who were periodically singled out for marketing purposes. It was appallingly poor scientific research, but inspired marketing. People read an abstract or summary and a headline and are totally fooled.

Within six years, the Grand Rapids trial was hailed as a roaring success based on spurious counts comparing numbers of decayed, missing or filled tooth surfaces of the monitored school children at the beginning of the trial and then after several years. Subjects should have been studied for an additional nine years—that was the study plan. When data were re-examined by independent researchers years later, they did not actually show the dental improvement that had been claimed, as reported in Dr Waldbott's book *Fluoridation, the Great Dilemma.* The manipulation of data to produce the pre-ordained outcome favouring the government narrative of safe and effective by ignoring harm remains the hallmark of government public health studies and dental fluoridation research to this day.

Fluoride intake studies attempting to verify the safety and efficacy of water fluoridation at one part per million rapidly got muddied. Control cities already dispensing fluoride supplements got fluoridated and kept giving supplements; dozens of other communities fluoridated at 1.2

ppm or even 1.5; fluoride toothpastes, tablets and vitamin drops with added fluoride were marketed; school fluoride rinse programs were instituted even in areas that already had fluoride in their waters.

Eighty years on, Google's AI Gemini, when asked, spews the same sales pitch that tricked those city fathers. Example: I asked, "What is the VOLUME of fluoridated tap water a six-year-old child must consume for dental benefit?" Gemini:

> ***Concentration Matters:*** *The most important factor is the amount of fluoride in the water. A child drinking water with the recommended concentration will receive the dental benefits regardless of the total volume consumed.*

How is that even possible! Magic? Dental benefits from a couple teaspoons or a gallon, all the same? Medical doctors don't give people a bottle of pills with instructions to take as many or few as you want. Dose matters!

Another answer from Gemini told me that water fluoridation works to prevent tooth decay by providing a "continuous dose." But Gemini, we don't consume water continuously and could not survive a continuous dose in an uncontrolled volume of plain water, never mind a physiologically damaging substance added to it! Volume consumed DOES matter! Even AI has been corrupted by the marketing copy.

Every industrialized nation in the world had populations with dental decay problems from the influx of devitalized flour, sugar, starch, margarine, hydrogenated seed oils and canned foods. Every industrialized nation also had fluoride pollution problems. America's problem was more intensely urgent because, in addition to its ramped-up wartime production of steel and aluminum, its secret facilities were emitting vast quantities of extremely toxic fluorinated gases in the race against time to produce fissionable uranium. The public could not be told of the true nature of the emissions; that was a wartime secret.

Fluoridation's industrial waste origins and toxicity had to be sanitized and sold to the masses as a vital public health policy—through deception, abuse of scientific and ethical principles and political machinations, and so it was.

Mom and Me

When fluoridation started in 1945, my mother was a vibrant, lovely 19-year-old student at Calvin College. Her hair was a mane of glossy cascading brunette waves. She had 32 straight white teeth and a beautiful smile. She had no allergies. According to the school pictures I have, her classmates and friends were well-built, healthy and good-looking. They were first- and second-generation children of Dutch immigrants, stable and prosperous. Many, including my mother, were the first in their families to get a post-secondary education. Graduates of Calvin did well in life. They were founders of corporations, entrepreneurs, politicians, clergy, and professionals.

These college students were too young to join the war, but in 1945 were too old to have their dental health monitored in the trial. There was of course zero interest in monitoring their reproductive, digestive, immunological, or neurological health.

Soon after the start of the fluoridation trial in Grand Rapids, my previously healthy mother had surgery for appendicitis. She had to get amalgam fillings in a few teeth. She developed scalp inflammation with itchy dandruff, treated with smelly coal tar shampoo. She started growing small brown lumps on the skin of her back and trunk that had to be regularly removed. She got hives when around animal or bird dander. Then she developed a severe allergy to penicillin, cheeses and fermented foods. She was diagnosed and treated by a colleague of Dr George Waldbott, who had begun to identify and treat patients for fluoride allergy and toxicity and would later work extremely hard for years to reverse fluoridation as a public health policy and paid a high price just as today's professional dissenters do. By 1950 she was married and expecting, but still very unwell.

My mother had excellent dental health in childhood and as a young adult. Her teeth were intact when she died at 97-years-old, thanks in part to the benefit of a charitable nutrition program in the 1920s, feeding nourishing meals to inner-city Grand Rapids pregnant women and toddlers. This was based on the work of Dr Weston A. Price, DDS.

Price, a practising dentist and author of the seminal text, *Nutrition and Physical Degeneration*, had studied primitive societies, documented their dental health, analysed the nutrients in their native diets, compared everything with the dental health and diets of Americans eating processed foods, and concluded that dental disease and malformations of the skull, teeth and jaws, as well as reproductive problems with fertility, pregnancy and birth, were preventable with nutritious foods, especially from animal sources.

Dr Price, a dental scientist, reported in the prologue of the seventh edition of his book that people who abandoned their native diets in favour of processed commercial foods, experienced results that were "disastrous for all groups studied. **Rampant dental caries** was followed by progressive facial deformities in children born to parents consuming refined and devitalized foods. These changes consisted of "**narrowed facial structure and dental arches, along with crowded teeth**" [emphasis added] (Price, 2009).

Price and other scientists had documented the evidence that fluoride ingestion from food and water caused dental fluorosis; chronic exposure caused debility, tooth loss, skeletal fluorosis, reproductive problems, and overall decline in health of adult humans and animals.

While children with dental fluorosis were observed to be apparently less prone to cavities, as adults they were more likely to lose their teeth. It was well known that poor nutrition made people and animals more susceptible to natural and industrial fluoride toxicity and subsequent tooth loss. The evidence from Price and his colleague Frank Pottenger was overwhelmingly in favour of avoiding fluoride for overall health and focusing on prenatal and childhood nutrition that excluded processed devitalized food to protect dental health.

Price had serious misgivings about the safety of topical sodium fluoride treatments for cavity prevention, writing: "Fluorine treatment, like dental extractions, cannot be a panacea for dental caries." He had no use for fluoridation, writing: "Adding it to food and water for general use is beyond the practice of dentistry." (p. 455, 456. 7th ed.) Prior to 1940, the idea that fluoride supplementation of any kind should be recommended for infants and children to improve dental health was not well supported, until the narrative was reversed to serve wartime purposes.

My mother did not connect her health problems, miscarriages, preterm births, or her children's ill health to fluoride overdose and nutritional deficiencies until I showed her years later what I had learned.

I was born small, a month early, in Grand Rapids in 1952. My older sister was born nearly two months early and required incubation. She failed to thrive initially. As per the modern "science-based" custom of discouraging mothers from nursing their infants, we were formula fed with boiled tap water and milk powder on a fixed schedule. We both had intractable colic, just as Dutch paediatrician Dr Hans Moolenburgh had found in his infant patients living in the fluoridated part of Amsterdam during the fluoridation trials in the Netherlands. Relief came from eventually moving out of Grand Rapids for a few years. But the damage had been done. I was forever made hypersensitive to fluoride from any source, and had no physiological resilience to cope with overexposure, whether from water, food, air pollution, anesthesia, medications, my father's chain-smoking, or drinking tea.

From 1959 to 1968 we lived in a small Ontario town with natural fluoride and arsenic from ground water. My mother's scalp problem and chronic fatigue flared again. She was hospitalized several times with pneumonia and gallbladder inflammation. My sister and I developed goitres. Our brothers had crippling bowel pain, I had intractable diarrhea, and we all had painful joints. Did we stop getting cavities? No!

When I moved to fluoridated Toronto from unfluoridated Kingston at age 21, I immediately developed allergies, asthma, rashes and digestive problems, but did not connect fluoridated water to my health problems for another ten years, when I had my first baby. He was born three months too soon because fluoride had suppressed my thyroid function. Through classic experimentation of exposure/withdrawal/re-exposure, I figured it out. I stopped drinking Toronto tap water in 1984.

There must be hundreds of thousands of people my age from all the early fluoridation trials who have been harmed like I am, but never counted. Fluoridation everywhere still practised is the big lie built by denying us.

My sister and I have very mild dental fluorosis on our incisors from the pre- and perinatal exposure in Grand Rapids. We both had thyroid problems, several mercury amalgam fillings due to cavities in our molars as children, and many restorations as adults while living in fluoridated areas. We both had delayed eruption of canine teeth due to fluoride, overbite and crowding that required extraction of adjacent teeth. We had impacted wisdom teeth removed under general anesthetic, and orthodontic braces around adolescence because of narrowed dental arch and too-small jaws, exactly as Dr Weston Price had documented in his book. We both had infected tonsils and adenoids removed as toddlers due to airway blockages from developmental malformation of jaws and palate. We both developed sleep apnea as young adults. Our brothers have similar problems. One has moderate dental fluorosis due to being given fluoride drops.

I still have 24 teeth instead of 32. I have been able to keep them free of decay with nutrition and hygiene for over 20 years. I wonder what my face would really look like if my skull and jaws had been allowed to develop fully, with good nutrition but without fluoride overdose, like my mother's lovely face.

I wonder what my life would have been like if I hadn't suffered with thyroid disease—if I hadn't been poisoned with industrial waste since before I was born.

Fluoridation is the policy of using drinking water systems and consumers as waste disposal systems for industry waste product; and people in positions of power are still enthralled to the glitzy snake oil patter that was developed in 1945 by the Father of Propaganda, Edward Bernays.

21st Century

It's uncomfortable and discouraging to make repeated public deputations giving reasoned and referenced scientific, ethical, logical, budgetary, and legal arguments as to why fluoridation should be voted out, to mostly hostile councillors and city-funded public health experts. They rarely read the handouts we provide; their faces and body language tell all, and often the people we want most to listen will rudely chat and laugh among themselves during our precious three, or if we're lucky, five minutes. Some deliberately make noise to attract attention to themselves and away from our words, as they pointedly leave the room in the middle of our speech. We may get a standing ovation from the citizens behind us, as some of us have, and that makes them furious.

My mother's generation would be the first to bear children poisoned by fluoridation from a scam performed by their own government. My siblings and I were the first to be fluoride-poisoned from conception by government order. Every generation since is more fluoride-poisoned than the previous, by government order. It is baffling beyond words that fluoridation is still here, eighty years later. Why? Why do they want this hardship, this suffering, this evil, for all of us?

The great Grand Rapids trial that started it all was unethical, ineffective, and inconclusive. It mocked science and coldly discarded the lives of the many workers fluoride-poisoned during the Manhattan Project while processing uranium for nuclear weapons. Redistributing fluoride to the rest of the world in drinking water as magic tooth medicine was a political cover-up, not a real clinical trial with informed consent. It should never have been conducted and fluoridation should not be allowed to continue.

The City that Refuses and Refuses to Drink Fluoridation Chemicals

By: Brent Foster, JD

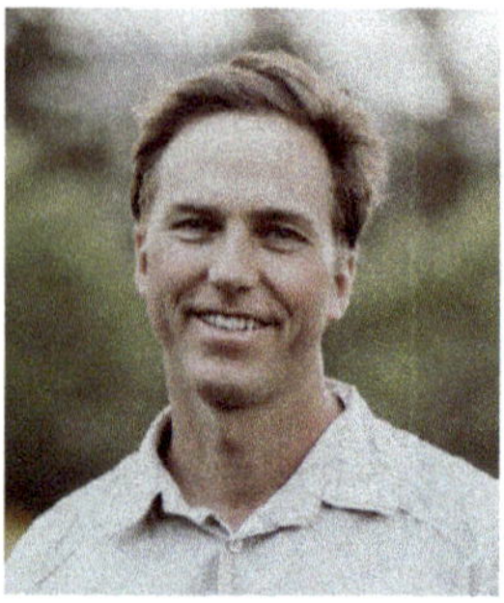

ABOUT: *Brent Foster lives in Oregon. He worked as a non-profit public interest attorney for over 20 years. He has been actively involved in state and local efforts to keep fluoridation chemicals out of drinking water efforts and was part of the campaign team that won a ballot referendum in 2013 in Portland, Oregon, overturning the City Council's vote to fluoridate. Brent also drafted and organized a ballot measure in the City of Hood River, Oregon, which blocked a push to fluoridate by amending the city charter to prohibit the addition of any industrial waste byproduct to the city's drinking water. Brent has a B.S. in Ecology and a B.A. in Environmental Science from the University of California at Santa Barbara and a law degree from Lewis and Clark Law School.*

CHAPTER 15

"Each time a man stands up for an ideal,
or acts to improve the lot of others,
or strikes out against injustice,
he sends forth a tiny ripple of hope."

—Robert F. Kennedy, Sr. (1966)

THE CITY OF PORTLAND long held the distinction as being the largest city in the United States not to add fluoridation chemicals to its drinking water. Portlanders, in fact, had already voted to reject fluoridation three times when promoters in 2012 made their most sophisticated and well-funded attempt yet to push through fluoridation.

Rather than risk losing yet another public vote, fluoridation backers instead attempted to pass fluoridation through a behind-the-scenes lobbying effort and a rushed vote from the Portland City Council. In August 2012, the news broke that a coalition of fluoridationists had quietly hired political consultant Mark Weiner to lobby the Council for fluoridation (Schmidt, 2012). Weiner was uniquely positioned since he had run the political campaigns for a majority of the then sitting Council members.

After a token public process, the Council unanimously approved fluoridation despite strong opposition at the one hearing where public comment was allowed. The strategy behind the rush was obvious—pass fluoridation before an opposition movement could form. Oregon law allows voters to refer a City Council vote to the public if they are able to collect the signatures of 6% of registered voters within 30 days. For Portland that meant collecting at least 25,000 signatures to ensure that 19,858 valid signatures were submitted.

This would have been daunting even for an established group with financial resources in a community where most prior referendum efforts had failed. But we were not well established and had almost no resources when we gathered in a small meeting room at a local restaurant in 2012t o consider our response to the City's fluoridation referendum. The prospect of collecting 25,000 signatures in four weeks felt impossible, but if we succeeded it would stop any immediate moves to fluoridate until there was a public vote.

We had a spirited debate about whether to even attempt a referendum or focus instead on running a stand-alone ballot measure many months later to prohibit fluoridation. This second option would have meant a longer window to collect signatures, but risked allowing the City to immediately start building fluoridation infrastructure which could make fluoridation seem like a fait accompli at a later election.

We decided to confront the City Council vote head on and attempt what many openly speculated was an impossible task. While our group came from many diverse backgrounds and interests, we shared a passion for clean water and decided to center that passion in our campaign by calling our group "Clean Water Portland." We knew what our goal was, but we had little idea how to pull it off.

Activist Advantage

Fluoridationists had a seemingly limitless budget and had spent nearly a year working behind the scenes to line up more than 50 local public health and civic groups in support of fluoridation.

While we had almost no money, we did have an incredible group of passionate Portlanders. The initial core was a tight-knit group who had worked together previously fighting efforts to pass a statewide fluoridation mandate. Founded by Lynne Campbell, a tireless activist who led the fight against fluoridation in Oregon for many years, Oregon Citizens for Safe Drinking Water coalesce the local group with activists such as Rick North, the former head of the Oregon American Cancer Society; Roger Burt, who had helped lead the 1980 campaign against fluoridation in Portland; and Kim Kaminski, who helped stop multiple statewide attempts to mandate all cities add fluoridation chemicals to their water. They knew the science of fluoridation's risks, were articulate speakers and understood grassroots organizing.

The Council's vote to fluoridate Portland's prized water supply also inspired a wave of new activists. Frances Quaempts-Miller, for example, quickly volunteered to be a Chief Petitioner for the referendum along with Kim Kaminski, who became the Executive Director of Clean Water Portland. Frances, a woman of African American and Muscogee Indian descent, was a powerful voice in rebutting the core message being pushed by fluoridationists that fluoridation was necessary to help children from low-income communities of color.

The Portland NAACP and their director Jo Ann Hardesty similarly came out in opposition to fluoridation, helping undermine one of the key pillars of the fluoridationists' talking points.

At one of the earliest organizing meetings, Zia McCabe, a Portland rock star and keyboardist for the Dandy Warhols, strolled into a meeting of less than ten people and declared she was ready to fight fluoridation. She proceeded to become another key part of our grassroots campaign, bringing a cool factor that was both uniquely Portland and critical in reaching younger voters.

Hundreds of other everyday Portlanders sacrificed their work, time with their families, their evenings and weekends to volunteer in our unprecedented effort to gather the close to 1,000 signatures a day we needed to qualify the referendum.

Push for Signatures

Within days after the Council's vote to fluoridate, we had raised enough funds to rent a funky old Quonset hut as our campaign headquarters. Some days over 100 people showed up to learn how to collect signatures. Volunteers who had little to no political experience eagerly trained other volunteers and we quickly had people standing in front of supermarkets, walking farmers' markets, and attending almost every public event in town collecting signatures.

If you have noticed lots of women's names at the campaign core, that is because women at all levels of the campaign significantly outnumbered men. From Kim Kaminski's tireless work as Clean Water Portland's director to the work of our office managers, signature collectors, door knockers, envelope stuffers and freeway sign wavers, women played an outsized role in the campaign.

But it was not only women attempting the impossible. Shortly after we started collecting signatures, Hiram Asmuth walked into the campaign office and asked if we needed any help organizing signature collectors. He turned out to be what can only be described as a petition signature gathering kingpin. He had years of experience running signature collection campaigns and knew which supermarkets and light rail lines would generate the most signatures. And, importantly, he had great contacts with professional signature collectors.

With meager but critical donations in hand, we started hiring signature collectors to create an integrated petition effort with both volunteers and paid collectors working side by side. That unique level of integration made the daunting task ahead seem a little more attainable.

Three weeks later we had gathered 20,000 signatures, still short of the 25,000 we needed to account for signatures from non-registered voters who had inadvertently signed the petition. It's time to "turn on the afterburners," said Kim Kaminski in a local news story covering passage of the 20,000-signature milestone (Korfhage 2012). And turn on the afterburners we did.

By the 29th day of the signature drive, we had collected a whopping 43,236 signatures, more than twice the number required. As a special message to the fluoridationists, we submitted the signatures a full day early. We were ecstatic that the City was stopped from immediately moving forward with fluoridation, but the campaign fight had just begun.

Overcoming the Odds

The petition effort had taught us that Portlanders were split on fluoridation. Soon after the referendum qualified, we commissioned a poll that found a solid majority of voters supported fluoridation while just over 30% opposed it, with the remainder undecided. These were not the numbers you wanted to see when facing an opponent with seemingly unlimited campaign coffers, one of the State's top political strategists, and a broad coalition of organizational supporters.

Our call with the pollsters to discuss poll results felt like they were delivering a cancer diagnosis. Given the lopsided resources, majority support for fluoridation, and limited public opposition, they made clear it would take a near miracle for us to win.

But what none of us were able to fully appreciate was the power of a campaign focused like a laser on protecting clean water from fluoridation chemicals.

The arguments against fluoridation were abundant. Fluoridation chemicals, for example, clearly met the legal definition of a drug* and adding fluoridation chemicals to drinking water plainly removed individual choice on whether or not to be medicated. The scientific evidence also presented compelling evidence that fluoridation posed a range of serious public health threats such as IQ deficits in children (Taylor et al., 2025). Furthermore, there was little credible scientific evidence that water fluoridation has a meaningful effect on cavity rates (Iheozor-Eljiofor et al., 2024).

Strong as any of these arguments can be, however, focusing on the message that we did not need *any* more chemicals added to our drinking water resonated with Portlanders and inspired a truly unique level of voter and volunteer engagement.

As a part of this messaging, we strategically avoided using the word "fluoride," for two reasons. First, there is not a city in the country that adds elemental "fluoride" to their drinking water. Instead, what they add are "fluoridation chemicals," such as fluorosilicic acid, and to a much lesser extent sodium fluorosilicate or sodium fluoride. Talking about the addition of "fluoride" to drinking water is simply not accurate. (Reeves, 2000)

But as importantly, as linguistic strategist George Lakoff has highlighted, the words we use to frame an issue are critical to determining how the general public perceives it (Lakoff, 2004). The term "fluoride" has a squeaky-clean image with a broad swath of the general public thanks to decades of promotion by fluoridationists and billions of advertising dollars by toothpaste companies. Starting a discussion with voters using a term that has so much public relations power behind it makes little sense. Convincing voters their positive impressions of "fluoride" were wrong may have been an impossible lift.

By focusing on the addition of "fluoridation chemicals" to the drinking water, we were able to lay the foundation for many voters to re-think fluoridation through a different lens. Time after time, our campaign volunteers would meet voters who started a conversation saying they supported adding "fluoride" to the drinking water, only to quickly start to re-think that support when asked if they knew that the chemical "fluorosilicic acid," an undisputed industrial waste byproduct, would be the chemical used to actually "fluoridate" the water.

This framing also tied into other questions such as: what were these fluoridation chemicals, where did they come from, and what was in them? Even fluoridation's most-high profile booster, the U.S. Centers for Disease Control, openly acknowledged that, "[a]ll of the fluoride chemicals used in the U.S. for water fluoridation, sodium fluoride, sodium fluorosilicate, and fluorosilicic acid, are byproducts of the phosphate fertilizer industry." Fluoridation proponents in Oregon put their own gloss on the issue by calling fluoride "a useful by-product of the phosphate fertilizer industry." Not even highly paid political strategists, however, could make adding waste byproducts to the drinking water sound good.

Additionally, there was substantial voter interest in the fact fluoridation chemicals commonly contained other toxic byproducts of fertilizer production, such as arsenic and lead (Peterson et al., 2016)). To highlight this, we asked the City of Philomath's water manager to test the source of fluorosilicic acid they used to fluoridate drinking water in their city just south of Portland. Not surprisingly, their tests confirmed the presence of arsenic in the fluoridation chemicals they were adding to their water and we highlighted this in a TV news conference. Voters that may have supported "fluoride" in their drinking water now had to consider whether they wanted some additional arsenic as well.

In this context, however, we did talk about the broad spectrum of "new science" showing that the fluoridation chemicals once thought safe were now associated with impacts such as the increased risk of childhood cancer (Bassin et al., 2006; Żwierełło et al., 2024). Like so many other chemicals, once thought safe, modern science now tells us that there are real reasons to be concerned about fluoridation. The difficulty of shifting people's long-standing beliefs is well-documented. Highlighting the "new scientific studies" about fluoridation's risks, however, was an effective way to meet educated Portlanders with a positive view of fluoridation where they were and then use the new science to encourage a second look.

To this end, the Fluoride Action Network's (FAN) website database of scientific summaries and source articles was invaluable. FAN's credible and user-friendly interface was perfect for voters and volunteers alike to do the type of independent research we saw building our support daily.

Grassroots Ground Game

Not long into the campaign, the fluoridationists were flooding the television, radio, and newspapers with propaganda. Every day it seemed a new pro-fluoridation mailer was arriving in mailboxes. Portland's largest newspapers were running regular editorials in support of fluoridation. Our only chance of winning over public support was an aggressive grassroots campaign. And aggressive it was. Hundreds of volunteers from across the political spectrum– Democrats, Republicans and Independents—worked tirelessly for months to educate Portlanders to reject fluoridation for the fourth time.

Campaign volunteers like Rick North, now on Fluoride Action Network's Board of Directors, and dentists such as Dr Jay Levy and Dr Bill Osmunson, as well as Kellie Barnes, Roger Burt, Clean Water Portland Director Kim Kaminski and many others made over 100 community presentations to virtually any group willing to listen. Armed with a message of clean water, the risks of fluoridation chemicals, and choice, they changed minds and built support one late night meeting at a time. Behind them were dedicated volunteers and donors, too many to name, that scheduled presentations, answered the phones, wrote donation checks, trained volunteers, and prepared the outreach materials essential to such a robust outreach effort.

In 2013, the importance of social media in campaigns was not well-established, but with extremely limited funding, the campaign focused on building thousands of followers on Facebook, which became a critical organizing springboard for everything from volunteer recruitment to fundraising. Some of the Facebook posts of photographer Mark Coleman's 2013 images with people holding their homemade signs about why they supported clean water got over 20,000 likes and were shared widely.

Very early in the campaign we also strategically deployed thousands of blue and white signs in front of supporters' houses on high-visibility Portland streets that read, "Vote No on Fluoridation Chemicals." Volunteers went door to door on the highest traffic streets and if someone was supportive, we asked if we could place a lawn sign in their yard. In just a one-week period, the city streets bloomed with our signs. They energized our base, inspired conversations among neighbors, and centered our message.

They also drove fluoridation promoters nuts and, after several weeks, our signs started disappearing at a scale that was difficult to explain as anything short of a coordinated effort. Despite this, our volunteers would put them back up as quickly as they came down.

Other visibility events, like regular sign waving along freeways and Portland bridges, helped create the visible momentum that we started to see reflected in our climbing support numbers and growing volunteer base.

Another critical component of our campaign was educating people at their front door about the threat fluoridation chemicals posed to clean water. But there are few things harder to recruit volunteers to do. Retired police officer and Democratic activist KC Hansen and others, however, tirelessly trained reluctant volunteers in how to have the type of high-quality conversations that can change minds and motivate your base.

We also organized weekly TV media events. Whether it was our "*Toast to Clean Water*" event we held with hundreds of people gathered at a local reservoir to drink up some un-fluoridated water or the unveiling of a building-sized billboard with Mark Coleman's portraits showing the diversity of Portlanders opposing fluoridation, we were a consistent presence on the local news.

As our list of supporters grew, we invested significant resources into tracking these supporters so we could make sure they voted when ballots were mailed out. We digitized data from the more than 43,000 voters who had signed our paper referendum petitions and added in supporters we had met from canvassing, community presentations, and repeated on-line supporter pledges.

Just as ballots were being mailed out, rockstar and volunteer Zia McCabe organized our biggest media event yet. It was a carnival-like march through the streets led by Portland's iconic March Fourth Marching Band, featuring everyone from baroque stilt dancers to moms pushing strollers. It was loud, energetic, and covered live by every TV news outlet in town.

Despite all these efforts, our post-election polling found that voters identified the voter pamphlet statements we had organized from a diversity of experts and perspectives as one of the most important things voters relied on in making their decision. While expensive and time consuming to prepare, our voter pamphlet statements were our chance not only to make the core argument that fluoridation chemicals were a threat to clean water, but also a chance to connect with voters about why fluoridation would deprive Portlanders of medical choice and to remind voters about the growing body of new science about fluoridation's health risks.

Sweet Victory

The final days of the campaign culminated in a major get-out-the-vote effort to drive our database of supporters to vote. By election day fluoridation promoters had spent just shy of $900,000 and outspent our campaign by a 3:1 margin (Mesh, 2013).

As we gathered in a local restaurant bar to watch the returns, we knew had done everything we could despite the outsized odds. When the first returns were announced, it was clear we had won; the crowd erupted with jubilation. Voters that had once supported fluoridation had now rejected it by a landslide margin, 61% - 39%. The communities of color which fluoridationists had framed their campaign around had rejected it by an even larger margin than the general public. Clean Water Portland had beaten the odds and done what once seemed almost impossible... even to us.

***Footnote**: 21 U.S. Code § 321(g)(1) provides: "The term 'drug' means: (B) articles intended for use in the diagnosis, cure, mitigation, treatment, or prevention of disease in man or other animals..."

My Struggle for a Serious Debate about Fluoridation

By: Dr Mark Diesendorf, BSc, PhD

ABOUT: *I was originally a theoretical physicist. However, my research expanded into interdisciplinary problems in energy, health and environmental sustainability. I am currently Honorary Associate Professor of Environment and Society at UNSW Sydney. My previous positions include Principal Research Scientist in Australia's national research organisation CSIRO, and Professor of Environmental Science and Founding Director of the Institute for Sustainable Futures at the University of Technology Sydney. My major research paper, that raised questions about the alleged benefits of fluoridation, was 'The Mystery of Declining Tooth Decay' published in Nature in 1986.*

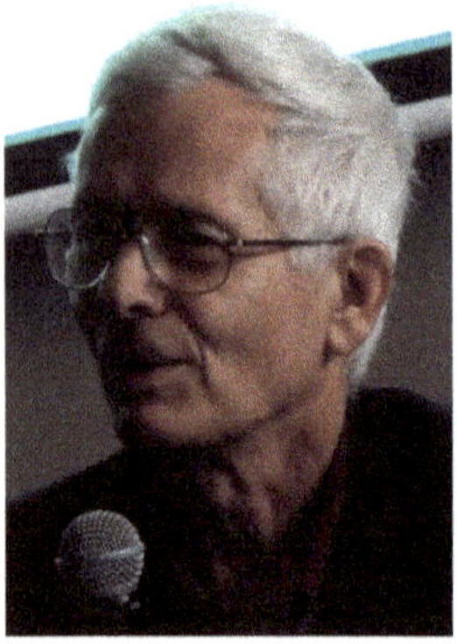

Photo Credit: Danimations - Own work, CC BY-SA 4.0, https://commons.wikimedia.org/w/index.php?curid=75319430

CHAPTER 16

"As soon as we abandon our own reason and are content to rely upon the authority of others, there is no end to our troubles."

—Bertrand Arthur William Russell (1872-1970)

MY PHD THESIS was focused on the physical conditions in the solar interior. When I learned to my dismay that my calculations were being used by the Lawrence Livermore National Laboratory to improve their design of nuclear weapons, I resolved to devote my future research to science for the people, not for the military or big business.

In the 1970s, I became secretary of, and public spokesperson for, the Society for Social Responsibility in Science (SSRS) in Canberra, Australia. Over that period SSRS had about 200 members, mostly scientists and academics. It aimed to inform decision-makers, scientists and the public about the social consequences and implications of science and technology. As secretary, I had an overview of almost all its activities, which were mostly on environmental issues, and was also able to introduce some of my own areas of interest: a critique of modern medicine, support for the new public health and community health movements, energy alternatives and opposition to the testing of nuclear weapons in the atmosphere. One of the issues that came before SSRS was fluoridation.

Becoming Involved in the Fluoridation Controversy

As a result of campaigning by pro-fluoridation dentists, supported behind the scenes by funding from the junk food industry, fluoridation was widely regarded as a 'forbidden' topic of public debate that was only raised by 'unscientific faddists and eccentrics'. Raising a debate was made even more difficult by some anti-fluoridationists in the so-called 'health' food industry, who claimed unscientifically that "natural fluoride is good for you while artificial fluoride is bad". Nowadays, some medical doctors, dentists, scientists, and members of the public worry that the anti-fluoridation case is weakened by its support by Robert F. Kennedy, Jr. who lost credibility with them by opposing vaccination on dubious grounds.

As a research scientist, it was natural for me to begin my investigation of fluoridation with a thorough review of the scientific literature on its health hazards and alleged benefits. I went back to the original papers in dental, medical and scientific journals, so as not to be restricted to official reviews and reports of inquiries.

By contacting leaders of the anti-fluoridation movement, I was put in touch with other scientists, dentists and medical doctors who had doubts about the safety and/or the effectiveness of fluoridation. In the 1970s and early 80s, my main professional and scientific advisers on fluoridation were Dr Philip R.N. Sutton, a retired dental researcher and senior lecturer from the School of Dentistry, University of Melbourne (Sutton, 1960), Dr Albert Burgstahler, Professor of Chemistry at the University of Kansas (Waldbott, Burgstahler & McKinney, 1978), and Glen Walker, a retired businessman with expertise in metal-finishing and electrochemistry, who was the coordinator of the grassroots antifluoridation movement in Australia (Walker, 1982). From the mid-1980s onwards, I benefitted greatly from regular correspondence with Dr John Colquhoun, a former chairperson of the Fluoridation Promotion Committee of New Zealand who became a leading opponent on the world scene (Colquhoun, 1984, 1987, 1994; Colquhoun & Mann, 1986, 1987).

I soon found several scholarly papers presenting evidence that skeletal fluorosis, a disease of the bones and joints, is endemic in several naturally fluoridated areas of the world. This contradicted the conventional 'wisdom' that low concentrations of fluoride in drinking water are safe. Subsequently, I also found studies that the observed decline in tooth decay in fluoridated regions in the 1960s (before fluoride toothpaste) was matched by similar declines in unfluoridated regions over the same period (Leverett, 1982; Multiple Authors, 1982).

When I proposed to publicise this research, I received strong opposition from fellow members of SSRS as well as others who were worried that I would question the so-called 'cornerstone of dental public health'. Challenging fluoridation was indeed the forbidden issue! However, as someone committed to democratic decision-making and open scientific debate, I decided to break through the silence barrier.

Before discussing my personal struggle to challenge the power of the vested interests in fluoridation, I must explain my strategy, which is based on experience in campaigning in the public interest (as I see it) in several major issues.

State Capture by Vested Interests

One of the first steps in changing a practice that is unhealthy, or environmentally destructive, or socially unjust, is to achieve a serious public debate about the issue. Often, one finds that the *status quo* or business-as-usual viewpoint on many important issues has been established by politically powerful vested interests, such as the junk food, fossil fuels and weapons industries, certain professional organisations, and big business as a whole. These vested interests gain enormous political influence by means of political donations, election expenditure, 'revolving door' jobs with government and the public service, concentrated media ownership, and so-called 'think tanks' that are controlled by, and lobby for, these interests. This well-documented process is known as 'state capture' (Australian Democracy Network, 2022; Diesendorf & Taylor, 2023, chapter 6). It can be defined as the exercise of power by private actors to shape government policies and/or implementation in service of their narrow interests.

State capture is a form of corruption that goes far beyond petty corruption where an individual person or business pays a government minister or public official to influence a government decision. State capture is systemic and well-organised. It involves repeated transactions, often on an increasing scale, and can involve corporate influence, even control, of all major political parties, public officials, mass media, social media and institutions originally designed to regulate the industry concerned. With the support of these institutions, the vested interests build up a 'culture' of thinking within the community that rejects deviations from their viewpoint as allegedly ill-informed, unscientific, eccentric and/or uneconomic. This has been the case, with varying degrees of success, for the following issues in which I've been involved in challenging the once dominant beliefs:

- the notions that nuclear power is a safe and clean technology and that an electricity system cannot be run entirely on renewable energy;
- the neoliberal ideology that governments and hence taxation should be small and that wealth trickles down from the rich to the poor;
- the belief that the poor are poor because they don't work hard enough;
- the public acceptance that the United States should have many more nuclear weapons than the rest of the world taken together and have around 750 military bases around the world;
- the belief that the fluoridation of water supplies is safe and effective in preventing tooth decay.

Of all these examples, the task of breaking through the cultural barrier established by vested interests and achieving serious public debate on fluoridation has, in my experience, been one of the most difficult.

Who are the vested interests in fluoridation? In the early years when fluoridation was first proposed to prevent dental caries, the principal vested interest was the aluminium smelting industry, whose emissions of fluoride into the atmosphere were responsible for substantial damage to the local environment and animal health (Waldbott et al., 1978). Nowadays, the junk food industry benefits from the incorrect notion that people can avoid tooth decay while eating foods high in sugars and other refined carbohydrates, provided they are protected by 0.7 parts per million of fluoride in their drinking water. Dentists, too, have gained status as promoters of public health, while they still get plenty of work treating tooth decay—for them it's a win-win situation. Another vested interest is the phosphate fertilizer industry, which sells one of its waste products, silicofluorides, to many fluoridated water supply authorities. These silicofluorides are not pharmaceutically pure—they contain low concentrations of toxic substances such as arsenic.

Based on this understanding of state capture and its methods, the first step in challenging the establishment, as I see it, is creating a public debate that is soundly based scientifically and ethically. Then, with at least minority public support, it becomes possible to campaign against the methods of state capture listed above and thus weaken state capture.

Breaking Through the Silence Barrier

As my knowledge of literature on the health hazards and alleged benefits for fluoridation increased, I began to publish scholarly papers (e.g., Diesendorf, 1980; 1986a,b; 1987; 1989; 1990a,b; 1995; 1996; Diesendorf & Sutton, 1986; Diesendorf & Varney, 1986; Diesendorf, Colquhoun, Spittle, et al., 1997; Diesendorf & Diesendorf, 1997) and give seminars and conference papers on the issue. These gave me some credibility for publishing popular articles in magazines and letters in local newspapers. When community opposition arose to proposals to fluoridate communities, I was invited to address them. Initially, fluoridation proponents agreed to debate me but, after a few such public events, they refused to debate.

Throughout my campaign, proponents of fluoridation attempted to suppress and discredit me with dishonest arguments, misrepresentations and personal attacks. In the present chapter, I outline two case studies. More examples and details are given by Diesendorf (1996).

The Australian and New Zealand Association for the Advancement of Science (ANZAAS) Symposium Gains Wide Publicity

My research on fluoridation was stimulated by the publication of papers by others reporting that there had been large declines in tooth decay over the 1960s and 1970s in several *unfluoridated* developed countries

(Leverett, 1982; Multiple Authors, 1982). I was also aware of evidence of similar declines in Australia—in prefluoridation Sydney and unfluoridated Brisbane. These declines had commenced before fluoride toothpaste was widely used and there was evidence suggesting that fluoride tablets had not played a major role. The obvious question, avoided by the dental researchers and fluoridation promoters, was: if similar large reductions in tooth decay were occurring over a similar period in both fluoridated and unfluoridated areas, is it not likely that the same factor was responsible in both cases? If so, that common factor could not be fluoridation.

In Australia, the promoters of fluoridation had not revealed in their official reports (e.g., NH&MRC, 1985) even a hint of the new scientific evidence. I thought that the new material would be of interest to the Australian scientific community and the media. So, I enlisted the collaboration of Philip Sutton and together we convened a symposium on fluoridation at the 1985 Festival of Science sponsored by the Australian and New Zealand Association for the Advancement of Science (ANZAAS). We invited Wendy Varney, who had just written an insightful political science PhD thesis on fluoridation (published subsequently as Varney, 1986), to join us as a speaker and then, to liven things up even further and to inject 'balance', we invited the profluoridation *Australian Dental Association* (ADA) and the *National Health and Medical Research Council* (NH&MRC) to each provide a speaker as well.

The ADA wrote back promptly, not to us, but to the organisers of the ANZAAS Festival of Science, declining to participate and questioning our motivations. The ANZAAS organisers interpreted this letter as an unsubtle attempt to stop the symposium and resisted it. The NH&MRC only replied about a fortnight before the symposium, stating that they would only participate under conditions which were by then essentially impossible to fulfil.

These establishment responses failed to stop the symposium. Indeed, when we explained the situation to the media, they found it to be 'news' and gave excellent advance publicity for the symposium. As a result, about 100 people attended, including the media and many scholars who were previously uncommitted on this issue. For the first time, widespread media publicity was obtained in Australia for the evidence that the benefits of fluoridation have been greatly exaggerated, that there are genuine health hazards from fluoridated water, and that the promotion of fluoridation and fluoride products has been funded in part by vested interests such as the aluminium and sugary food industries.

In the subsequent media coverage, the fluoridation proponents were forced to come out and debate. Unaccustomed to discussing openly the issue, which they had labelled as 'beyond scientific debate', they did not offer meaningful answers to many of the points raised at the speakers at the symposium but instead tried to disparage us personally. In participating in this symposium and in the media reports, I was described as a CSIRO scientist, as I was entitled, but I was careful to state that my conclusions were not necessarily those of any organisation with which I was associated. (CSIRO is the *Australian Commonwealth Scientific and Industrial Research Organisation*.)

The real counterattack by the proponents of fluoridation took place behind the scenes. The ADA wrote to the chairman of my employer, CSIRO, and the Minister for Science and Technology, who is responsible for CSIRO, complaining about my 'activities', describing them as 'misleading, verging on fraudulent' and attacking me for allowing myself to be identified as a CSIRO scientist (Henry, 1985). Fortunately, neither the Chairman of CSIRO nor the Minister was impressed with these heavy-handed tactics. A CSIRO administrator informed me about the complaints and I was then able to obtain the correspondence under Freedom of Information. The Minister, Barry O. Jones, had annotated one ADA letter with the following comment: "Had the possibility of countering his argument occurred to their collective minds? Perhaps unfamiliar with the concept of scientific debate."

Dentists and medical doctors are more vulnerable to this kind of pressure than I was. Cases of intellectual suppression of dentists, scientists and medical doctors concerned about fluoridation are described by Waldbott (1965), Martin (1991) and other authors of the present book.

Publication in '*Nature*'

Following the success of the ANZAAS symposium, I felt that it was time to foster an international scientific debate on the alleged benefits of fluoridation. So I assembled all the data I could find on the decline in tooth decay in unfluoridated areas, summarised it in a form comprehensible to scientists who are not dentists, incorporated new data from the Australian School Dental Services, posed the obvious question about the mechanism of the decline in tooth decay in unfluoridated areas, gave the paper the catchy title of 'The Mystery of Declining Tooth Decay', and submitted it to what is arguably one of the two the leading general science journals in the world, *Nature*.

A few months later, the editor of *Nature* sent back a referee's report which presented the usual profluoridation line. I pointed out to the editor that my original manuscript had already answered most of the referee's criticisms. To account for the remaining points, I made minor revisions and resubmitted the paper. To my delight, the paper was published in July 1986 (Diesendorf, 1986). I think it must have helped my credibility as a serious scientist with the editor that over the previous 16 years I had already published peer-reviewed research papers in *Nature* on three different 'hard science' topics: astrophysics, space physics and wind power. The publication of such a substantial, controversial paper in *Nature* gained media coverage around the world. It was a major breakthrough for the anti-fluoridation case.

The counterattack of the fluoridation establishment was to circulate covert critiques misrepresenting my paper, to spread the false statement that my paper had not been refereed (see Martin, 1991, p.76), and to pressure the editor of *Nature* not to publish any further articles by me on fluoridation. I only learned of the last move several years later when someone in the USA sent me a copy of a letter and an attached unpublished critique of my *Nature* paper, which had been addressed to the editor of *Nature* by one of Australia's then most vocal pro-fluoridation campaigners of the 1980s, Graham Craig. Contrary to the normal scientific practice of encouraging open debate, the letter (dated 15 August 1986) commenced: "This letter and its enclosures are not intended for your correspondence columns." I had not previously seen this material, although the way in which it reached me suggested that it must have been circulated widely around the world. Craig's material is very easy to refute, so it did not surprise me that he did not submit it for publication.

Someone also sent me a copy of a letter, dated 18 September 1986, from the then head of Dental Health in the Federal Department of Health, Dr Lloyd Carr, to Dr David E. Barmes, Chief of Oral Health, World Health Organisation. Carr's letter was obviously a response to a request to "Please explain and counter the Australian data used in Diesendorf's *Nature* paper". There could be no doubt that the publication of my *Nature* paper had upset the international fluoridation establishment.

Conclusion

In challenging the establishment 'experts' on fluoridation and other issues, I have found that both grassroots opposition and anti-establishment 'experts' are necessary. Without the former there is no community base and no political pressure for stopping fluoridation, and without the latter the movement would have much less credibility with the media, other professionals, scientists and decision-makers.

The profluoridation establishment is aware of the danger to their power and influence from anti-establishment experts. My own experience and research have exposed the following techniques used by the establishment for suppressing scientific and public questioning of fluoridation and for damaging the credibility of anti-establishment experts:

- the production of misleading information for distribution to decision-makers and the public;

- *de facto* censorship of scientific, medical and dental journals, by pressuring editors to send manuscripts which raise awkward questions about fluoridation to hostile referees, who are establishment 'experts', or to reject the manuscripts without review;
- intimidating into silence dentists, medical doctors and scientists who have concerns about fluoridation, by means of personal attacks, and misrepresentation of the fluoridation critics' work, in the media and professional journals, and by damage to the career prospects of critics through professional associations and employers;
- keeping informed opposition out of the press/media by informing journalists and editors that opponents are either cranks, right wing extremists or alternative health 'faddists'; the issues being raised have already been considered decades ago and are therefore not news; publishing or broadcasting anything on the issue would be damaging to public health; and fluoridation is endorsed by numerous national and international medical, dental and public health organisations. (Actually, it is mainly small elites within the listed organisations who have actually endorsed fluoridation.)
- if critics of fluoridation somehow manage to get media coverage, ensuring that a pro-fluoridation 'expert' always has the right of reply and the final say, and then publicly attacking the motivations and qualifications of critics;
- circulating covertly, to decision-makers and media, dossiers and reports attacking opponents personally or by association and misrepresenting their work on fluoridation.

For many years, these tactics by the profluoridation establishment have successfully stereotyped the opposition to fluoridation and intimidated some opponents, thereby creating a barrier of silence in the dental and medical literature and in the popular media. However, the tide has, very slowly, begun to turn. The implementation of fluoridation of community water supplies has almost ground to a halt as a consequence of the efforts of the community based anti-fluoridation movement, assisted by non-establishment experts.

Further progress in rolling back fluoridation could come from building alliances with the consumer, environmental, community health and social justice movements. Such alliances can campaign together on the common goal of strengthening democratic decision-making on a wide range of issues by targeting the methods used by vested interests to influence and 'capture' nation-states (Diesendorf & Taylor, 2023; Diesendorf, 2025). These methods include political donations, election expenditure, revolving door jobs, concentrated media ownership, reports and lobbying by so-called 'think tanks', and neoliberalism.

An important first step is breaking the silence barrier. However distasteful it may seem, the public exposure of intellectual suppression is the best way of countering it (Martin et al., 1986). As the suppression is illuminated and destroyed, the fluoridation of drinking water will come to be recognised as the harmful aberration it is.

EDITORS' NOTE: Despite many mischaracterizations, opposition to fluoride is nonpartisan and nonideological. It is grounded in the evidence of harm backed by rigorous science. Other subjects in scientific controversy, obviously, have different science, and anti-fluoridationists hold different views on these items based on their familiarity with that body of science, as well as their personal bias.

Kyle's Story

Fluoride Hypersensitivity and Autism

By: Audrey Adams

ABOUT: *Audrey Adams and her son, Kyle, were named plaintiffs in the "Fluoride Trial" (FWW et al. v EPA et al.) which concluded in the plaintiffs' favor in September 2024. Audrey and Kyle have multiple chemical sensitivities and suffer multiple symptoms from fluoride exposure, though Kyle's reactions are far more severe. Audrey gave up her banking career to be a full-time "autism mom" and advocate for children with special needs in schools, councils, and legislative activities. Eventually, the need for anti-fluoridation activism became a priority and Audrey became a board member of Washington Action for Safe Water in 2010.*

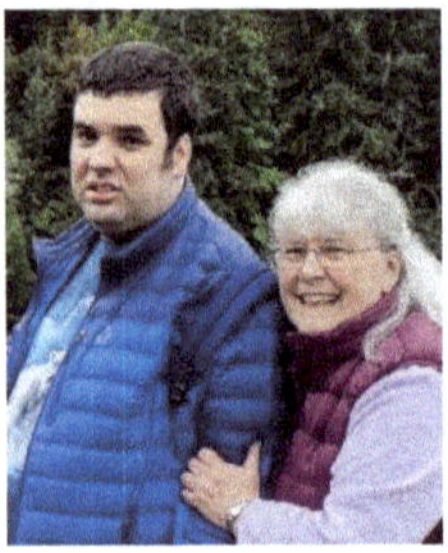

CHAPTER 17

"Fluoride is capable of producing any number of symptoms. They include drowsiness, profound desire to sleep, dizziness, nasal congestion, sneezing, runny nose, sore throat, coughing, wheezing (asthma), chest pain, hives, and various intestinal symptoms. Most of the information concerning specific reactions to fluoride, as seen in private practice, never reach publication."

—Hobart Feldman, MD (1979)

WHERE HAVE ALL the years gone? It feels like the fluoride fight has both sucked the life out of me and invigorated me. I'm 70, very tired with care responsibilities for three disabled family members, but I can't be done with this fluoride business yet. There are so many others who have waged this war without the personal need to do so that I have because of my son. These are my angels and my heroes because they fight for what's right simply because they are extraordinary, intelligent, caring human beings. I love them all.

Kyle Growing Up

My son Kyle, age 40, has autism and is severely hypersensitive to fluoride, but I didn't know about it for the first 14 years of his life. We have traveled a very long and painful road together, his pain physical and profound, my pain emotional. My Fluoride Action Network (FAN) friends have given me advice, knowledge, and a helping hand when I needed it, though they mostly didn't know it, then or now.

I don't claim to know to what extent fluoride affected Kyle as a baby, or if fluoride reduced his IQ, as many studies have found, but it seems plausible that a child who has multiple chemical sensitivities (as do I) and a specific hypersensitivity to fluoride would be at greater risk of neuro-developmental injury. Kyle's vulnerability to fluoride might be genetic since I am also sensitive to fluoride, but I didn't recognize my own fluoride-induced reactions until I was forced to figure out the source of Kyle's pain. I consider fluoride among a large stack of environmental assaults and chemicals that stole Kyle's future, but fluoride has remained the worst of that long list because, added to tap water, it's so damn hard to avoid.

Abundant Sensitivities

Being a skeptic of the bizarre myself, I understand when people are Incredulous when faced with Kyle's story of such severe hypersensitivity to fluoride that he can't drink tap water, can't tolerate food cooked in tap water and can't shower in fluoridated water. I do not judge skeptics of my son's story. Honestly, I absolutely did not want to believe it myself because it made my life profoundly more difficult.

I have been telling Kyle's fluoride story for a quarter of a century because I must pay it forward and thank two different moms of teens with autism—at different times and living in different states—who advised me to investigate fluoridated water as a possible cause of Kyle's suffering.

What suffering? Let me explain. When he was 13, Kyle was in pain constantly, all over, but especially the back of his neck and his extremities (hands, feet, lips, tongue). None of the many doctors we took him to had any answers—a specialist doctor would do his tests, find nothing, and send us to the next specialist...and so on, and so on. And the agony continued with no solution, no treatment, no known cause and no end in sight.

Kyle cried inconsolably when the pain in his fingers got so bad that he couldn't play his beloved cello in the orchestra at school. He had to quit playing piano, too, and he could barely hold a fork to eat. There were mysterious pain "peaks", especially in the middle of the night, but other times, too. He screamed and raced around the house as if pursued by killer bees. His school sent him home repeatedly with horrific headaches. Pain relievers were useless. Tylenol caused him kick-back migraines.

At night the house shook wildly with the leg-pounding on the bed that seemed like grand mal seizures, but weren't. I wouldn't have noticed an earthquake. His screaming was deafening. We got very little sleep.

It was the autism biomedical treatment conferences in the late 1990's that awakened my awareness of chemical sensitivities. I learned so much from both the presenters and the many smart parents in attendance about the clash of chemicals and autism. In time, I realized Kyle was completely intolerant of chemicals in the air and his food, so I switched his entire diet to organic, stopped using any cleaners or scented products and got the school to cooperate with a low-chemical environment... and so much more. He only drank water—nothing else.

With all of these changes, he improved, but still had pain every day, with screaming, racing, jumping, sweating, heart racing—gasping from the exertion... and crying. My nearly non-verbal son begged me to "Make it go away!"

Kyle Was Not the Only One

An autism mom from Oregon was the first who encouraged me in 2000 to eliminate fluoridated water for Kyle. After switching to reverse osmosis water for drinking and cooking, Kyle had a profound improvement in 3 days. His pain drained away, and our lives got better.

No, he was not (is not) completely free of all pain—sadly, unexpected chemicals lurk everywhere. But by providing Kyle with fluoride-free water—his only drink—chronic pain was no longer the 24/7 "norm", so detecting the other chemical triggers was finally more achievable and allowed much greater success at avoidance. Fluoride remains the worst, and most difficult, to avoid. It took me many years to understand the many sources of fluoride, and to fully realize the extent of Kyle's sensitivity to it.

A Focus on Fluoride in Water

By 2006, I had started talking to various officials about the injustice of water fluoridation for people like Kyle and the families who care for them. It simply is not fair to add a drug—or, for my son, a poison—to something as life-sustaining as water, regardless of any potential benefit to others. Kyle and I attended a public meeting of Seattle Public Utilities (SPU) to explain that unfairness. SPU didn't want to hear what I had to say, and when a dentist in the audience introduced himself, I thought, "What bad luck!".

But it turned out that the dentist was Dr Bill Osmunson and he *did* want to hear our story, and he wanted me to tell it again and again. Bill cast the line, and I caught the bait and the bug of anti-fluoridation activism. In 2008 Bill and I spoke with over 50 state legislators or their aides requesting a review of fluoridation.

There are many who believe that acute transdermal fluoride poisoning by showering or bathing in fluoridated tap water is impossible. I used to be one of them. After 8 years of hauling thousands of gallons of reverse osmosis and spring water to my home, and after 2 years of political activism in opposition to fluoridation, I was still a non-believer that a fluoridated shower could harm Kyle. I used a carbon shower filter to protect him from chlorine fumes, and although I knew fluoride would not be filtered out, I naïvely thought it could not be absorbed through the skin.

Compared to those insanely hard, painful years prior to our initial "fluoride discovery," Kyle was doing decently in 2008 and I thought I was an expert at protecting him from chemicals by then. Oh, but I had a lot to learn!

More Detective Work

Kyle's vastly improved quality of life had enabled him to work a part-time office job at Highline Community College. But I was stumped about morning headaches he'd been having for many months and had had multiple conversations with his doctor about it. We investigated various possible causes—was it mold? Or something in his completely organic, highly specialized breakfast? My detective skills failed me. Each morning, he woke up without a headache, but before he left for work his head was throbbing.

Another mother of an autistic teenager contacted me after reading my letter to the PCC Market Editor that I had written about fluoridation and my autistic son's reactivity. That mom told me about her son's fluoride hypersensitivity, and her own which was even much worse. She told me of a visit to Seattle, and one bath in fluoridated water here that resulted in nasty red, itchy welts at the bath water line and below, which then bled and peeled over the next 2 weeks. I began to wonder about my mysterious itchy rash of tiny red bumps on my scalp, chest and back and began to wonder about Kyle's morning headaches.

The next day I had Kyle skip his morning shower. No morning headache. Then I had him shower before bed. Oh, Lordy—déjà vu! It had been many years since Kyle's once-common, middle of the night bedroom "earth-shakes"—legs wildly pounding and hours of yelling and screaming. Seeing it again, I remembered that back in those old days I gave him Epsom Salt baths before bed for pain... in fluoridated, but de-chlorinated water.

I stopped the showers entirely and heated bottled water on the stove for my 220-pound, man-size son to sponge bathe. No morning headaches. I conducted several more "shower trials", still using the carbon shower filter (that removes no fluoride), and all were followed by head pain around 5-15 minutes after showering, even before he had eaten. I tried the evening shower only once more, with the same screaming aftermath.

When we'd go camping for a week or two, I'd call ahead about the fluoridation status. Campgrounds almost never have added fluoride, but do have chlorine. Kyle does not get headaches when showering at campgrounds with no fluoridation, but with chlorination. Likewise, in non-fluoridated cities, even in the absence of a chlorine filter, he did not get headaches after showering.

After months of bottled water sponge baths, I finally found an expensive shower filter that removes enough of the fluoridation chemicals for Kyle to be able to take short, low-pressure showers. After all these years, it still infuriates me that we have to go to such lengths and expense to filter the fluoridated water that we pay for.

The Injustice of Fluoridation — Sensitive People Cannot Avoid Fluoride

Water fluoridation is a particular injustice to all children and adults with chemical sensitivities, a condition that affects those with autism more than the general population. Children with autism and their families are often the ones who suffer the most at the hands of an uncaring government that is more interested in protecting their outdated and unscientific beliefs when it comes to adding a toxic chemical to public water.

This may sound prickly to some, but a drug (poison) added to public water for someone else's teeth is active discrimination against people like Kyle. He can't go ANYWHERE without a fluoride-free bottle of water and fluoride-free food packed from home. This discrimination-by-fluoridation is particularly hurtful coming from the dental community (that avidly supports fluoridation) because I painfully remember the two dentists who refused to treat my son (at age 3 and age 39) for no reason other than his autism.

After the EPA denied a 2016 petition to end fluoridation, Kyle and I were asked to join a legal suit against the EPA as plaintiffs. We won, with Judge Edward M. Chen's ruling that fluoridation poses an "unreasonable risk" of developmental neurotoxicity. With the expected delays and EPA appeals, our water still must be filtered, but I am hopeful (Chen, 2024).

Kyle is not the only one affected by fluoridation. Several studies have found that autism behaviors are associated with early fluoride exposure. The Florida Medicaid study found that, when living in fluoridated areas, the database of 73,254 children continuously enrolled for their first 10 years of life had significantly greater incidence of autism spectrum disorder symptoms, attention deficit-hyperactivity disorder, intellectual disability, and specific delays in development (Geir & Geir 2025). A study of mother-child pairs in Los Angeles documented that exposure to 'optimally fluoridated' water during pregnancy is associated with more neurobehavioral problems in offspring, including emotional outbursts and symptoms of autism spectrum disorder (Malin et al., 2024).

I believe that the studies have found these behavioral outcomes because many children with autism suffer pain from fluoride as Kyle does. Kyle's behavior "on fluoride" is wildly different from "off fluoride." When exposed to fluoride, he displays many times more problem behaviors that are associated with classic autism, but those behaviors are driven by pain, not by the neurological factors of autism. This story has a happy ending. First, without fluoride or chemicals, Kyle is a calm, considerate, helpful, loving, happy man who enjoys going to church on Sunday or going on a hike in the woods. In other words, having a relatively normal life. And second, fluoridation is going to stop thanks to the countless brilliant and dedicated fluoride fighters who won't quit until it's out of our water.

Shooting the Messenger

The dental profession's attempt to silence me for publicly opposing fluoridation.

By: Dr Hardy Limeback, BSc, PhD, DDS

ABOUT: *My career is a little different in that I earned a BSc and PhD in Biochemistry before I earned a DDS, all at the University of Toronto. This is because I always wanted to be a biochemistry research scientist, and research on dental tissues just happened to be the topic of my PhD. I was inspired to help my future dental patients and saw the realworld implications of scientific research and its application in dental practice.*

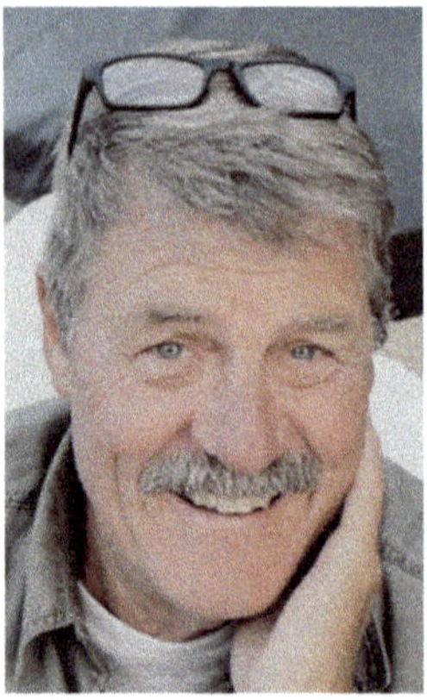

However, an odd thing always struck me. Even though I was a "Doctor" while studying dentistry, I was routinely addressed as "Mister" or by my first name until I earned my DDS. That is indicative of the phenomenon of giving more credence to even small-town dentists than to scientists with deep subject matter knowledge and impeccable credentials. That is a big mistake and the biggest obstacle in trying to make a paradigm shift in dentistry—a critical number of practicing dentists need to become more educated in science and demonstrate enough personal and professional fortitude in order to change ingrained belief systems that are not based on evidence.

More of my background is in the 'Introduction' of this book.

CHAPTER 18

"There is no doubt in my mind that fluoridation
has next to no benefit in terms of reduced dental
decay and the risks for harm to several organ systems,
including the brain, are so significant as to make fluoridation
a practice that can now be considered ineffective and unsafe."

—Dr Hardy Limeback, BSc, PhD, DDS

AFTER AN HONOURS BSc in Biochemistry, I yearned for even higher education in this most comprehensive field. I was accepted by Dr Jaro Sodek in the University of Toronto Biochemistry Department who was cross-appointed with the dental school. He was one of five PhD supervisors in a special Medical Research Council Group led by Dr Tony Melcher, a well-known periodontist and dental researcher.

Other researchers in our group included dentists studying for their specialties such as periodontics, oral surgery, and orthodontics. I remember distinctly working beside an oral surgeon whose research project of two months had failed completely. He was furious. He turned to me in the same lab and said, "Do you realize how much money I could've made in two months as an oral surgeon?" He continued, "Hardy, how can you stand to do this kind of work and why did they want to make us do research for master's degrees?" I told him, "I just love research. You discover things that no one has ever discovered before. You're the first one in the world to report a new finding. You are permanently entered in the scientific literature. You make history. How can you not like that?"

They all asked me in the group what I was planning to do after my PhD. I said I would probably have to do a few years of postdoctoral research and leave Toronto. They all said, "Why don't you get a Doctor of Dental Surgery and stay in Toronto then start a career in dental research? Our dental school needs dental researchers." So, I applied to dentistry in my final year of the PhD. The admissions committee interviewed me and one prof asked me the standard question: "Why do you want to be a dentist?" I said I didn't really want to be one, but I wanted the DDS degree to get grants, my own lab and do dental research. With that answer I thought I would be rejected, but I got in.

Initially, I hated being a dental student with a PhD. I questioned everything. I wanted to read studies that supported why we did things the way the dental instructors taught us—and they often didn't have any answers. By the third year, when we started working on patients who thought they were getting deals while being treated by inexperienced dental students, I had learned to keep my mouth shut. After all the instructors knew best. They were skilled and knowledgeable, or so I thought.

But there were times I thought clinical instructors were wrong and sometimes that maybe they loved the power they held over dental students. As an example, we were working in the Pediatric Specialty clinic where we were learning how to do fillings on young kids. I disagreed with the instructor (a grey-haired Pediatric Dental Specialist) saying that there wasn't a cavity where he wanted me to drill and fill.

I asked, "Please show me where it is. I can't see it." He got annoyed. "It's obvious," he said. I told him that's not what we were taught in our cariology and restorative classes. Then he said, "Push harder with the explorer. It'll get stuck. Even if it doesn't, you need practice. Drill there." I'll never forget the experience. My ten-year-old patient heard everything and got really upset.

By the time I was close to graduating, I was way behind. I failed to learn the tricks of the trade. I would overhear "I'll trade you two patients who need crowns for your patient who needs a partial denture. I just need one more partial denture and then I have all the credits they want us to get."

This kind of bargaining of patients, like they were valuable hockey trading cards, was typical of the negotiations I heard in the locker room near the end of fourth year. After nearly all the patient charts were handed in by my classmates, I was asked to finish some cases because I did not have all my credits. I finished what *my* patients needed and took on more while my classmates went home or on holidays.

I continued to work well after the summer deadline in the clinic. I started to love doing dentistry. I enjoyed treating patients, understanding their health and personal problems. Treating them as real people and not 'procedures' to be traded and bargained for in order to graduate faster. I tried to be compassionate, understanding and caring. (Still to this day, I have dental phobia myself from dentists who used to torture me as a kid). I was truly interested in helping patients in the dental school to NOT have to come back to be handed over to incoming fourth year dental students, who would invariably look into their mouths for more credits.

With that realization, I had found my calling: it was preventive dentistry.

Fast forward many years and I realized with crystal clarity, as an experienced dental professor who was trying to do my best caring for the patients that my students were treating, that the current dental school system was highly flawed. I learned how dental schools benefit from the clinical teachers and profs working there. Patients were a source of income. Empathetic patient care was at the bottom of the list of priorities. Dental schools had to provide clinical experience to their students. They also had to be profitable, and profit trumped comprehensive and compassionate patient care.

My Early Days as an Assistant Professor in University of Toronto.

Immediately after graduation, I became an assistant professor. I got a prestigious national grant for my salary and for running a new lab to do research on enamel proteins. It was an exciting time—lots of fun. At the same time, I was given one day practice privilege of the five working weekdays (weekends were not work days for the dental schools). That was traditional because dental schools wanted their profs to be clinically experienced. I was assigned to be the chief dentist for a city-run group of nursing homes, and I started working part time for a dentist Wednesday evening as well as Saturdays. I spent the rest of my time working in my lab, writing grant proposals, publishing papers, preparing lectures for two courses and, of course, rushing home each night to be with my wife and two young sons.

Even back then, as a new dentist, I wasn't getting much experience to treat patients with a lot of dental decay. I took three months off to travel to remote northern Ontario to work in one of the Indian reservations. That was quite an experience. I was really exposed to some serious dental decay.

Because I was inexperienced, I started to extract the teeth that looked the worst. But even the teeth with the most serious decay had cavities where the exposed dentin was hard to the touch of my dental explorer. It didn't take long to discover that the kids who were put to bed with a bottle when they were infants or even toddlers, who didn't get infant formula or cow's milk (that was too expensive to get to the reservation because all supplies had to be flown in) but instead either soda pop, or tea sweetened with a lot of sugar, had the most horrible decay.

That was "Baby Bottle Tooth Decay." Professional fluoride therapy was irregularly provided to the community because so few dentists visited northern Ontarian communities, but that is immaterial because no amount of fluoride can stop baby bottle syndrome.

Stopping the habit of putting the baby to bed with a baby bottle filled with sugary liquids and stopping the habit of sticking a baby bottle or a sippy cup in the mouth of a young toddler during the day are the only ways to stop the bottle-mouth decay. Once the causal factor is halted, the teeth may repair on their own and become very hard, painless and functional to use.

Basic Lab Research to Clinical Research: Dental and Bone Fluorosis

In my part-time dental practice and as an instructor teaching dental students to provide dental care to children in the dental courses I provided, I noticed far too many kids had dental fluorosis. Where was all the fluoride coming from? My first 'anti-fluoride' paper was "Fluoride accumulation in teeth and bones. Is dose adjustment now required?" published in 1993 in the *Canadian Journal of Public Health*. Fluoride came from tap water (at the time fluoridated at 1.0 mg/L), fluoridated toothpaste, supplements, foods, and pollution. I developed a simple micro-abrasion technique to remove the unsightly streaks and spots of dental fluorosis that the kids hated and were embarrassed about. I was familiar with the literature of fluoride in bone and reasoned that if fluoride can harm teeth, it would likely harm bone.

Together with a well-known bone researcher, we applied for federal funding to conduct a clinical trial that would look at whether fluoridation affected bone as well. By comparing the femoral heads donated by patients getting new hip joints in Toronto (fluoridated in 1963) with those getting the same procedures in Montreal (never fluoridated), we showed that Montrealers had far less fluoride in their bones than Torontonians. The levels were so high in Toronto bone that for some there was serious risk for bone fracture. Our engineering graduate student tested bone mechanical properties and found significant and alarming differences but, apparently, they weren't remarkable enough to convince public health that fluoridation should stop.

That's when I publicly apologized to the student body for not looking into the negative effects of fluoride and for simply accepting public health's claim that fluoridation was 'safe and effective.'

I realized the science was NOT settled as claimed. I had always told my students that science progresses when so-called settled facts are questioned and tested, and this was a first-class example of that.

Going Public about Fluoride Toxicity

While working in my dental clinic, a woman who I hadn't seen since childhood days walked into the clinic and asked me to read a binder full of papers on fluoride toxicity. She was part of an organized anti-fluoridation movement. Because of my work on bone fluoride (my first publication questioning fluoride levels in drinking water (Limeback, 1993) I agreed. I was blown away. She had proof that they were using toxic waste from the phosphate fertilizer industry to add to the drinking water instead of pharmaceutical fluoride. After looking into it myself I uncovered more evidence of harm. Our research project showed that fluoride (mostly from fluoridation) was harmful to skeletal systems of Torontonians. In 1999, I was interviewed by the *Toronto Star* (one of three national newspapers in Canada). The story blew the lid off fluoride safety—and my career.

The article mentioned the bone and dental fluoride effects (our research). A line in the article indicated an end to my interview. Then the reporter provided speculation from other sources that fluoride caused all kinds of other ill health effects. I never said those things that were included in the article but my colleagues thought I did. They blamed me for their patients asking that their kids skip fluoride treatments which were profitable for their dental practices.

I was interviewed by a reporter from the Canadian Broadcasting Corporation (our primary national TV/radio corporation). The video is still in their archives (Fluoride: How Much is Too Much? 1999). The director of the Fluoride Action Network, Dr Paul Connett, and his son Michael, traveled from New York to my dental practice in Mississauga Canada (a bedroom community of more than 750,000 people west of Toronto) to interview me. That was when I still thought fluoridation was effective and 'relatively' safe. Back then, I thought the concentration in drinking water just needed to be lowered as I had published in 1993 (Limeback. 1993). Because of pressure from many sources, it eventually **was** dropped to 0.6 ppm in Ontario from 1.0 ppm.

A Career Change

My reputation as a dentist and dental researcher willing to speak out against fluoridation spread. I was invited to talk to groups that were considering continuing, ending, or commencing fluoridation.

In 2001, I was invited to take part in a public debate about fluoridation in the British Columbia city of Kamloops. An elderly resident had been able to get the necessary ten percent of the population signatures on a petition to force a plebiscite. I was placed in the awkward position of opposing my good friend and colleague, a prominent dental public health researcher. He had warned me not to come to his province (BC) in an email. "Don't come to Kamloops, Hardy, this is my backyard." Well, I did, and I informed the public about the risks of fluoridation, even in a TV interview.

Kamloops voted to end fluoridation. Sometime later, while I was trying to get my dental office in a new location underway, I got the dreaded letter from the Royal College of Dental Surgeons of Ontario (RCDSO) saying a complaint had been lodged against me by a public health dentist in BC, not only to the RCDSO but to the president of the University. My dean got a copy of the complaint, cornered me in my office and told me if I lose my dental license, he'd "nail me to the wall" and I'd lose tenure (my tenure was based, in part, on me being a qualified dentist). It took me one year to defend myself but my name was never cleared. The RCDSO simply said they didn't have enough evidence to take my license away.

Because of my public opposition to fluoridation, my new dental office was getting calls from dentists all over complaining to my receptionist how awful I was to oppose fluoridation. The receptionist was my wife Lynne, and she was in tears for quite some time actually fearing for our livelihood and even our lives (there had been documented 'coincidences' of bad things happening to prominent people opposed to fluoridation).

Was the gas line leak in my brand-new VW Jetta just a coincidence?? I thought, nah, no one would try that.

But this fired me up.

They wanted to silence me, but instead, it only made me more determined to educate health professionals (doctors and dentists) about the harm that fluoride ingestion can cause.

I had organized an international symposium on fluoride (Limeback, 1999) and published quite a bit on the topic by that time. (Limeback, 1999; Brothwell & Limeback, 1999; Limeback, 2001; Brothwell & Limeback 2003)

My first big talk was to the Irish Ministry of Health Committee on Fluoride (along with Paul Connett). Despite learning about fluoride's harmful effects, they did not stop mandatory fluoridation—but eventually they *did* lower the level to 0.7 ppm.

I went to San Antonio, Texas to give a CME (Continuing Medical Education) course to residents and MDs in the Christus Santa Rosa Medical Center. I remember an orthopedic surgeon, concerned about negative bone effects on his fluoridated patients, was threatened with losing his hospital position if he continued to publicly oppose fluoridation.

The 2006 NRC Report on Fluoride — a Landmark Review

In 2003, I was invited to join the National Research Council of the US National Academy of Science (NRC/NAS) committee to study fluoride in drinking water. They needed a 'balanced committee' and I was known as a researcher who studied harmful effects of fluoride. It took us three years to review the fluoride literature and come up with a report. Our committee was given a very specific charge to NOT look at the benefits of fluoridation, but only consider fluoride harm and whether the EPA maximum contaminant level goal (MCLG) had adverse health effects.

Our report to the EPA was published in 2006. We advised the EPA that its MCLG of 4 ppm was definitively unsafe and should be lowered. Fluoride at a water concentration of 4 ppm, which was also the EPA's actionable concentration, would cause moderate and severe dental fluorosis in consumers which included loss of dental function as well as mild skeletal fluorosis.

Furthermore, we advised the EPA that there was no evidence of safety at any concentration for susceptible subpopulations who could be expected to suffer ill effects at concentrations below 2 ppm which the scientific evidence we examined suggested would include damage to bone, thyroid, liver, guts, kidneys, and the immune system. We even recommended the EPA determine a safe reference dose. The EPA failed to act on any of our recommendations or findings.

That 2006 NRC Report is still considered a landmark book in fluoride science today, but it is woefully out of date. So much new research has come out since then—research which has validated not only our recommendations, but our concerns about the harm to vulnerable consumers.

Spreading the Word

I continued to give talks to nurses, MDs, and dentists, but most of the time I addressed the public. I found I was singing mostly to the choir at public presentations, to people who opposed fluoridation and wanted validation from a university professor. I traveled a lot, luckily with the blessing of my family (my wife Lynne was reassured I would not lose my university job).

I have been to Cork Ireland, Wellington Florida, Wooster Ohio, Toronto Canada, Regis New York, Hannover and Keene New Hampshire, Cortland New York, San Antonio again, Dunedin New Zealand, Escondido California, Fort Saskatchewan Alberta, Hood River Oregon, Juneau Alaska, Madison Wisconsin, Salem Oregon and Salt Lake City Utah. They were all great experiences where I met really nice people—hard-working, dedicated local activists opposed to fluoridation. It was gratifying, but ultimately, it wasn't enough to eliminate fluoridation, but it was enough to damage my professional career.

Trouble at the Dental School

It took far too long to be promoted to full professor. I was *persona non grata* in my own faculty. The same dean who was bent on kicking me out of the dental school took my lab away and gave me more teaching duties.

The grants that I helped secure to study fluoride in bone were taken over by my co-principal investigator as well as our shared PhD student who was no longer 'shared.' She defended her PhD thesis without me. It took 10 years to publish her paper (Chachra, 2010) about her PhD work and I was not invited to help revise the publication. The paper downplayed her results—that fluoride exposure alters the biomechanics of bone.

All that did not deter me. I attended University of Toronto seminars on how to retire early on a full pension from the university and bided my time by writing my last 'hurrah'. It was a textbook on comprehensive preventive dentistry with the most up-to-date fluoride mechanisms, benefits, and side effects (Limeback, 2012)

When it was published, I took early retirement in 2012. Some of my colleagues are still working at the faculty at full professor salaries even as I write this chapter—13 years later. This financial setback was something I was willing to accept to keep my sanity and independence.

It Ain't Over 'Til It's Over

During the years of my early retirement, I prepared my small part-time practice to be sold. After it was gone, I worked a little as a part-time associate dentist in my own dentist's office but then gave clinical dentistry up altogether in 2019. From 2012 to 2023, I continued to teach dentists and hygienists in preventive dentistry continuing education classes and at dental conventions. I was welcomed at the Pacific Dental Conference in non-fluoridated British Columbia, but not at the Ontario Dental Association meetings in fluoridated Toronto.

I have spent the last five years focusing on hydroxyapatite toothpaste with a little group of like-minded researchers who feel hydroxyapatite is a clinically proven alternative to fluoride. I am proud to say that Kinder Karex is the first fluoride free hydroxyapatite toothpaste to get 'validated' by the Canadian Dental Association.

While the ADA currently only recognizes oral care products that have fluoride, I believe we will soon see toothpaste companies remove fluoride from their toothpastes targeting toddlers. They will likely not do it on their own; they are being pushed to do so by the Attorney General in Texas and in a class action lawsuit launched against them by Attorney Michael Connett who successfully sued the US EPA to better regulate fluoride in drinking water.

Conclusion

It takes time for change. Authorities don't like to admit they were wrong, but they must so that we can finally take the necessary actions to protect our children, our parents, and ourselves from fluoride harm.

Everything I Learned in Life, I Learned from Fighting Water Fluoridation

By: Carol Kopf, BS, MA

ABOUT: *Carol Kopf spearheaded the effort which reversed 29 years of fluoridation in Levittown, NY in 1983 when a young mother. Inspired by her deep dive into both the science and politics of fluoridation, she earned a BS in Biology and an MA from NYU's Science and Environmental Reporting Program. She is currently a media liaison for the New York State Coalition Opposed to Fluoridation. Her blog is:" fluoriodedangers.blogspot.com". Carol prides herself on her continuing activities as a keyboard activist and a social media influencer. Her goal is to provide education to anyone who cares to listen about the evidence that fluoridation is neither safe or effective. She does it for her grandchildren.*

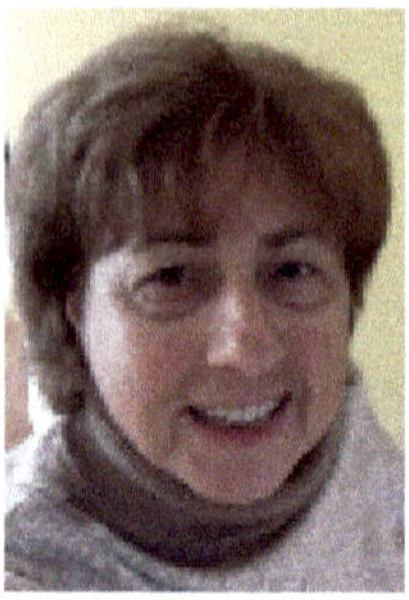

CHAPTER 19

"While four out of five dentists may be enough to pick a gum, all should agree before we force-medicate the public."

—Judge Peter Vallone, Jr. (2012)

"YOU'RE A BABY KILLER," a dentist called out to me as two cops whisked him into the annual Greater New York Dental Meeting in Manhattan. I was picketing with a group against fluoridation; he was attending the meeting. WINS 1010 Radio carried the story all day. We were elated because it was near impossible, at that time, to get media attention about anything damaging to fluoridation. But it hardly caused a ripple to the pro-fluoridation mafia and the journalists who trusted them.

The seed to focus on educating the media was planted in the 1980s when a New York City council member organized a fluoridation meeting with experts testifying against fluoridation. If we didn't get the press, he said, he would back off. We couldn't and he did. In 2012, New York City Council Member Peter Vallone tried again. He sponsored a bi-partisan bill to ban fluoridation in New York City and held a rally on City Hall steps (Queen's Gazette, 2012). This also went nowhere. As was and is the norm in the media, he was vilified for it. Now he is a judge.

Name-calling was and is a favorite tool of fluoridationists and, unfortunately, is very effective in swaying public opinion. Besides "baby-killers," we were called lunatic fringe, fluorophobes, poison mongers, John Birchers, health-food fanatics, anti-science, conspiracy theorists, quacks, little old ladies in tennis shoes, and/or pseudo-scientific (none of it true).

We were and are mostly mocked by journalists who reveal their own biases by including an excerpt from the satirical movie "Dr Strangelove." The word conspiracy isn't far behind. Rarely, if ever, is science discussed, investigated, or validated. And never are studies promoting fluoridation dissected, examined, or denigrated. Are they all perfect?

Because he accidentally included me in an email to Potsdam, NY, legislators and the media in 2017 (Kopf, 2017), fluoridation lobbyist, dentist Johnny Johnson, American Fluoridation Society President, who often sports an "F yeah to fluoridation" t-shirt, falsely accused me of attempting "to use smoke and mirrors to influence local Community

Water Fluoridation (CWF) decision-makers into thinking that CWF is some evil sinister conspiracy to dumb down the masses." He falsely implied that I embraced CWF as a communist plot, the notion it was a Nazi concentration camp tool used against the Jews, a John Birch Society crusade, or a modern-day conspiracy theory against everyone in the world that's done CWF research. He more recently showed his true nasty, vulgar personality in an email, obtained from a freedom of information request, where he tried to strong-arm a small North Dakota town to retain fluoridation (Baletti, 2025a), Before him, dentist Michael W. Easley bragged: "To the antifluoridation folks, I'm public enemy number one" (Baker 1999). He wasn't. His tactics were science deficient and he mischaracterized fluoridation opponents, including me.

How I Got Into This Nasty Battle

After my kids started grade-school, I entered college. Journalism 101 semester's assignment was to report on a controversial issue. About a year earlier, a Nassau County PTA member, Joy Grand, wrote a 3-part series in our Local weekly, *Levittown Tribune,* which concerned me. But, when 2 dentists rebutted her with the magical but unscientific phrase, "safe and effective," it allowed me to remain blissfully ignorant. With all those letters after their names, how could they be wrong? So, I ignored the warnings. But it was a perfect choice for my class assignment.

At first, I wanted to hand in a pro and con article. My professor said I had to pick a side and I had a moral obligation to tell the truth. So, I dug even deeper.

I wrote, called, and/or visited government agencies, health and water departments, legislators, researchers, scientists, the media, and libraries and fact-checked each side as best I could; I read books and articles both for and against fluoridation. When I learned the NYS Dept of Health lied to me, I was shocked. Dr. Taimi Carnahan of the NYS Department of Health told me a 1978 fluoridation lawsuit in Pennsylvania was thrown out of court for lack of evidence. I wrote to Judge John P. Flaherty, chief justice of the PA Supreme Court. He wrote back and said that I was told a "mistruth." The case stands on its merits, but the judiciary branch of government doesn't have the power to stop fluoridation—only legislators do. From Judge Flaherty:

> *"Nothing I have seen changes my view of the serious hazards occasioned by public fluoridation. To the contrary, what I have read convinces me all the more that in depth, serious, scientific effort should be undertaken before further expanding a questionable practice. Those who belittle critics of fluoridation do the public a mis-*

service, yet it seems in the face of strong, uncontradicted prima facie evidence, that is the tactic most often employed." (Flaherty, 1988)

"My decision regarding the fluoridation of the public water supply, made during my tenure as a trial judge almost twenty years ago, was on appeal, purely a jurisdictional issue... That the practice is deleterious is more and more accepted —its utility doubted." (Flaherty, 1996)

Fluoridationists had no evidence of fluoridation safety, except for the scientifically invalid and inconclusive 1945 Newburgh NY human experiment (Schlesinger, 1945). The Newburgh experiment was so bad, an entire book was dedicated to its flaws and other fluoridation human experiments (Sutton, 1960).

The most-used fluoridation chemical is never-safety-tested hydrofluorosilicic acid (HFSA), a toxin laced industrial waste product of phosphate fertilizer manufacturing (NSF, 2019). Surely, when the active environmental movement of the time learned this, they would be eager to join us. But no. The fluoridationists' PR was so good at vilifying us that most environment activists feared associating with us. They had their own problems.

Back then, I believed fluoridation reduced cavities. But I couldn't get past the lack of safety evidence for drinking HFSA, especially since it contained traces of lead, arsenic, and other toxins. Environmentalists were fighting to get industry's wastes OUT of our environment. Levittown was purposely putting it INTO the water. Fluoridationists had no information to quell my fears. They generally said "fluoride is fluoride is fluoride" without telling people, especially the water works employees, that HFSA will eat through metal, concrete and, of course, skin and bones.

So many entities and organizations gave me glossy PR paraphernalia, a list of endorsing organizations (which is much shorter these days) and *Consumers Reports* magazine articles dated 1978 (with no byline) which looked suspiciously like an article written by a fluoridationist copied from a dental publication. I informed each of the Consumers' Union Board of Directors (*Consumer Reports* publishers) about this apparent plagiarism, detailed the similarities to no avail. They also ignored Edward Groth III, PhD, Senior Scientist with the Consumers' Union who admitted fluoridation was adopted more by politicking than by science (Martin, 1991).

I also received too many copies of Stephen Barrett's crazy science-deficient name-calling article "Fluoridation: Don't Let the Poison Mongers Scare You" (1st or 2nd edition). At that time, Barrett was the media go-to guy whenever journalists wanted someone to debunk anything that wasn't accepted by the mainstream (or their advertisers, I presumed).

Those opposed to fluoridation answered, with evidence, all my many suspicious questions or easily debunked fluoridationists' criticisms AND were good people and mostly volunteers. Fluoridationists typically dismissed me, avoided me, name-called those who I was learning from, and couldn't produce any primary evidence that fluoridation was safe. One dentist said that fluoridation was punishment for not taking care of our teeth.

Fluoridation is like the fairy tale "The Emperor's New Clothes" by Hans Christian Anderson which told of a supreme ruler who walked the streets naked, yet believing he was clothed in beautiful garments. He wielded so much power that no one dared tell him the truth. That tale inspired the title of my Journalism 101 report, "Fluoridation: The Emperor Has No Clothes."

The Battle of Levittown Begins

I worked closely with the New York State Coalition Opposed to Fluoridation (NYSCOF) whose volunteers guided me to be diplomatic, respectful, non-inflammatory, and, above all to be absolutely accurate in what I say and do. We followed a code of ethics that fluoridation-promoting dentists, and the government officials they influence, fail to follow. NYSCOF incorporated in the 1970's to successfully thwart a bill to mandate fluoridation by getting its members around the state to contact their legislators to sign onto a bill to ban fluoridation. NYSCOF also created a home rule legislation which generated many letters of support which required fluoridation decisions be made by governing bodies, not just one person after Suffolk County's Health Commissioner attempted to mandate fluoridation. Besides Suffolk County, NYSCOF aided many communities across New York State to reject or stop fluoridation. Out-of-staters, also, often called for information.

We petitioned in public places and door to door. We put flyers in stores, libraries and anywhere that would allow us, got professionals to speak before local groups, asked for and received endorsements from PTA's, soccer clubs, school boards, etc. We wrote letters to the editor and took out ads in local weekly papers. Our assemblyman was a big help when he sent out a pro/con mailing to every home.

Although the weekly *Levittown Tribune* instigated fluoridation in 1954, it was very supportive in presenting our side of the issue which mostly went unreported by the major daily newspaper, *Newsday*. A *Newsday* reporter, B. D. Colen, put me on speaker phone and laughingly accused me of being with the John Birch Society because I used the phrase "Occam's Razor" which my professor spoke about. It was the first time I ever heard about the Birch Society; but not the last. It's amazing how glib journalists were and still are as they protect fluoridation based on their unscientific beliefs and fluoridationists' PR. They will soon learn, that they and government institutions have been manipulated by organized dentistry to publish misinformation.

I was inspired by the citizen environmentalists who fought and won battles against industries that left their toxic residue behind, sickening residents. Lois Gibbs, another mother from New York state, was one of them. She brought public attention to the environmental crisis in Love Canal that resulted in the evacuation of over 800 families. She was a mother fighting for her children's health. So was I.

Gibbs formed the Citizens Clearinghouse for Hazardous Waste (renamed Center for Health, Environment & Justice in 1981). I followed its activism manual. One suggestion: if interviewed, create a photographer-appealing scene. Pictures garner more attention. Newsday finally covered our fight but not the issue. My 5-year-old and I stood in front of a skull and crossbones poster, and behind a table full of glass gallon bottles of water obtained from a nearby natural non-fluoridated spring. We were instructed to frown. After the article and photo were published in 1983, the phone rang off the hook with people ready and willing to help or just give words of encouragement.

A town effort began. Karl, the artist, created the flyers. Joan's printing store made the flyers. Mary called those who signed petitions, asking for donations for advertisements, bumper stickers, and stamps.

The two Pat's, Joanne, Harriet, and others went door-to-door delivering flyers or getting petitions signed. Three Carols ran the Levittown Safe Water Association. Joy, Evelyn, NYSCOF President, attorney Paul Beeber, and Dr. Carlton spoke before many Levittown groups. We wore "Stop Fluoridation" sweatshirts to the 50's dance with Barbara and Annette. Our kids made posters together.

Shut the Tap

Then Presiding Supervisor Tom Gulotta gave us the opportunity to end fluoridation by opening the door after we showed him a fistful of signed petitions; but, educating residents was our burden.

First, he set up a citizens advisory committee (seven against fluoridation; seven for - including six dentists). No opinions changed. The only science the dentists provided was a Tasmanian report which I doubt they ever read. They didn't bother to read or refute our information.

With enormous help from NYSCOF volunteers, especially, its founder, Eleanor Krinsky, and attorney Paul S. Beeber, NYSCOF President and Levittown community members, we reversed 29 years of fluoridation in 1983 by a 2-1 vote of water customers.

Martha Bevis, Carol Patton, Betty Fowler, Pat Jacobs, Darlene Sherrell, Maureen Jones, Lynne Campbell, Elaine Chesley, Ellie

Rudolph, Dr. Deb Moore, were unsung heroes fighting fluoridation in other states who lent us support too.

Gulotta asked me to stand beside him as he proudly flipped off the switch to the hydrofluorosilicic acid tank dripping toxic industrial residue into Levittown's drinking water.

Then, the major media took notice. Interviews followed on National NBC news and some local outlets. *NY Times* reported it. But the *NY Daily News* editorialized that Levittowners' teeth would rot because of me. They failed to report that New York City, totally fluoridated since 1965, has a higher decay rate than neighboring non-fluoridated Nassau County which includes Levittown.

In 1996, Gulotta played a major role in stopping fluoridation in the towns bordering New York City which received NYC's fluoridated water. Also testifying, along with NYSCOF and residents, was Phyllis Mullenix, PhD, author of one of the first rodent studies to show fluoride's neurotoxicity (and was condemned for publishing it).

Also, in the 1980s, I authored a PTA resolution from my local PTA in Island Trees to stop fluoride mouthrinses in schools, which was formalized into a position of the NY State PTA (Dempsey, 1983). At least 2 schools stopped their mouthrinse program as a result. Now there are none.

As more adverse fluoride studies were published, a reporter told me our leaders were not credible. Then came a very credible, accomplished, and popular environmental activist, chemist Paul Connett PhD, who became Executive Director of the newly formed science-based Fluoride Action Network (FAN) in 2000. But he was vilified, too—even after he authored a scientifically based book proving fluoridation wasn't safe or effective.

I naïvely thought reporters just didn't understand science. So, I became one. I majored in Biology with a minor in journalism. I earned a master's degree from NYU's Science and Environmental Reporting Program in 1999, which is now called the Science, Health, and Environmental Reporting Program.

Money Players and Propaganda

Then reality hit me. Among the first items I received at NYU was Stephen Barrett's article "Don't Let the Poison Mongers Scare You" from his 1993 book *Health Robbers*. The fluoridation chapter was adapted from a 1980 American Dental Association (ADA) article that refers to "fluoride deficiency" as a common form of malnourishment in America. The ADA is the single strongest force behind fluoridation. The ADA influences government bureaucrats and legislators and apparently universities. Why? It's all about the money (Kopf, 2014). A *NY Post* editor who spoke to our class said that anyone who pitches an article against fluoridation not only would not get it published, but she wouldn't accept anything that person (me) pitched to her on any subject. Even the controversial *New York Village Voice*, suggested by the program's director, would not publish a fluoridation article by me because I was opposed to water fluoridation.

However, a new NYU Science Health and Environmental Reporting Program (SHERP) director, whom I never met or spoke to, Pulitzer Prize winner Dan Fagin, wrote a very good article in *Scientific American* magazine, published in 2008 called "Second Thoughts About Fluoridation," quoting the chairman, John Doull PhD, chair of the NRC 2006 report as saying: "The thyroid changes worry me." (Fagin, 2008)

After Levittown's success, I felt powerless since legislators ignored non-constituents. But, in 1995, the world opened to me when I connected to the internet. Since mainstream media wouldn't have me, I could bypass jaded editors and compromised journalists to pass on scientific evidence directly to consumers. I became a keyboard activist.

My first comment received a, soon-to-be-routine, onslaught of negative replies, which was good, because it gave me the opportunity to educate them as well as any lurkers with links to the evidence. I was involved in discussion groups, social media, commented on media articles, and started free websites and blogs. Sometimes I was censored from the right **and** the left, e.g. DailyKos, Reddit, Facebook, even though I never was abusive. Just being an "anti" was enough for some outlets to censor me.

Then the fluoridationists set up a Rapid Response Team that included NY State DoH employees. They would not only suggest comments be made, but they would report unfavorable comments in order to make them disappear. This Rapid Response Team became the American Fluoridation Society. Its self-imposed President, dentist Johnny Johnson, is the one I previously mentioned as sending inappropriate and inflammatory emails to decision-makers.

Before the internet, it was letters. When I went to TV show tapings, I asked hosts like Phil Donahue to do a fluoridation show. He patronizingly shook my hand, looked away and said "we should." Loved the guy; but was crushed at his indifference

Similarly, Gabe Pressman, a prominent NY city reporter for WNBC-TV, gave me a hand-shake and a cold shoulder. I got the same reception from News 4 TV national medical reporter (when I interned at 30 Rockefeller Avenue) and from *Sixty Minutes* producers who came to my undergrad school.

Despite the unearned media condemnation, Robert F. Kennedy, Jr. awakened a sleeping giant of opposition when, in November 2024 during the Trump second term election, he weighed in against fluoridation. As of July 4, 2025, over 70 communities and 2 states stopped fluoridation. Using CDC data, the Associated Press (Stobbe &

Pananjady, 2025) reports that 734 municipalities or counties stopped fluoridation in the last six years, based on only 36 states. Some communities quietly stopped without informing the CDC, which suggests that any studies using CDC fluoridation data should be suspect.

I was kicked out of the Nassau/Suffolk Oral Health Coalition. They changed the rules to require joiners to agree with their objectives—which was to get fluoridation legislation passed. So, I walked out the door and wrote a News Release about their intentions. I think they have since disbanded. But there is a NY State Oral Health Coalition.

I also was invited to leave a fluoridation strategy meeting held by fluoridation's PR guy, Matt Jacob, in nearby SUNY Farmingdale. It was free and near my home. I was quiet and respectful. Their efforts to fluoridate would affect me. They knew who I was when I signed up and asked NYS Department of Health Dental Director J.V. Kumar if they should kick me out. They did. But I did receive copies of Matt Jacob's slides which recommended avoiding talking about fluoride's risks because they have no good retort for that. A subsequent FOIA request revealed that the organizer said I must have been stupid to use my real name (Kopf, 2015). But I, unlike them, had nothing to hide.

Since our side was rarely included in news reports, in 1995, we organized a protest against fluoridation at the Grand Rapids 50th birthday celebration and got a mention (Kopf, 1995). Few people knew opposition existed because the media and public health officials failed them.

In 2005, along with FAN, we protested fluoridation's 60th birthday four-day-long celebration in Chicago. Our news release began:

> *"While Chicago children suffer with dental pain, limousines delivered dignitaries to a large white tent, ringed with yellow-shirted security guards, where dentists and others, on government payrolls, kicked off a four-day 60th birthday party for water fluoridation replete with ice sculptures, free duffle bags, food and specially made fluoridated bottled water, on July 13, 2005, in Chicago's Millennium Park, hosted by the American Dental Association (ADA) and the U.S. Centers for Disease Control (CDC)."* (Beeber, 2005)

Attendees came, from many states and seven foreign countries, for continuing education credits, to learn political fluoridation strategy and/or for a free trip to Chicago. But first they had to pass through us. We handed out a timely Washington Post article entitled, "Professor at Harvard is being investigated: fluoride-cancer link may have been hidden," by esteemed science journalist, the late Sharon Begley

(2005), described as "science writing royalty," who happened to be married to Consumer Union's Ted Groth, PhD.

There was no 80th birthday party for fluoridation this year. Was it something we said?

END IT

The Perversion of Science and Journalism

My Involvement with fluoride

By: Dr Paul Connett, MA, PhD

ABOUT: *I was a full-time teaching professor at St Lawrence University and most of my spare time was dedicated to fighting trash incineration, which by 1996 had already taken me to 49 states in the USA and four Canadian provinces when my wife Ellen persuaded me to read some fluoridation literature. I had unthinkingly accepted the conventional "wisdom" that fluoridation must be "perfectly safe" and fluoridation opponents were a little crazy. Like many other scientists and journalists, I had drunk the Kool-Aid of the pro-fluoridation propaganda machine.*

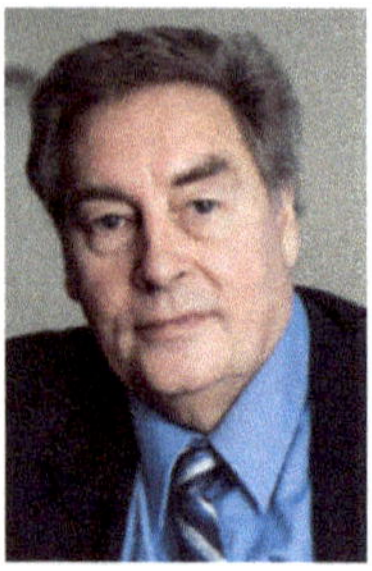

Alarmed at the scientific evidence against fluoridation, I helped form the not-for-profit Fluoride Action Network (FAN), and was its Executive Director for many years. FAN is dedicated to objectively sharing the truth about fluoride's toxicity and documenting its health effects. In 2003 I was the only scientist opposed to fluoridation to give in-person (Connett PH and Connett MP, 2003) testimony to a National Research Council panel which produced a landmark review in 2006 (Doull et al., 2006). In 2010, with two other retired professors, James Beck, MD, PhD from Calgary and Spedding Micklem, D.Phil (Oxon), we wrote the book "The Case Against Fluoride: How Hazardous Waste Ended Up in Our Drinking Water and the Bad Science and Powerful Politics That Keep It There."

CHAPTER 20

"There are people who will protect fluoride no matter what the cost, no matter what the evidence says. They will disregard the evidence and continue to say that it is unequivocally safe and effective. We've seen this over and over by people who have strong interests in promoting fluoridation."

—Christine Till, PhD (2020)

I HAVE BEEN FASCINATED by the science involved in the water fluoridation debate and disturbed by the politics involved in promoting the practice since 1996. But I have been appalled at the misuse of governmental power and dishonesty in so many professional spheres that has kept this practice going for nearly eight decades when, from an ethical point of view, it should never have started!

Dr Christine Till's assessment of the way many proponents of fluoridation ignore the science is rapidly gathering acceptance among the professional community. Dr Till is one of the key authors of two US government-funded studies which have found a strong association between fetal and infant exposure to fluoride and lowered IQ studies (Green et al., 2019; Till et al., 2020). The American Dental Association, American Academy of Pediatrics, and the Oral Health Division of the CDC who dismiss, deny, and misrepresent those studies are among the fluoridation proponents.

The Science

Fluoride serves no beneficial function in the soft tissues. As a result, fluoride—despite its natural abundance—is not an essential nutrient. Far from it, it poses a toxic threat to many fundamental biochemical processes. There is no need to swallow it and it is unwise to do so. If it works at all in fighting tooth decay, it does so predominantly on the outside of the tooth after it has erupted (CDC, 1999). Modern studies and reviews confirm it does very little good when you swallow it.

When I got involved in 1996, it coincided with the publishing of the first two Chinese studies on fluoride and IQ published in English and one year after the landmark animal behavior study on rats the previous year (Mullenix et al., 1995). I—and FAN—have followed the issue of fluoride's neurotoxicity closely ever since.

But there were many other things which Ellen shared with me that I found revealing and disturbing:

- The earliest opponents of fluoridation were biochemists, including two Nobel Laureates, who knew that fluoride inhibited many enzymes (the substances that catalyze nearly every chemical reaction in the body);

- Fluoride interfered with hydrogen bonds which are fundamental in determining the shape and function of key biochemical molecules like proteins and nucleic acids;

- The natural level of fluoride in mother's milk (baby's first meal) is very low—at least 100 times lower than the level added to water. In other words, mother's milk protects the baby from fluoride, but water fluoridation removes that protection;

- Fluoride at the same concentrations that supposedly lowered tooth decay actually damaged the growing teeth causing a condition called dental fluorosis.

A key question for me became: if fluoride interfered with the normal development of the tooth enamel by some biochemical mechanism, would it not also interfere with the development of other issues by interfering with similar biochemical mechanisms?

I was surprised by how little attention was paid to this key question (it was what I called in our book "the fluoridation gamble"). Instead, the early dental researchers only seemed concerned with being able to reduce tooth decay using fluoride without causing too much dental fluorosis. It was as if teeth were the only tissue in the body that counted. Indeed, soon after the fluoride trials appeared to show that fluoride lowered tooth decay, in 1950 the US Public Health Service (PHS) endorsed fluoridation before any of the trials had been completed and before any serious impacts on health (either short-term or long-term) had been considered.

Soon after those early trial results were published, key researchers swiftly moved from an investigative mode to outright promotion of the practice, using many of the same propaganda techniques still used today, including how many bathtubs of water you needed to drink before it killed you! And more seriously, using the absence of study to conclude absence of harm!

Ever since establishing its website in 2000, FAN has studiously and comprehensively reported all the studies it could find, detailing the animal and human studies that have found harm to any tissue in the mammalian body (the FAN Health database, which can be found at FluorideAlert.org). Beyond the brain, we know that the teeth, bone, connective tissues, thyroid, kidneys, and essentially every system in the body is damaged by fluoride. This is not surprising because fluoride attacks biochemical systems at a fundamental level!

A huge boost to our efforts came in 2006 from a review by the National Research Council (NRC) on the toxicology of fluoride, which took three years to produce. We in turn used this landmark review to communicate these health risks to the public in 2010 in our book, *The Case Against Fluoride*.

Instead of recognizing these risks, the governments practicing fluoridation continued to produce what I have called "dummy reviews" of the literature, using hand-picked pro-fluoridation "experts". These include the Fluoridation Forum in Ireland (2002, 2005), Health Canada (2008, 2009, 2024) the National Health and Medical Research Council (NHMRC) in Australia (2007, 2017), and the Ministry of Health in NZ (2014). None of these could find anything wrong with this practice! We discussed the earlier examples of these in chapter 24 of our book. Because of these activities, fluoride has been called the "protected pollutant."

In parallel with these government efforts, various dental lobby groups have conducted a campaign of ridicule and abuse of fluoridation opponents in a fairly successful effort to keep mainstream scientists, doctors, and dentists away from the scientific literature which indicates that fluoridation is neither safe nor effective.

To my dismay, the mainstream press, instead of championing the truth on these matters, decided to treat fluoridation as a major plank in public health policy and even joined in the ridicule of opponents—as many chapters in this book sadly attest.

Politics of Fluoridation

Fluoride has been called the protected pollutant, and fluoridation policy is apparently privileged and profitable. Moreover, the perversion of science by the pro-fluoridation lobby involves very powerful organizations. In the USA, these include the *Oral Health Division of the Centers for Disease Control and Prevention* (CDC) and the *National Institute of Dental and Cranial Research* (NIDCR).

Also misusing their power and influence are professional bodies like the *American Dental Association* (ADA) which have stooped to outright propaganda in their promotion. The ADA simply works backwards from the desired result to a conclusion that it is perfectly safe. If a study is published that finds harm, it simply must be bad science. Readers can see many examples in the ADA's frequently re-issued booklet, "Fluoridation Facts." A glimpse of its long-standing unprofessional attitude to scientific research can be seen in the advice it gave to dentists in a 1979 white paper, where they wrote:

> *"Individual dentists must be convinced that they need not be familiar with scientific reports and field investigations on fluoridation to be effective participants and that non-participation is overt neglect of professional responsibility."*

Unfortunately, the ADA's propaganda extends to the US Congress where it has a huge lobbying presence and the US population where it is perceived as an objective source of information. Unfortunately, for the ill-informed, the combination of the ADA and CDC represent as a "safe" and "reliable" authority on this controversial issue.

Other chapters in this book will give first-hand accounts on how powerful and brutal the "pro-fluoride lobby" can be. Dental researchers, dentists, and even doctors and scientists, have been intimidated, threatened, bullied and even fired for speaking out. The phrase that I coined to describe this behavior is "Not all the thugs wear black hats, some wear white coats."

A Soul-Crushing Fight

I don't mind a good fight or a healthy debate, but **grappling with dishonesty combined with the arrogance of power has been debilitating.** For some of the key players, all that matters is winning, never mind what harm it causes to our children. For example, proponents often claim that they are doing this on behalf of poor children. While it is true that tooth decay is more prevalent in children from low-income areas, the last thing they need is to have their brain development impaired. That will make it even more difficult for them to escape the poverty trap. To continue to use this emotionally-appealing argument in 2025 is dishonest.

What these children need is targeted education, a good diet, and access to affordable dental care. The Childsmile program in Scotland has provided a cost-effective example of how this can be done. This program involves supervised toothbrushing in schools as well as working with parents to provide better nutrition. It has not only reduced tooth decay but has improved overall health. By reducing consumption of fizzy drinks and other sugar-laden products, it also fights obesity and diabetes.

Two Important Scientific Findings

Before I talk about the perversion of science and the media, there are two important findings which I believe are very revealing.

The first occurred in the 1990s, when Chinese research on aborted fetuses in areas endemic for dental and skeletal fluorosis, found that fluoride could interfere with both brain and bone development. It took me many years before I grasped the significance of this. In fact, it was not until the publication of the first mother-offspring IQ study that the penny finally dropped (Bashash et al., 2017): fluoride could cross the placenta! From the first day of pregnancy, a baby's developing tissues are exposed to any fluoride that the mother ingests. Neither the fetus nor the fetal brain is protected from fluoride.

The second occurred in 2012, when Ron Breaker at Yale announced the discovery of proteins that pump fluoride out of bacteria and fungi. These were christened FEX or Fluoride exporting proteins. Others have reported similar systems since. This indicates that very early on, nature—or evolutionary forces— knew that basic biochemical functions needed to be protected from exposure to fluoride. In essence, key biochemical functions are incompatible with fluoride exposure. In retrospect, this makes the introduction of fluoride into drinking water even more reckless than I had thought. Nature knew about fluoride's toxicity long before we did.

I would like to conclude my story by providing two recent examples of the perversion of science and the media by fluoridation promoters.

Dummy Review from New Zealand

In 2014, the New Zealand government recruited prominent scientific figures to write a "dummy" review of the current science of the fluoridation debate. The prominent figures chosen were Sir Peter Gluckman and Sir David Skegg. Gluckman was the Prime Minister's top scientific adviser and Skegg was the director of the Royal Society of NZ.

They were recruited to write a short scientific review of the risks and benefits of fluoridation. At the time, scientific reports of fluoride's lowering of IQ were emerging from China and several other countries which have regions with high natural levels of fluoride in the drinking water. In particular, in 2012, an important review (a meta-analysis) was published by scientists from Harvard and China (Choi et al., 2012).

Of the twenty-seven studies Choi analyzed, twenty-six showed a lowering of IQ. This was a remarkable consistency considering that the studies had been performed in different geographical areas by different research teams over a period of 20 years. The authors reasoned that it was unlikely there could have been any other environmental factor like arsenic which would explain these results, because of the variety of geographical locations.

Choi reported an average loss in IQ of 0.45 SMD (Standardized Mean Deviation) which is approximately 7 IQ points. However, Gluckman and Skegg, wrote:

"Recently there have been a number of reports from China and other areas ... that have claimed an association between high water fluoride levels and minimally reduced intelligence (measured as IQ) in children....the claimed shift of ***less than one IQ point*** *(my emphasis) suggests that this is likely to be a measurement or statistical artifact of no functional significance."* (Gluckman & Skegg, 2014)

Gluckman and Skegg had confused a drop in IQ, measured *in points* with a drop measured in terms of *a standard deviation on the population IQ curve*. Confusing a drop in IQ of seven IQ points with a drop of less than one IQ point is a huge error.

When the mistake was pointed out to them, Gluckman and Skegg could have given a corrected version which would have made it clear that instead of a drop in IQ which was of "no functional significance" (half an IQ point) it was in fact one of very large significance (7 IQ points).

But Gluckman and Skegg chose not to do that, instead they simply changed the words "less than one IQ point" to "less than one standard deviation." This is technically correct but by failing to explain the significance of their mistake and leaving the rest of the sentence intact, they deceived the public. **In other words, Gluckman and Skegg changed the premise of their sentence but did not change their conclusion.**

For those who know the issue the final result is preposterous: a drop of seven IQ points is **NOT** "likely to be a measurement or statistical artifact of no functional significance." A downward shift of seven IQ points in a population would actually more than half the number of very bright children (IQ greater than 130) and increase considerably the number of children who would require special assistance (IQ less than 70).

As far as the politics is concerned, Gluckman and Skegg's report was successfully used by the NZ government to push through mandatory fluoridation in parliament, despite clear warnings from scientists like myself. Sadly, only three Members of Parliament attended the presentation I delivered in the parliament building itself (NZ Fluoride Feud: Paul Connett's Presentation to the New Zealand Parliament, 2017).

Critics' Concerns Vindicated on Fluoride's Neurotoxicity

Meanwhile, the IQ studies kept rolling in. By 2025, over eighty studies linked fluoride exposure to a significant IQ loss in children while only twelve haven't (Connett E, 2025). These included three high quality studies from Mexico and Canada, which were funded by the National

Institute of Environmental Health Sciences (NIEHS) (Bashash, 2017; Green, 2019 and Till, 2020).

FAN's Contribution to the Issue of Fluoride's Neurotoxicity

I am proud to say that the Fluoride Action Network has made a massive contribution to securing an honest evaluation of these IQ studies. For example, FAN has been making available on our website each IQ study as it has appeared in English, and translating others that appeared in Chinese and other languages. FAN made this literature available to the US National Toxicology Program (NTP), when we asked this important body to review the literature on fluoride's neurotoxicity. Also, in 2016 FAN made this same literature available to the EPA in a petition to ban the addition of fluoride to drinking water under provisions in the Toxic Substances Control Act (TSCA).

What both of these initiatives ultimately did was to find a level-playing field on which the science of fluoride's neurotoxicity could be judged on its merits, not by the self-serving "authority" of regulatory bodies beholden to promoting fluoridation.

These initiatives culminated in the publication of a state of the science monograph on the neurotoxicity of fluoride by the NTP in 2024 and using this same report, an 80-page ruling produced by a federal judge from a 7-year-long TSCA trial that the deliberate addition of fluoride to the public drinking water posed an "unreasonable risk" to the developing brains of children.

The Big Lie: Fluoride Only Causes Harm at Very High Levels

The three words that fluoridation promoters fear most are: "Margin of Safety." The world was lucky to have both a lawyer and a judge who understood the significance of those words in the TSCA trial. In short, once a scientific study has established some harm, determining a level which does not present an "unreasonable risk" requires the application of a safety (or uncertainty) factor to protect the whole population, including the most vulnerable from harm. The factor is a multiple of ten. Most EPA safety factors are around 100. The role that "margin of safety" plays in formal Risk Assessment calculations is covered in Chapter 20 of *The Case Against Fluoride* (Connett et al., 2010).

Meanwhile, fluoridation promoters are working overtime to prevent the public from understanding what the words "margin of safety" mean and the role they play in health risk assessment.

The giveaway words to look for in any pro-fluoridation piece today is the erroneous claim that fluoride is only a threat to children's brains at levels "much higher" than used in fluoridation programs. That is not true. Applying a minimal margin of safety to the findings of harm at 1.5 mg/L from the NTP would result in a determination of presumed safety at a fluoride water concentration of no higher than 0.15 ppm. If we used the EPA 4 ppm MCL as our scientific point of departure, safety would be assumed at no higher than 0.4 ppm. If we used the benchmark concentration level of 0.3 mg/L, the threshold would be 0.03 ppm. All of these "assumed safe" thresholds are much lower than the 0.7 ppm promoted by fluoridationists. Judge Edward M. Chen clearly spelled this out in his verdict (Chen, 2024).

Not only are proponents of fluoridation conveniently ignoring the concept of margin of safety but they are also ignoring—or downplaying—the three NIEHS-funded studies that were done in communities in Canada with fluoridated water (Green et al., 2019; Till et al., 2020) or in Mexico City which uses fluoridated salt (Bashash et al., 2017). The Mexican mothers' urine levels in the mother-offspring study were equivalent to the levels in pregnant women in fluoridated Canadian cities (NTP, 2024; Taylor et al., 2025).

Perversion of Journalism

I would like to turn now to how the pro-fluoridation lobby has captured some respected media sources including the *New York Times* and the *BBC*. For some inexplicable reason these trusted news services seem hell-bent on keeping news of fluoridation's potential to harm the developing brain away from the public. This kind of censorship is tragic and thoroughly unprofessional.

Elsewhere in this book, the veteran BBC health journalist, Michele Paduano, explains when he submitted a long piece documenting the evidence of fluoride's neurotoxicity, he was told by his superiors that it would only be published if he dropped a discussion of the NTP's seven-year review and the judge's decision in the TSCA lawsuit. Dropping these two key pieces of evidence essentially gutted his story and forced him to resign in disgust at the blatant and outrageous censorship of his work being exercised by the BBC.

Professor Emeritus Vyvyan Howard and I wrote to the BBC Director General regarding their unprofessional coverage of this issue especially at such a critical moment for the practice of fluoridation in the UK. Currently, the UK government is increasing the number of communities proposed for fluoridation, after mandatory fluoridation was slipped through in a parliamentary bill in 2023. (Appendix D).

There were two giveaway paragraphs in the response we got from the complaints department at the BBC:

1. In this podcast we also reflected the majority view – from the World Health Organisation, US Centre for Disease Control, the American Dental Society and others – that adding fluoride to water is safe and reduces dental decay. But we also clearly explained that the practice is controversial because others take a different view – we explained in detail what some of their concerns are. The BBC's health reporter was also very clear that fluoride can be harmful in some situations.

2. The reporting of risk can have an impact on the public's perception of that risk, particularly with health or crime stories. We should avoid worrying our audiences unduly and contextualise our reports to be clear about the likelihood of the risk occurring. This is particularly true in reporting health stories that may cause individuals to alter their behaviour in ways that could be harmful.

Readers should note that the censored BBC reporter we cited above presented two key pieces of information to his superiors to satisfy the need to "contextualise" the validity of the neurotoxic risks involved in his report:

- The NTP (2024) state of the science review. Surely a review by a top agency in the USA (the National Toxicology Program), which had spent seven years researching the world's scientific literature on this question, should have satisfied this demand?

- A federal law judge's conclusion after carefully reviewing the scientific evidence presented in a seven-year trial by experts from both sides, along with the NTP (2024) review, ruled that fluoride poses an "unreasonable risk" to children's brain development.

However, the BBC censored both these "authorities," preferring instead to rely on the World Health Organization (which has not recently reviewed fluoride's neurotoxicity), US Centers for Disease Control (one of biggest promoters of fluoridation in the USA), and the American Dental Association (the other major promoter of fluoridation in the USA) to be the arbiters of the risks involved!

The ignorance and arrogance of the BBC on this serious matter is literally breathtaking!

Clearly, the "harm" that the BBC was trying to avoid was not to the mental development of thousands of offspring or infants, but harm to the UK government's fluoridation program.

Conclusion

For many authors of this book, opposition to fluoridation has cost them dearly in terms of their employment and career. This has not been the case for me. My opposition to fluoridation came well after I had tenure and my colleagues were not only supportive of my efforts but were actually key in ending fluoridation in my hometown.

However, where I have been hurt by this issue is witnessing a lack of scientific integrity where I expected to find it, namely in those government and professional bodies most responsible for overseeing the health of the public. Without truth there is no science and without honest science, there is no public health measure we can trust. There will be a huge price to pay when the public no longer trusts the government on health issues. In addition, I would add that for me personally, as someone who starts each day on the BBC webpage, losing trust in this body has been extremely painful. I know that fluoridation is only one issue, but integrity is indivisible; if you lose your integrity on one issue, it makes it very hard to keep it with others.

Birth and Growth of the New Zealand Fluoride Action Network

By: Mary Byrne

ABOUT: *I am an ordinary citizen with no health or science qualifications. In fact, I worked most of my working life as a computer programmer, a field which requires an ability to deal with complexity, logic, and tenacity. However, one of my children had a serious health condition that led me to find out, first hand, that while so-called "modern" medicine is fantastic at treating emergencies and performing surgery for certain things, it is not usually good at fixing chronic issues. And worse, it is often scathing and dismissive of natural modalities that can have a huge positive impact on people's health. This is what led me into the fluoridation issue where I used my aforementioned professional skills.*

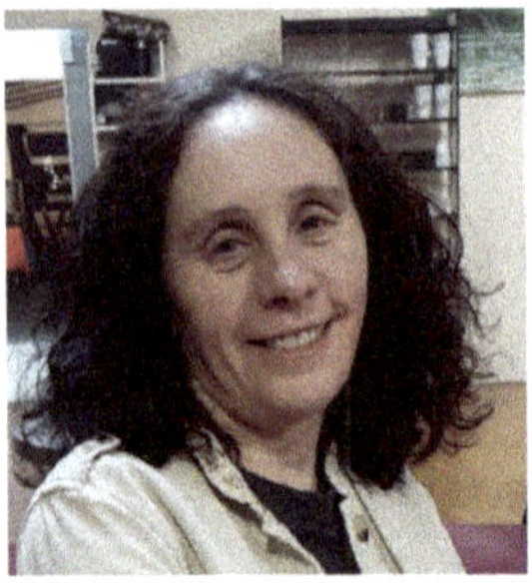

Once I realised the extent of the harms caused by fluoridation, I felt compelled to actively work on trying to stop it for the whole of New Zealand.

Despite all the setbacks, it has been a great journey where I have felt my efforts go into something I have truly believed is a very important and good cause. I have met so many brave and intelligent people with integrity, right across the social spectrum (too many to mention) and it led me to exploring other health issues that have benefited me personally. If I could go back in time and do it all again, I certainly would.

CHAPTER 21

"It is my best judgement, reached with a high degree of scientific certainty, that fluoridation is invalid in theory and ineffective in practice as a preventive of dental caries. It is dangerous to the health of consumers."

—Dr John Colquhoun, BDS, PhD (1993)

IN 1983 I WAS SITTING on a bus and saw a headline in the local evening newspaper that said, "Department of Health says Fluoridation is Safe".

About a week before, I had read an article in that newspaper questioning the safety of fluoridation. That article was probably written by Dr John Colquhoun. He had been the Principal Dental Officer of Auckland and then the head of the Fluoridation Promotion Committee from 1980 until 1983 when he publicly changed his mind. He did this following his world study tour on fluoridation commissioned by the New Zealand Department of Health where he found, much to his dismay, that fluoridation was not effective and probably not safe. The full story of this brave and principled man can be found at fluoridefree.org.nz/dr-colquhoun/.

I had thought the article, from the week before, questioning fluoridation raised very good points but after seeing the Department of Health saying it was safe, I thought "that man that wrote that article must have been mistaken. The Department of Health couldn't possibly be wrong." I also thought "That's good. You wouldn't want to be wrong about fluoridation, would you?" We all make mistakes in life, but finding out you promoted, and therefore are partially responsible for, giving a poison to the entire population would be a very hard pill to swallow and I didn't want the people in our Department of Health to have that burden.

I didn't think about fluoride again until about 1995 when I saw, for the first time, a tube of toothpaste on a supermarket shelf that said "low strength fluoride for children." Knowing that companies do not lower the levels of things unless there is a serious reason to, and that the usual trajectory is to gradually lower levels until it is gone and all forgotten, I thought "they will ban fluoride one day".

I once again gave it no more thought. I was actually living in non-fluoridated Petone from 1981, although I worked in fluoridated Wellington.

In 1999, I was browsing a book shop in my lunch hour when I came across a book by a New Zealand author, Toni Jeffreys, called "Your health at risk". This book was the catalyst for changing my life. Each chapter in the book contained a different topic such as mercury amalgam fillings, vaccines, cholesterol, margarine, mammograms, and of course fluoridation. It was the fluoridation chapter that had the most impact on me, as it really hit home that there was serious doubt about its safety. That was enough to convince me that we shouldn't continue fluoridation because putting something into the water supply is not something we can afford to take risks with unless it is absolutely necessary, such as making the water safe to drink.

As destiny would have it, about two months later our local council announced that it was going to fluoridate our beautiful, naturally clean artesian water supply. So, I visited a friend who I knew was into alternative health and would be bound to know about the risks of fluoridation. I said to her "we should do something about this" and she agreed. Her husband got involved too and we printed a flyer that said "The Council wants to add toxic fluoride to our water supply". Then we added some information into the body of the flyer and invited people to attend the Community Board meeting that was happening in a few days' time. We put the flyer in every letter box in our suburb. Consequently, about 70 people turned up to the meeting, overflowing into the hallway. This kicked off our campaign. We were ultimately successful, and that suburb is still not fluoridated. In fact, hundreds of people come every week from all around the region to fill up water containers from our public fountain.

Since I became the unofficial spokesperson for our local group, I read everything I could get my hands on. I became more and more convinced that fluoridation had to stop for the whole of New Zealand. In fact, the feeling I had when they were trying to fluoridate our suburb was "over my dead body".

I learned that there had been many people before me who had stopped fluoridation in other towns and people who had kept fluoridation out of their town. I learnt about Dr John Colquhoun and all the great fluoridation fighters from around the world.

Mark Atkin, now our Science and Legal advisor, joined me, and we started going to councils in our region—trying to get them to stop.

In 2003 Prof Paul Connett visited New Zealand for a speaking tour. He knew we needed to be organised so he gathered active people from around the country who could come to Taupo (a town in central north island) to an inaugural meeting at which we decided to form Fluoride

Action Network New Zealand. We contacted a number of long-time successful campaigners from around the country to join the committee.

Our group progressed and we became more determined and focused on getting fluoridation stopped. We built a website and sent regular newsletters, which we are still doing today. Ross Forbes from Kerikeri started an internal email for those of us in the core group. We've had an Annual General Meeting every year since 2003. In 2009 we started our Facebook page.

In 2009 to 2010, we helped locals in the Far North towns of Kaitaia and Kaikohe. Their council had agreed to a two-year trial of fluoridation (March 2007 to March 2009), promoted by the local district health board and funded by the Ministry of Health. The agreement was that after the towns had been fluoridated for two years, there would be an assessment of whether there were dental health benefits.

The agreement required that if the towns stopped fluoridation before ten years the council would have to repay the Ministry of Health the $232,700 it had been given for the infrastructure unless the council held a referendum.

Due to lobbying, fluoridation was turned off after the two years and in 2010 the mayor and councillors agreed to a mail-in consultation of the community to decide whether or not to restart fluoridation. However, the council staff decided to only send the consultation forms to people who were paying the water rates. Households with more than one person only got one vote which took us back to a time when only land owners could vote. Many people living in social housing or rented property completely missed out as often their water rates were being paid by the house owner. Residents of retirement homes did not receive a form.

The situation was completely undemocratic, but we were unable to change it. A four-week window was given for people to send in their forms. It took two full weeks for the council to release the vote count which we suspect was because they were trying to invalidate as many votes as they could. Despite all this, 56% of votes from Kaitaia were against fluoridation, and 67% of the votes from Kaikohe were against fluoridation.

There are 67 local councils in New Zealand with nearly half of them having some fluoridation. These councils tend to be the large councils such as Auckland and Wellington thereby resulting in over 60% of the population supplied fluoridated water.

Fluoridation was started in Hastings in 1954 after the Hastings Fluoridation Experiment. This experiment was originally designed to compare non-fluoridated Napier to fluoridated Hastings as the two towns are only twelve miles apart and have basically the same water supply. However, dental decay rates declined just as rapidly in Napier as they did in Hastings so Napier was dropped as the control so that the drop in decay rates in Hastings could be used as "proof" that fluoridation worked. Dr John Colquhoun and Prof Robert Mann uncovered this deception. Another reason decay rates seemed to decline so precipitously was because the criteria for diagnosis were changed so that fillings could no longer be placed for prophylaxis.

Hence, fluoridation in New Zealand had rested on fraud for the entire past 70 years.

The 1956 Royal Commission of Inquiry held that fluoridation decisions should be made by local councils following the statutory "special consultation" process with residents, and this is how it was until 2016 when the Government introduced a Bill to shift decision making to the local District Health Boards. Up until then, we used the Councils' annual plan process to raise the issue.

Through our newsletter and Facebook page, we started organizing people to give feedback to their local council's draft annual plan if they lived in a fluoridated area. Lots of people started putting in submissions and turning out in order to speak to it.

Having lots of feedback on a topic meant that the council had to take notice, especially when people turned up to speak in person and even more importantly, when our good dentists and doctors spoke with us. However, it was, and still is, very difficult for dentists to speak against fluoridation in New Zealand. Dentists, Dr Lawrie Brett, Dr John Jukes, Dr Stan Litras, and Dr Russel McLean joined us at various council meetings and public talks despite the ridicule they received from other dentists in the profession. They were also attacked by the NZ Dental Council.

We found that in just about every local council there would be some councillors who were opposed to fluoridation. These councillors were able to lobby within the council to have special consultations or referendums. We started holding film evenings where we would show the half hour documentaries *Professional Perspectives on Fluoridation* and *The Fluoride Deception*, followed by a talk and a discussion. It was difficult to get people to these events as most people didn't know that much about fluoridation plus it was hard for us to reach people. However, we were reaching enough people through the newsletter and Facebook page that these evenings allowed us to connect to the people in an area that were engaged in the issue and we then coordinated with them to host speaking tours around New Zealand.

Professor Paul Connett's speaking tours have been a crucial part of raising awareness and providing inspiration for people to actively campaign to have fluoridation stopped.

Our next big success as Fluoride Action Network NZ was when the city of New Plymouth stopped fluoridation in 2011. The New Plymouth

City Council agreed to host a Tribunal on fluoridation as was the advice of the Ministry of Health at that time. The tribunal allowed representatives from both sides to give 1.5 hours of expert testimony followed by five-minute oral presentations from people who had submitted to the process. It ended with half an hour of each side giving closing arguments. A near record 400 people had submitted to the process and of them, 50 chose to speak. Because of the numbers, the Tribunal took two days to hear all the submitters. Whangarei dentist, Dr Lawrie Brett and Hamilton GP, Dr Peter Scanlon presented expert testimony on behalf of Fluoride Action Network NZ.

We then moved on to a small town, Taumarunui, where locals had spoken at the council during their draft annual plan process. This allowed Prof Connett to speak to the council while he was on tour. The councillors put the issue out to public consultation and subsequently stopped it. The same happened that year in another small town, Waipukurau.

However, we were not so lucky with some other small towns in Taranaki. The Ministry of Health (MoH) was providing funding for the South Taranaki District Council (STDC) to upgrade its water supplies but the money was only provided if they included fluoridation of two small towns, Patea (population 1200) and Waverley (population 800). This has historically been a standard tactic of the MoH. Regardless of the hundreds of submissions the council received against fluoridation, the council voted to start fluoridation. [note: Patea still not fluoridated as of May 2025].

This financial coercion of communities against their will led to court action. A non-profit organization, New Health New Zealand (NHNZ), embarked on a Judicial Review of the decision, on a range of grounds.

The first hearing was in the New Plymouth High Court in November 2013 and a ruling was given in March 2014. The judge rejected all the arguments made by NHNZ. He even said. "While I accept that fluoridation has a therapeutic purpose, I conclude that the means by which the purpose is effected does not constitute medical treatment." This boggles the mind for most logical people. So, if a doctor gives you a pill for a therapeutic purpose that constitutes a "medical treatment" but if your council puts a substance in your water supply for a therapeutic purpose then that does not constitute a "medical treatment". The sort of logic that comes straight out of George Orwell's 1984.

NHNZ appealed the decision. While waiting for this next hearing they took another case, this time against the Ministry of Health seeking a Declaratory Judgement on whether Hydrofluorosilicic Acid (HFA) and Sodium Silico Fluoride (SSF) were medicines under the Medicines Act 1981.

In October 2014, the judge ruled that HFA and SSF satisfied all the key elements of a medicine in that they are used for a therapeutic purpose, and they achieve their intended action on the human body by a pharmacological means. Despite this, the judge ruled they were not medicines since they were added to the public drinking water at a concentration lower than 10 mg/L. The judge had made a patently obvious error as he had referred to a section in the Medicines Act that regulates Prescription, Restricted and Pharmacy only medicines. Not meeting the classification for one of these types of medicines, does not mean it is not a medicine; it just means it is a *general sale* medicine. He then went on to say, "While I am confident my conclusion is correct, the Ministry may wish to consider recommending a Regulation that exempts HFA and SSF from the definition of 'medicine' when those compounds are used to fluoridate water."

Despite 1300 submissions, the Government moved quickly to approve an exemption for fluoridation chemicals from the Medicines Act in February 2015, proving the point that they must actually be medicines otherwise there would be no need to exclude them.

You start to get the feeling that the courts are working hand in hand with the Government, when the courts are supposed to provide some safeguards against Government overreach, don't you?

The NHNZ case against STDC carried on to the Appeals court, where they lost again with the Appeals judges ruling there was no substantial difference between fluoridation and chlorination. NHNZ then carried on to the highest court in the land, the Supreme Court. This Ruling was given in June 2018 and found, by a majority (four of the five judges), that fluoridation was medical treatment and, being unavoidable once added to the public water supply, constituted compulsory medical treatment. Hence, this ruling engaged our right to refuse medical treatment. This was a landmark decision internationally as courts had previously ruled that no one was forced to drink the water supplied to their homes or businesses. Sian Ellias, the Chief Justice at the time, ruled that councils had no legislative right to fluoridate but the other four ruled they did. Sian Elias and three of the other judges ruled it engaged section 11 of the Bill of Rights (the right to informed consent to medical treatment). However, Section 5 of the Bill of Rights Act allows a "get-out-of-jail-free" card for situations that breach fundamental rights but are "enactments considered to be justified in a free and democratic society". Two of the four judges ruled fluoridation was justifiable, one ruled it depended on the area, the chief Justice ruled it was not justifiable and the last didn't rule on it as he has already ruled it was legal, Hence, fluoridation was found to breach our fundamental right to refuse medical treatment but did not become illegal as there was no majority ruling on Section 5 to say it was not justified.

Tribunals, Referendums, and Reversals

Over these years, our Fluoride Action Network NZ group was still working hard on trying to stop fluoridation by educating the public as much as possible and by lobbying the local councils.

In 2013, resident Pat McNair managed to persuade Hamilton City Council to hold a Tribunal as New Plymouth had done two years prior. This one ended up even bigger with 1500 submissions. It had the same format as the New Plymouth Tribunal but took four days to complete since so many people wanted to speak to their submission. It was person, after person, after person explaining, in 5 minutes or less, why they did not want fluoridation.

Amazingly, it was never boring and every person provided another important piece of information. Once again Dr Lawrie Brett and Dr Peter Scanlon represented Fluoride Free New Zealand along with Dr Andrew Harms from Australia. The Summing Up was given by Dr Peter Scanlon, Dr Anna Goodwin, Dr Jane Beck and Prof Robert Mann.

There were seven councillors on the Tribunal panel. The vote was seven to one to stop with the one councillor who voted for fluoridation saying that he had talked to his wife the night before and she said we put iodine in salt so therefore it must ok to put fluoride in water. Astonishing, that four days of testimony, as well as expert testimony, could be tossed out in favour of someone who did not even attend the Tribunal.

The New Plymouth and Hamilton tribunals go to show that most people will be opposed to fluoridation once they have had the time to listen to the whole argument and they are not subject to competing monetary or political interests, even if those in positions of power find irrational reasons to justify fluoridation schemes.

Hamilton is the fourth largest city in New Zealand so its decision was a big blow to the fluoridation promoters. One of the councillors, who was not part of the panel, did not attend the Tribunal (it was open to the public), and was conflicted by being a District Health Board member, was vying for the mayoralty and 2013 was election year. He decided to champion a petition to get fluoridation on the ballot box and with the help of the dentists and the local district health board, 68% of the 34% of people that voted chose to restart fluoridation.

That same year Jon Burness from Whakatane had managed to get the issue on the ballot box there and Angela Hair had managed to get it on the ballot box in Hastings. Unfortunately, neither of these referendums were successful, due to what can only be described as propaganda blitzkriegs by the Ministry of Health, with 61% and 56% of people voting in favour of fluoridation respectively.

We continued on though. Kane Titchener had joined us and was instrumental in rallying people to go to the Auckland council, even holding a protest outside the council chambers. Combined with a big talk in Auckland by Prof Paul Connett, the council started asking some serious questions. The CEO was then obliged to contact the Prime Minister's Chief Science Advisor asking for clarification. Were the anti-fluoridation people right? Did fluoridation work? Was it safe?

Prof Peter Gluckman (chief science advisor) contacted Prof David Skegg of the Royal Society of New Zealand and the two of them devised a plan to do a review of the science. Emails obtained under the Official Information Act show they had no real intention of seriously reviewing the science as it appears their dogmatic belief in fluoridation did not allow for that. Instead, they chose a quasi-scientific review that took two and a half months. They employed a writer who farmed out the various aspects of the topic to researchers they (we believe) considered to be favourable.

The New Zealand Review *Health effects of water fluoridation: A review of the scientific evidence* became the go-to, last word for anyone supporting fluoridation. It relied heavily on the soon-to-be-published study from Otago by Prof Jonathan Broadbent to claim that fluoridation did not cause lowered IQ in children. This study compared the IQ of people who had grown up in fluoridated Dunedin with the then non-fluoridated nearby suburb of Mosgiel. It used data from the world-renowned Dunedin Longitudinal Study, but it did not account for which children were taking fluoride tablets. Hence, it was subsequently considered a low-quality study when the US National Toxicology Program undertook their review of all fluoride-IQ studies.

There were many failings of the NZ Review (which was internationally critiqued), but the most egregious was a mistake they made when discussing a meta-analysis that had been published in 2012 by Harvard researchers. The NZ Review stated that the meta-analysis only found a lowering of IQ by "less than one IQ point" which they considered to be "a statistical artefact of no functional significance". However, we quickly pointed out to them that the meta-analysis had described the loss of IQ in terms of standard deviation, rather than actual IQ points. What they had actually found was a seven IQ point drop which is just less than ½ a standard deviation for IQ. [standard deviation for IQ is 15]. This was internationally known 2 years before this "scientific review" was penned.

The authors of the review duly changed two words so that the sentence read "less than one standard deviation" but they did not change the conclusion! This review still reads today that the drop was "a statistical artefact of no functional significance".

This is hugely important because it misled the whole country into believing that no significant drop in IQ had been found. Had the correct conclusion been given i.e. if the Review concluded "a drop of 7 IQ points.... Which is functionally significant" the whole conversation around fluoride and IQ would have been different.

We Were Not Deterred, Neither Were They

During these years we were gaining traction, and more people were becoming active. Our campaign in the Kapiti Coast in 2014 nearly saw fluoridation stopped there. Six of the 11 councillors were onside ready to vote to stop it. According to one councillor, she asked the CEO when the issue would come up next on the agenda as she needed to go to Australia for work. She was told it would not be until after she was back, but once she was gone the issue was put into the agenda and we lost the vote since it was a 50/50 split which meant the status quo remained.

We were also making progress with the other councils around Wellington - Hutt City Council, Wellington City Council, Wellington Regional Council and the local district health board. District Health Board members were quoted in the media saying that the anti-fluoridation campaign was winning, and the proponents needed to do something if they wanted to keep fluoridation. So, they did.

The Chief Executive Officers (CEO) of the local councils in New Zealand are suspected of actively working for the Government apparatus rather than the people. From what we can gather, at our last attempt to stop fluoridation in the Kapiti Coast (we had three goes at it in total), the CEO suggested to the mayor that the decision should be made by the central government rather than the local councils. Their reasoning was that they were not the experts, yet they were being made to make a health decision. We have always rejected that argument as we believe that there was no need to be a health expert to know that compulsorily medicating people through a public water supply was unwise and a violation of fundamental rights.

This council chose to take the issue to the other councils through a shared body (Local Government NZ) to lobby for the central government to take the decision away from them. 60% of the councils agreed.

In 2016 the National Government (National is one of the two main political parties) introduced legislation to shift decision making away from the local councils to the local district health boards. This legislation was introduced by Member of Parliament, Peter Dunne from United Future, who was in coalition with the Government. In his opening statement he said "So I say—for the benefit of the tinfoil-hat-wearing, UFO-abducted, anti-fluoride campaigners out there still peddling the same old pseudo-science myths—there is nothing left to debate on this issue. It is over; science has won."

That's what we were dealing with in 2016. All parties that were in Government at the time—Act, Labour and the Greens—voted in favour of the Bill, with only the New Zealand First Party voting against it, maintaining that the decision should be made locally.

The Bill went to a Select Committee process where the public could make submissions and speak to those submissions. 1300 people gave feedback and over 100 spoke to their submission. The vast majority (over 90%) were opposed to fluoridation.

The Bill was then due to go back to Parliament for its second reading. All bills go through three readings in Parliament before they become law. Once again, despite overwhelming opposition, the Select Committee was not going to recommend any changes to the Bill. But because it was election year, the Bill was delayed as the Government knew it was unpopular.

As fate would have it, the National Party did not get back into Government and instead a Labour, Greens and New Zealand First coalition was formed. The following year we were able to secure a time for Prof Paul Connett to speak at Parliament. However, only three MPs turned up. But one of them was NZ First MP, Clayton Mitchell. Clayton listened intently and completely understood the argument. He went back to his caucus and got agreement to make a deal with the Labour party not to progress the Bill. We don't know the details of that but presumably NZ First had to compromise on something for that to happen.

We then spent the next few years in a stalemate. The councils wouldn't do anything as they said the Government was taking over and the Government wasn't doing anything saying the councils were responsible.

Then came COVID in 2020. Our Prime Minister, Jacinda Ardern, had become very popular as happens in times of crisis. Her Labour Party was then voted back into power without the need for any coalition partners. The following year they progressed the Bill, but because they disbanded the local district health boards in favour of one centralised unit, the issue was handed to the Director-General of Health (DGH) to be the sole decision maker on whether places in New Zealand were required to be fluoridated.

In July 2021, the then Director-General of Health Ashley Bloomfield, directed 14 councils in New Zealand to start fluoridation. This has taken the total number of councils from 22 to 32 with four more still to start. The legislation allows for the DGH to enforce fines of $200,000 plus $10,000 per day for every day a council fails to comply with the directive by the stipulated date. This has resulted in every council so far bowing to the demand even though most of them did not want it and they faced serious public opposition. The Whangarei District Council went as far as court action seeking an Interim Injunction until a Judicial Review could be heard. The Interim Injunction was unsuccessful with the judge ruling "Although it (US Federal court case) concluded that water fluoridation (at the level applied in New Zealand) posed an unreasonable risk of injury to the health of the public in the United States, it did not conclude that fluoridated water was injurious to public health." Obviously, the judge is either claiming an "unreasonable risk" is acceptable, or that the people of New Zealand are fundamentally different than Americans.

The Whangarei District Council subsequently dropped its legal case as not enough of the councillors were willing to spend rate-payers money fighting an obviously corrupt system. However, New Health NZ, who achieved the 2018 Supreme Court ruling through its action against the South Taranaki District Council, has lodged a judicial review against the DGH's directives. That case is ongoing.

As part of our public education campaign, we invited US attorney Michael Connett to New Zealand for a speaking tour in early 2025. Michael had won the groundbreaking case against the US Environmental Protection Agency proving that fluoridation poses an unreasonable risk to human health. Michael's talks were packed to overflowing in many places and he received standing ovations. His talks provided the last nail we needed to get recognition of the issue at central Government level (Water Fluoridation, 2025).

Our group initiated a petition to the NZ Parliament in the last months of 2024. We collected 4131 signatures on paper and another 20,619 online. The speaking tour helped generate public awareness and support, so much so that the New Zealand First political party, which is currently a coalition partner in the NZ Government, agreed to accept our petition. We, including Michael Connett, were met at Parliament steps by the Deputy Prime Minister and four other members of parliament and invited to a meeting with four of the MPs. NZ First then submitted a Members Bill to the Ballot Box, which would repeal the Amendment to the Health Act that gave decision making to the DGH and put it back into the hands of the local councils. The Bill also requires the fluoridation be decided by binding referendum in each local council area. We don't know when this Bill will be drawn from the Ballot box.

In the meantime, the Rotorua Lakes Council has agreed to write to the Prime Minister calling for a Commission of Inquiry into fluoridation. Fluoride Free New Zealand (as we are now known) is in the process of lobbying all councils to join with Rotorua Lakes Council and call for an Inquiry.

We are heartened, and relieved, to see what is happening in the US. While the fight is not over there, we believe the issue has turned a corner and fluoridation is on its way out in the US. The New Zealand Government took 26 years after the US to stop lead being added to paint and petrol, so we are not waiting until the NZ Government finally catches up. We will be applying pressure for it to end in this country once and for all. We expect to succeed.

Storm in a Teacup

My battle to get tea recognised as a major dietary source of fluoride in Ireland

By: Declan Waugh, BSc, CEnv, MCIWEM

ABOUT: *Declan Waugh is a professional scientist from Ireland with over 30 years experience managing environmental challenges across multiple disciplines. Since 2011, Declan has devoted considerable time and resources to independently assess the environmental and health risks associated with fluoride exposure, in addition to undertaking due diligence examination of community water fluoridation. Declan undertook the first risk assessment of fluoride intake from tea in the Republic of Ireland, addressing its implications for water fluoridation. In addition, Declan published a similar study of fluoride intake from tea in New Zealand. This comprehensive study also reviews the international evidence regarding chronic fluoride intake and its association with chronic pain, arthritic disease, and musculoskeletal disorders and provides insights into possible association between fluoride intake and the high prevalence of these disorders in New Zealand. Declan has also published several other studies addressing the molecular mechanisms of fluoride toxicity, which have been widely referenced in scientific literature and has been a leading figure and significant voice in the fight against fluoridation in Ireland.*

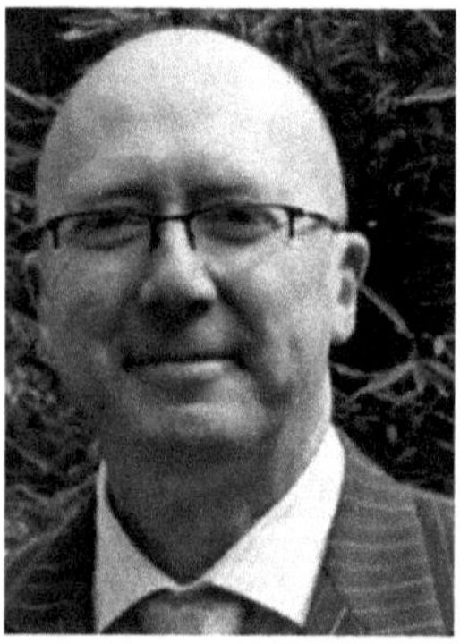

CHAPTER 22

"Dead with tea and dead without it."

—Irish Proverb

TO BEGIN, I DON'T THINK I will ever forget the Saturday morning in the summer of 2011 just a few weeks before the birth of our first child when I was approached at our local farmers market and asked if I knew anything about water fluoridation and whether I had any concerns about the possible adverse health risks with the adding fluoride to public water supplies.

Prior to this I had spent a large part of my career focusing on heavy metal pollution in the environment related to mining activities, including impacts on surface and groundwater; participating in environmental research, undertaking environmental impact assessments, conducting environmental due diligence assessments, and actively engaging in efforts both in work and the community to promote a more sustainable world. Despite my varied career, I wasn't sure how to answer the question, as up to that moment I had never had a conversation about water fluoridation or fluoride with anybody. I was aware it was a public health measure against tooth decay but, apart from that, I knew very little, if anything at all.

The last time water fluoridation had ever been mentioned in the media in Ireland had been a decade earlier when the "Report of the Forum for Fluoridation" was presented to the then Minister for Health, Mr. Micheál Martin TD, who is currently the Taoiseach or Prime Minister of Ireland. The Forum's report published in September 2002 was the first major review of water fluoridation in Ireland since it was introduced in 1964. However, prior to its publication, in my lifetime, the debate, or controversy surrounding this topic received little, if any, media coverage in Ireland.

When the report was finally published, Ireland was experiencing a period of rapid economic growth often referred to as the "Celtic Tiger" years. My generation was in the midst of a soaring housing inflation and the Irish mainstream media was, to a large degree, singularly focused on promoting the housing and commercial property market, thereby playing an important role in the property bubble and ensuing crisis. In addition, other events, like the outbreak of the foot-and-mouth disease in March 2001, focused the attention of the media and public when the State went into lockdown to save Irish agriculture over fears the disease would spread. In many respects, it was a prelude to the COVID-19 pandemic.

Many sporting and social activities came to a halt, troops were deployed to border crossings, and, by the end of the outbreak in September 2001, the world's attention was focused on the loss of human life following the September 11 attacks against targets in the United States, which would change the course of world history. Such events framed the narrative of media coverage, so it's not surprising that the release of the Forum's report did not spark widespread discussion or debate.

On a personal level during this period, I had recently started a new career, got married, and was trying to support my unwell mother, as well as cope with the distress and emotions of her diagnosis with a terminal illness. Now, let me fast forward to 2011 when Ireland was in the grasp of the worst financial crisis in its history: property prices had collapsed; banks went bust; public finances were out of control; unemployment soared along with emigration; and cuts in public expenditure, particularly in those areas providing care services, deepened social inequalities. Within this context, you may imagine how peculiar the fluoridation question seemed. Being unable to answer it effectively, I told the individual that I would look into it and get back to him.

If I recall correctly, my first port of call was reading the US National Research Council's (NRC) *Scientific Review of Fluoride in Drinking Water* published in 2006. I was astonished by many things I read in the NRC report, including the dearth of reliable scientific research examining the long-term impacts of chronic fluoride exposure on human health. I was equally alarmed to read in the NRC report that where tea drinking is common, such as in the United Kingdom, people can consume up to 9 mg of fluoride a day from tea alone! And that fluoride content in consumed tea will be higher if the beverage is made with fluoridated water.

This was the first time I was made aware that tea was a major dietary source of fluoride. To say I was astonished to learn this would be an understatement. It immediately set alarm bells ringing because the decision to introduce mandatory water fluoridation in Ireland in the 1960s was based on the premise that, at a population level, dietary fluoride intake via food and water were deficient, requiring the State to mandate the addition of fluoride to drinking water through water fluoridation. But how could this be the case given that for the last two centuries, tea has been Ireland's national drink and Ireland has had the highest per capita consumption of tea in the world, six times the global average?

Over the course of the following years, I read every major review, scientific study and publication related to fluoride and tea. I wrote numerous letters and reports to every politician, Government Official, and State Agency in Ireland responsible for maintaining the policy of water fluoridation, as well as to EU Agencies and European Commissioners responsible for Health Policy and Food Safety—expressing my concerns about potential harms to public health, the lack of any meaningful research in Ireland on exposure data, and highlighting inconsistencies and the reluctance of the regulatory agencies to correct them. I also devoted countless hours to research and campaigning both at the local and national level to ending fluoridation in Ireland.

This is my story as it relates to tea. But first, a brief history of tea and its rather unique, and some might say unhealthy, relationship with Ireland.

The Global History of Tea

The history of tea drinking in English speaking cultures dates back over 300 years to the time of the British Empire. The origins of the British Empire began with its conquest of Ireland, and it was the Irish above any other nationality in modern times that developed a special relationship with tea. Historically, tea has been valued not only for its flavour but also for its caffeine content that is produced as a natural pesticide and makes up close to four percent of the content of the younger leaves of the plant.

China is considered to have the earliest records of tea consumption dating back thousands of years. The culture of drinking tea spread from China to Japan around the sixth century. Thereafter, tea rapidly underwent global expansion moving from China and Japan, onto Vietnam and Korea, and then the Western World. Two principal varieties of the species are used in the cultivation of tea: the small-leaved Chinese variety (Camellia sinensis sinensis), also used for green tea and white tea, and the large-leaved Assamese variety (Camellia sinensis assamica), which has traditionally been used only for black tea (Waugh et al., 2017). Whether a tea becomes black, green, oolong, pu-erh, or white depends on the variety of tea grown, the method of harvesting, the degree of mechanical processing after withering, and how long the leaves are allowed to oxidize, or ferment, before they are dried.

Most of the tea produced worldwide is black tea, which represents 78 % of the tea produced and consumed worldwide and over 90% of all tea sold in the West. Black tea is principally consumed in North America, Western Europe, Africa (except Morocco), Western Asia, and

Australia. Moroccan green mint tea is popular in the northwest African countries of Morocco, Algeria, Tunisia, Libya, and Mauritania. In Asia, green tea and Oolong tea leaves are more popular. Tea sold in tea bags represents approximately 95% of all tea consumed in western countries, while orthodox loose tea is still the predominant type of tea consumed in many Asian and Middle Eastern countries. During the Ming Dynasty which lasted until the mid-17th Century, Chinese production met both Asian and early European demands for tea.

The Dutch were the first to commercially import tea to Europe and the British colonies in America. However, it was the British East India Company's rise to dominance from 1700 that led to the spectacular expansion in the tea trade growth from the mid-1700s, culminating in the 18th and 19th Century when the trade in tea contributed to the rise of global capitalism and consumerism.

Tea also played a pivotal role in the genesis of America as a nation-state. The monopoly rights of the British East India Company led to colonies boycotting the commodity, culminating in the Boston Tea Party on December 16, 1773, when colonists boarded tea ships anchored in the harbour and dumped their tea cargo overboard. Punitive laws introduced by the British Parliament to punish the Massachusetts colonists for their defiance led to the outbreak of the American Revolutionary War in April 1775. Against this backdrop, tea became associated with pro-British loyalties among many Americans, and coffee became the beverage of choice.

Until the 1840s, China was the sole supplier of tea to the world markets. At this time, the British purchased tea from China with silver. In order to have enough silver, the British sold opium to China, causing rampant addiction. In the 19th century, opium was Britain's most profitable single commodity trade. The British opium was produced in India and controlled by the East India Company which managed hundreds of thousands of poppy plantations generating immense profits for British merchants—profits were used to purchase tea. Britain's trade in opium destabilized China and China's resistance to the opium trade led to the Opium Wars, a series of mid-19th century conflicts between Britain and China. The wars severely weakened the Qing dynasty contributing to its downfall.

China was forced to pay war reparations, to legalize the import of opium, to cede Hong Kong to Britain, and to grant Britain the right to transport Chinese indentured labour to America and European colonies, so as to supplant the loss of slave labour. Thus, it can be said that in the 18th and 19th Centuries, the trade in tea contributed to the downfall of the British Empire in its colonies in America, the creation of the United States, and the collapse of the Imperial dynasty in China.

Key Observations About Fluoride Levels in Tea Beverages

It has been known from scientific studies dating back to the 1930s and early 1940s that tea is a hyperaccumulator of fluoride and that the consumption of tea is a major dietary source of fluoride. From the 1960s the preponderance of scientific evidence from all of the major tea consuming regions in the world unequivocally demonstrated high levels of fluoride in black tea products. Interestingly, it is also acknowledged that the fluoride level in tea is one of the best parameters to reflect the quality of tea, with finer qualities of teas having lower fluoride contents (Kavanagh & Renehan, 1998).

There are many factors that influence the fluoride content in tea including climate, the chemical nature of the soil, hydrology, the source of water for irrigation, use of fertilizers and pesticides, the age of the tea leaf, and methods of tea harvesting, and processing. Black tea generally contains higher levels of fluoride than green tea as green teas consist primarily of the earliest spring growth, made up of small buds and young leaves. The fluoride levels in tea infusions from tea bags are greater than in loose tea, as the smaller particle size of tea dust used in tea bags increases the rate of diffusion of tea constituents into water.

How Tea Became the National Beverage of Ireland and Britain.

In stark contrast to the United States, tea consumption in Great Britain and Ireland grew exponentially in the 19th century. This rapid growth in availability and consumption of tea in the Victorian period, especially prevalent from the 1860s onwards, coincided with the introduction of tea plantations in British India which significantly lowered the price of tea such that it was no longer considered a luxury item. By 1900, about 58% of the world's tea market was sourced from British India, while 40% came from China and Japan, and 2% from the Dutch East Indies.

One of the factors that helped promote the drinking of tea in Ireland was, undoubtedly, the climate which was cold, wet, windy, and damp; drinking warm tea provided a perfect antidote to the weather. Tea was also used by the working class to suppress appetite and quell hunger pangs. Another factor was that raw milk, a staple of the Irish diet, was contaminated with pathogens which caused tuberculosis. In the late 19th and early 20th centuries, tuberculosis was endemic in Ireland being responsible for more deaths than any other single cause. By 1906, one in every six of the total death-rate of the country were attributed to the disease (Boyd, 1908). As a consequence, the consumption of tea may be seen as an attempt at reducing the risk of tuberculosis by replacing milk with tea. Indeed, in 1908, the "Report on Tuberculosis in Ireland" noted this dietary change amongst the Irish, but also suggested that the replacement of milk with tea may account for much of the malnutrition, and dyspepsia from which the poorer classes in Ireland suffer.

The significance of tea in Irish culture is further reflected in the fact that in 1941 the Irish Government established a private company, Tea Importers (Eire) Ltd, for the purpose of purchasing and importing tea for the Irish market. After WWII, these responsibilities were transferred to a state-owned tea company and legislation was enacted making it compulsory to only import tea from the country of origin, thereby avoiding the need to purchase from the UK. In 1959, Tea Importers Ltd imported 8.28 million kg of tea rising to 9.3 million kg in 1963 and 14,951 million kg in 1977, when per capita tea consumption reached a staggering 4.57 kg per person. It is important to be aware that this peak occurred approximately 10 years after commencement of water fluoridation in Ireland. Coincidentally the same year, a study addressing the fluoride intake from foods reported that the average daily intake of fluoride will be much higher in countries with a high consumption of tea. Because of this, the authors cautioned that it is important to pay attention to the fluoride content in foods, especially in countries where drinking water is fluoridated (Kumpulainen & Koivistoinen, 1977).

At this time, and for decades after, one of the most senior politicians in the national parliament of Ireland was a prominent tea merchant and owner of one of the biggest tea brands in the country. Over the course of his long political career, he held numerous Ministerial positions including that of Minister for Environment, where he oversaw, among other things, water-related topics including water fluoridation, before eventually rising to the position of deputy Prime Minister or Tánaiste.

Almost a decade earlier, an article published in the Lancet Medical Journal reported on the tea consumption habits and fluoride levels in tea in the UK. It highlighted that tea was by far the single most important dietary source of fluoride in adults and children in Britain. Having analyzed the most common brands of tea sold in the country, it reported that the average fluoride content was 0.52 mg per cup (Cook, 1969). These results were comparable to a study conducted in Canada, published in 1976, which also highlighted that tea is an important dietary source of fluoride and that tea consumption can influence serum ionic fluoride levels (Husdan et al., 1976). However, it was a study published in 1983 on fluoride content in food and dietary fluoride intake in the UK that really set the cat among the pigeons. Not only did it report that tea was the main source of dietary fluoride exposure in the UK population, contributing over 70% of dietary fluoride intake, but of seven brands of tea tested the mean fluoride level in infusions was 3.2 mg/L (ranging from 2.0-4.7 mg/L). The authors reported that depending on the brand of tea consumed, above average tea consumption, as recorded in Britain, could result in fluoride intakes as high as 9.4 mg per day from tea consumption alone; and if water used to prepare infusions was fluoridated, the exposure from tea would exceed 10 mg per day. The report also noted that while less tea is consumed in the UK than in the 1950s, the fluoride content in tea infusions is higher (Walters et al., 1983).

In this regard, it is important to mention that, prior to the Second World War, the primary countries of origin of black teas in European markets were India, the Dutch East Indies (now Indonesia), and Ceylon (now Sri Lanka). In the years after the war, the trade in black teas was dominated by India and Sri Lanka with smaller imports from Indonesia. However, the volume of tea since the early 1980s imported from the main tea producing countries showed a complete paradigm shift with Kenya rapidly emerging as the largest provider of tea to the Irish and UK market. In 1982, Kenya became the main supplier of tea to the Irish and UK markets. Other countries to which Kenya is now the primary supplier of black tea include Pakistan, Egypt, and Afghanistan. In contrast, in the United States, China and Argentina are the primary suppliers of black tea where the majority of consumption is iced tea. In 2011, just 0.02% of the tea imports to the USA, 5% of the tea imports to Canada, and 8% of the tea imports to Russia were sourced from Kenya. It is also important to mention that the majority of Kenya's tea-growing regions are found in the Kenyan Highlands, on both sides of the Great Rift Valley, a high-fluoride region comprising volcanic geological formations with large deposits of fluorite. This means it is one of the places in the world where fluorides occur in the highest concentrations, not only in rocks and soils but also in surface and groundwaters (Manji & Kapila, 1984).

This may also explain why teas sourced from Kenya contain higher fluoride levels than those from other tea producing countries such as India, Sri Lanka, or Indonesia.

In addition to the change in the geographic origin of tea imports, another major change in tea consumerism occurred in the early 1980s with the rise and dominance of tea bags in the marketplace over the traditional orthodox loose tea, which continued to be the primary tea consumed in the UK and Ireland till the late 70s. Since the early 1980s, about 97% of tea is sold in tea bags, while the orthodox loose tea market is very small, about 3-4% according to the 2014 "Product Factsheet: Tea in Ireland" produced by the Centre for the Promotion of Imports from developing countries.

This brings us to the years 1987-1989 when, yet again, Ireland was reported to have the highest per capita tea consumption in the world (3.04 kg per capita); 5-fold higher than India, 10-fold higher than the United States or China, 17-fold higher than France or Germany, and 50-fold higher than Italy. For the same period, the second highest per capita consumption was the UK (2.81 kg), followed by Turkey (2.19 kg), New Zealand (1.59 kg), Tunisia (1.43 kg), Egypt (1.33 kg),

Australia (1.12 kg), Morocco (1.11 kg), and Japan (0.96 kg) (Graham, 1992). Yet, quite remarkably, despite Ireland having the highest per-capita consumption of tea in the world, no study had been undertaken to measure the fluoride content in tea products in Ireland. This gap in knowledge was first officially acknowledged in 1998 when the Principal Dental Surgeon of the Eastern Health Board and dental researchers at the School of Dental Science, Trinity College, and Dublin Dental Hospital highlighted that no data exists on the fluoride level in popular brands of tea available in Ireland and recommended that a research project be carried out to analyse the fluoride content in tea infusions available on the Irish market. Coincidentally, this recommendation came exactly one year after the prominent tea merchant retired from national politics. Yet remarkably, over a decade later no such studies had been undertaken in Ireland (Kavanagh & Renehan, 1998).

Then in 2011 came the bombshell revelation in the form of the findings of the first ever Total Dietary Fluoride Intake Assessment undertaken in Ireland by the Food Safety Authority of Ireland (FSAI). Quite remarkably, the FSAI reported that the average intake of total dietary fluoride from food, water, and beverages, including tea was just 1.99 - 2.09 mg/day. These values were based on tap water having a fluoride content of 0.8 mg/L. Somehow, against all odds we were supposed to believe that the dietary fluoride intake in Ireland was less than the reported for the USA, when in 2012 it was reported that the per-capita consumption of tea in Ireland was 14-fold higher than the United States (Beresniak et al., 2012).

It is pertinent to mention that the 2011 National Adult Nutrition Survey by the Irish Universities Nutrition Alliance found that tea was the most commonly consumed beverage in the whole population—consumed by 81% of individuals aged 18-64 and 94% of those aged 65 and over. It is also worth noting that the National Longitudinal study of Children in Ireland (2010) reported that 8% of infants at nine months of age were drinking tea from a bottle. Among the lower socioeconomic group, the percentage was 10%.

Two years later the European Food Safety Authority reported that drinking just two cups of tea per day (with a fluoride level of 5 mg/L), combined with an average consumption of fluoridated drinking water and use of fluoridated tap water in the preparation of food, but excluding all other sources (including solid foods, toothpaste and dental products), would provide a daily dietary intake of 6 mg per day. Clearly, where researchers in the UK found that above average consumption of tea, as occurs in the UK, could result in a fluoride intake of greater than 10 mg per day when prepared with fluoridated water and where the per-capita consumption of tea in Ireland was 20% higher than the UK and where the same branded tea products were available in both countries, it was inconceivable that the dietary intake would be so much lower in Ireland. Something about the evidence wasn't adding up.

Into the Fray

In April 2013, I wrote to the FSAI requesting a copy of the measured analytical data in respect of the Total Diet Survey. On receipt of the data, it was immediately evident that the fluoride content in foods was measured by preparing/cooking the foods using deionized water, rather than fluoridated tap water. This was extraordinary considering that it was known for decades that the fluoride content in foods and beverages increased significantly along with dietary intake when artificially fluoridated water was used in the processing, cooking, or preparation of foods or beverages. Further examination of the data revealed that the fluoride content in black tea infusions was estimated based on just two measurements undertaken in 2003 and 2005, which reported a fluoride content in black tea infusions of 0.70 mg/L and 0.40 mg/L, respectively. In other words, the fluoride content in tea infusions was less than the fluoride content in drinking water used to prepare tea. To put this in context, the values reported for tea products in the UK in published literature from multiple authors for the same time period were up to 10-fold higher than those reported for Ireland.

Accordingly, I wrote to the Minister for Health; Minister for Environment, Minister for Agriculture, Food and the Marine; The Office of the Taoiseach; and Chief Medical Officer of the HSE in May 2013 to inform them of these discrepancies, noting that the FSAI data was flawed and significantly underestimated dietary fluoride exposure in the general population. I subsequently wrote to the FSAI requesting that they provide information on the chain of custody regarding initial sample taking/preparation and delivery to the laboratory, explaining how the samples were taken, what tea products/brands were analyzed, the product packaging serial identification code, and any other details that were recorded. In addition, I requested details on who authorized/signed off on the laboratory reports as well as who signed off on sample preparation and delivery to the laboratory.

Two months later, the FSAI informed me that they were unable to identify the chemist/analysts who undertook the analysis of food samples or who signed off on the analytical report. Moreover, laboratory records were no longer available since the data was produced 10 years previously and records are required to be kept for a minimum of 6 years, in line with their legal obligations. You see, unlike the other food samples included in the study, the tea samples were selected and tested in 2003 and 2005 by someone unknown. How convenient, one might say. Notwithstanding this, the FSAI informed me that my concerns regarding the data included in the Total Diet Survey (TDS) were best addressed by the new TDS, which they were currently undertaking, and that this updated assessment of the exposure of the Irish population to fluoride would be completed by the end of 2013. Relief, finally they would correct their data. However, by the end of 2014 and early 2015, the TDS remained uncompleted.

Given the inordinate delays, in mid-2015, I proceeded with colleagues with a record in research to conduct a study to measure the fluoride content in tea products available in Ireland, which was published in a peer-reviewed journal in February 2016. In this, we found that the total cumulative dietary fluoride intake in the general population could readily exceed the levels known to cause chronic fluoride intoxication due to the high levels of fluoride in tea and the culture of habitual tea drinking; and we cautioned that the excessive fluoride intake may be contributing to a wide range of adverse health effects. To respond to these concerns, a number of recommendations were cited in the study, including that public health authorities should inform pregnant women that excessive fluoride intake from habitual tea drinking is unsafe for the developing child and that tea should not be provided to infants as a beverage. A month later in March 2016, the results of the long-awaited updated TDS were published by the FSAI. Despite the previous commitments, no data was included for fluoride exposure or fluoride levels in food products. One has to wonder why they decided to pull the plug on including fluoride. Could it have had anything to do with our published research?

Notwithstanding this, the FSAI reported that a separate project was currently underway to assess population exposure to fluoride, and it would be published as a separate study in 2016. It was not until April 2018 that the FSAI published the results of this study in which they finally acknowledged the contribution of tea to the total fluoride intake in the population.

Among adults, black tea consumption was found to provide more than 75% of their total fluoride intake, with tap water contributing just 12%. Crucially, the updated TDS study confirmed my earlier concerns regarding the first TDS in that the fluoride content in teas were found to be 10-fold higher than those reported in 2011.

In August 2018, I was invited along with Dr Vyvyan Howard and Dr Paul Connett to New Zealand in order to participate in a number of public engagements organized by Fluoride Free New Zealand. This afforded me the opportunity to present the findings of my more recent study which measured the fluoride concentrations in commercial black tea products available in New Zealand, as well as reviewing the international evidence regarding chronic fluoride intake and its association with chronic pain, arthritic disease, and musculoskeletal disorders. This study also provided insights into the possible association between fluoride intake and the high prevalence of these disorders in New Zealand. I should mention here that one of the co-authors of this paper was the late Dr Mike Godfrey from Tauranga, New Zealand. Mike was a warrior for medical freedom, a dedicated medical physician, gentleman, and scholar. Over the last decade of his remarkable life, we communicated frequently by email and it was a joy to finally meet him in person on our NZ tour.

Serendipitously, one of our New Zealand speaking engagements was the University of Otago in Dunedin. Among the participants present were perhaps a dozen university students who entered the lecture hall wearing tin foil hats, cheeks flushed with boyish pleasure, who promptly sat in the front row, arms folded in defiance. It was apparent that their intent was to ridicule the speakers and those in attendance; however, their boyish grins turned to blushed embarrassment and humiliation when I openly challenged and questioned them during the course of my presentation. In further humiliation, I informed them that the very first biomonitoring studies undertaken anywhere in the world examining fluoride intake from tea were conducted in Otago Medical School and published in the *British Journal of Nutrition* (Harrison, 1949a; Harrison, 1949b). These pioneering studies concluded that tea was the major source of fluoride intake in the New Zealand population. Yet, despite the high consumption of tea in NZ, drinking water was fluoridated in many of the major cities and communities including Dunedin. It was not until 2017 when our study was published, some 68 years later, that anyone reevaluated fluoride intake from tea in NZ (Waugh et al., 2017).

Conclusion

Data shows that throughout the 20th century Ireland had the highest per-capita intake of tea in the world and tea was the major source of fluoride intake in the population before commencement of water fluoridation. New Zealand also numbers among the world's high per-capita consumers of tea.

Prior to and after implementation of water fluoridation, both the Department of Health and Public Health Agencies and Food Safety Authorities in both countries concealed from the public the importance of tea as a dietary source of fluoride. They were negligent in their duty of care by ignoring and misrepresenting the contribution of tea to fluoride intake in order to protect the state policy of water fluoridation.

It is further evident that changes in the geographic origin of tea imports, along with the rise in popularity in tea bags, increased use of fertilizers and pesticides, and the mechanization of harvesting of tea contributed to increased fluoride exposure among consumers which went undocumented due to a total lack of appropriate regulatory control measures or population exposure monitoring.

To end, one of the reasons I got involved in fluoride research was because of my own health issues which were related to fluoroquinolone toxicity (Bennett et al., 2022) and aggravated by fluoridated water and tea. I found that by reducing my fluoride intake, my body could heal some of the long-term disabling side effects I experienced from my exposure to fluorinated antibiotics. I also pursued my interest in fluoride research to protect my children, wider family, and community from fluoride harm.

Fluoride Activism in Massachusetts

Accidental Involvement, Lifelong Reverberations

By: Dr Deborah E. Moore, MEd, MA, PhD

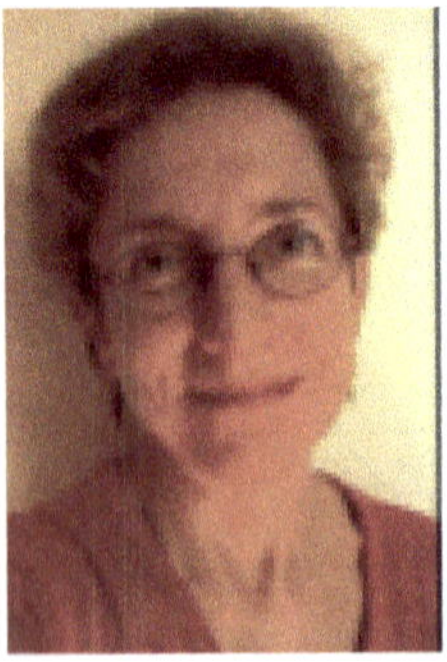

ABOUT: *Deborah Moore now lives in Central Vermont, and is very involved with various environmental health-related issues. She is mostly retired from her organization, Second Look, although she still supports the website, www.SLweb.org (looking forward to a major update). She still gets positive feedback from those the website continues to help, and she still occasionally answers questions and guides poisoned individuals who seek her out. Throughout her active tenure as Second Look's Executive Director, she organized several successful initiatives, all inspired by fluoride and other toxins, while writing commentaries for various publications on these issues. She continues to write on these topics through commentaries and in a forthcoming book. Deb has had unusually varied past work and life experiences including: special ed teacher; living and working in Switzerland; zookeeping; producing a successful 2-year series of environmental lectures; editing submissions and reviewing books for a scholarly journal; creating and teaching three unique interdisciplinary college level courses; academic advising for college undergraduates; ghost writing journal articles for a veterinarian; serious organic gardening; and always increasing her knowledge of holistic healing practices, among many other things. She is a passionate proponent of holistic medicine and holistic thinking, firmly believing that everything is very literally connected to everything else.*

CHAPTER 23

"Our deeds determine us as much as we determine our deeds."

—George Elliot (1819-1880)

IN 1996, WHILE on a long, strange trip toward my atypical later-in-life PhD, I was stuck in the construction of my dissertation proposal. I had all the pieces, but they weren't coming together and I was frustrated.

In the middle of this, on a visit to Living Earth, my health food store oasis in what I perceived to be the desert of the big city of Worcester, MA, where I lived, I saw something unusual: an informal petition to the City Councillors asking them to reject water fluoridation in the city. Until then, I had no idea that I had been consuming unfluoridated Worcester water, and the only things I vaguely thought I knew were the persistent narrative that fluoride was good for your teeth, and that people who opposed fluoridation were a bunch of misinformed kooks. But since I trusted Frank, the manager, for being on top of this kind of thing, that petition piqued my interest.

I signed the petition, understanding that the City Council meeting was the next day, spoke briefly with Frank about it, and headed off (pre-Internet) to the University of Massachusetts Medical Library in nearby Shrewsbury to see what I could find in the stacks. My big questions at the time were: Is there a scientific controversy about putting this stuff in the water? If there is, why not use the Precautionary Principle and wait until this controversy is settled?

After only a couple of hours in the stacks, I easily found that there was, indeed, a "scientific controversy" about fluoridation. That evening, I spoke with my then-husband who was the health agent in another Massachusetts town. He knew that there was a fluoridation law in MA and informed me about that and what I needed to do, as a citizen, to fight back. At that point, all I wanted was ammunition for the City Council public hearing the next day.

My eyes were opened and my innocence lost at the very beginning of my adventure with water fluoridation when I went to the City Council meeting that next evening. I had never been active in local politics and had never been to such a meeting, so I naïvely assumed a "public hearing" meant that the public would actually be listened to. I was first astonished, and then disgusted to witness many of the Councillors very obviously and rudely ignoring the testimony of the motley crew of individuals from the public. However, when the dentists and doctors presented with their slick graphs and charts and prepared speeches, I saw some of the Councillors excitedly twittering about seeing their own practitioners in front of them. It struck me as incorrect that the agenda put the opponents' testimonies before the proponents. With no discussion whatsoever, the Councillors voted to allow the Health Commissioner to order the water fluoridated. End of story. Or so they thought.

The next morning, Frank called me and asked if I wanted to speak with Nancy, whom I didn't know. She contacted him hoping to connect with someone who wanted to fight the impending fluoridation in Worcester, which had never been fluoridated. Before the end of the day, I made a decision that I didn't know at the time would change the course of the rest of my life.

Going into this effort with immense naïveté, never before having done any community organizing or running anything like a campaign, and unintentionally having to drop the work for my dissertation for the next eight months, I embarked on this adventure with equally naïve Nancy. We became the two lead organizers in a city of around 200,000 residents.

The learning curve here was very steep concerning: the reality of city politics; what's required to do such organizing; and, especially, the dangers of the stuff they wanted to put in the water "for our health." The more I learned, the more horrified I became. The story started to come together for me: why this push to fluoridate everywhere was so contentious; why it was happening in the first place; why the general public was so misinformed; what were the real motivations for pushing this chemical into people's bodies, etc.

The one Worcester City Councillor who opposed this effort to fluoridate approached us, offering very sage political advice on certain things to say and do, and on what wouldn't work. She also connected us with other politically-savvy folks who not only gifted us with more helpful advice but also made political signs and offered to kindly make ours at a much-discounted price when the time was right.

Connecting with fluoride opponents from around the country, I learned a great deal about what could work and probably wouldn't work. By the time the 90-day deadline to submit signatures (on the proper petition) approached, our army of about 100 volunteers had collected more than enough that hot summer to get our question on the ballot at the next election. And I had informed myself enough about fluoride and the fluoridation issue to feel that I was on fairly solid ground, enough to educate the rest of the city on what I had learned.

Meanwhile, I made some surprising and interesting observations that were subsequently confirmed, over and over, in all my years with this issue. When I first became involved, I went right to a friend who was the leading environmentalist in Worcester. He was head of the only environmental organization in this big city, of which I was a Board member. Coming from a liberal, environmentally-aligned orientation, I presumed he would help in a heartbeat. Explaining to Ted what was happening in his native city, when I asked if he would help, I was greeted with a very long pause, after which he said, "I'm not sure fluoridation is such a bad thing." I believe my jaw fell on the floor at that moment. How could this major environmentalist think putting this chemical in the drinking water was a good thing? He then said, "What about the poor children who need it?"

It actually took quite a few years for Ted to finally come around and get what this was about. The blind acceptance of the false narrative was one of my first shockers. Another revelation occurred to me while gathering donations for our campaign: our greatest supporters were Right-leaners! Prior to that, in predominantly Democratic Massachusetts, I don't think I had even met a Republican. So, it left a huge impression on me when I made the realization that those on the Right tended to be more on our side than those on the Left. Admittedly, the reasons they gave were often different from those that motivated me, which were chiefly about the well-documented science-based health concerns. For the most part, the concern from the Right at that time was a very emphatic, "I don't want the Government putting that stuff in my water!" When I confirmed those observations with other activists around the country, my reaction to these revelations was - amusement!

Once we made it to the ballot, we had just a few months to educate the public. From that first Worcester "public hearing" and throughout the months of my personal edification on fluoridation, I became aware that an ongoing problem in fighting this issue was the *appearance* that the only professionals who knew anything about it were the dentists and doctors who were pushing it. In any situation, such as that hearing or in articles in the paper, ordinary people who were not health professionals were judged against these "experts." The science was settled, and there was only one narrative on the science. It took little time to realize that this playing field was so *not* even!

Very quickly, I knew we had to fight fire with fire. By then, I had familiarized myself with most of the major fluoride opposition players in the US. These were activists as well as academicians, scientists, authors and other professionals. I was able to round up several of the best for a debate I was organizing at Worcester's Clark University, my PhD stomping ground. When the time came, we had no takers from the other side for a debate, so we went ahead with an informational forum. The bad news: in spite of our advertising, hardly anyone showed up, not even the local paper. After all the work putting it together, this was a huge disappointment. The good news: one of the participants of the forum had the foresight to make sure we had invited someone to videotape the whole thing, and that was done.

I'm so grateful to these professionals, and very proud of this forum. What emerged was "The Clark University Fluoridation Video" featuring a scientist, a scientist/professor, a dentist, an investigative author on the subject, and a lawyer. It is *still* traveling around the world, making a difference! This professional forum was the very first of its kind on the fluoridation issue and was the inspiration for other communities to follow this lead.

The other thing we did to educate the public was create an easy-to-read trifold brochure listing the best reasons to vote against fluoridation, including references to the latest science and other pertinent information. I believe handing these out at supermarkets and post offices was the best winning move, along with all the other ways we attempted to get out the word via letters-to-the-editor, commentaries, public meetings, etc.

In the end, we won handily in the November vote. An ironic side-effect was that my dissertation proposal fell into place coherently as a result of an insight I gained via the work I had done that year in my "fluoride time-out," allowing me to quickly finish that proposal. BUT this was not the end of my fluoride story....

2001

The fluoride fight of 1996 was not the first one in Worcester, which had turned down fluoridation twice before, many years prior. However, the difference in 1996 was that Worcester had just completed a new water treatment center. I learned that state funding of the facility came with conditions requiring that the city enforce fluoridation and provide a room for the necessary equipment. This had been the impetus for the push that year.

Those who presumed this would be an easy task were taken by surprise that there was any organized opposition at all. The fluoride chemicals were already waiting in the fluoridation room of the brand-new water treatment plant. In Massachusetts, it is the Boards of Health that issue the order to fluoridate. In the cases where the citizens have done the work to get it on the ballot and then have voted it down, Boards of Health can order it again in only two years. I knew the clock was ticking. As for the unused hydrofluorosilicic acid? Stay tuned....

After our win and the insight that informed my dissertation proposal, I finished my PhD in a few years, all the while knowing that "they" might start this up again at any time after 1998. Upon graduating in 1999, I organized what I had decided must be done at this point in my life: creating the first 501(c)(3) non-profit dedicated to fluoride. After some initial refocusing, I realized it needed to be a non-political, educational endeavor, concentrating on presenting the science on fluoride toxicity that was not reaching health professionals, scientists, or the public.

I raised some seed money from some very generous fluoride opponents, researched the foundations most appropriate for receiving start-up money, outlined what I would be doing and when, and felt good about where things were going. Just a few months prior to my organization *Second Look*'s official birth in January of 2001, I heard the news that "they" would be once again trying to fluoridate Worcester. That was the last thing I wanted to hear at that time, so I asked a former fluoride buddy to go with me to speak some sense to the City Councillors, one at a time. By that time, there was so much more information out there than in 1996, and we were well-versed on the logic of the argument. We were succeeding very nicely with persuading the Councillors, with the idea that we would head off this threat at the pass and thwart another full-fledged fluoride fight.

That plan worked well until the City Councillor who was pushing the effort made the decision to take it out of the hands of the Councillors and give the decision directly to the Health Commissioner. I knew immediately that another fight would be unavoidable, and this time much bigger....

From the amount and intensity of the work I had done five years earlier, I knew I didn't want to engage at that level again while nursing my new organization. I first called Nancy, who wanted nothing to do with this fight, still burnt out. I also called Deirdre, who had been one of our leaders but was now about to start law school. She said she'd help as best she could, and did, thank goodness. I couldn't find anyone else I thought might be capable of leading it up, and I didn't want to be drinking fluoride out of my tap, so I decided I'd better get started and hoped someone else would come along.

In 1996, I learned the hard way to trust my organizational judgment and stand up for it. I had reluctantly agreed to a complicated fundraising project, conceived by an industrious fellow activist, that I strongly felt would not be worth the time and energy. My instincts were correct; it was a waste of time. So, at the first community meeting in 2001, when a young man with no previous organizational experience or fluoride knowledge came on strong, trying to assume a leadership role, I knew enough to firmly resist. He soon realized he was in over his head and just disappeared, much to my relief. So, once again, I was the lead organizer, by default.

By then I was well ensconced in the logistics of gathering ten percent of registered voters' signatures, again, while trying hard to keep up with my plans for *Second Look*. And I knew that this time, "they" were determined to win and would put up a major fight. I learned they had the backing of a foundation that was created when a healthcare facility folded. (After it was over, we learned we'd been up against $600,000 the foundation had originally allocated for improving the health of "poor children." Instead, it went into the pockets of a very nasty PR firm.) So, this time around, I wasn't just leading a battle; I was fighting a war while also trying to sustain the work I needed to do for my new organization.

Meanwhile, I had been experiencing symptoms of what I later learned was a serious hypothyroid condition, brought about ironically (I later surmised), by exposure to fluorinated anesthesia and greatly exacerbated by the stress I was under dealing with two intense, time-consuming, more-than-full time jobs. I managed to do most of what I needed to do for my organization, except write grant proposals for start-up money. This would have great repercussions later....

The War

The great Worcester fluoride fight of 2001 was quite the battle. While I managed to round up sufficient supporters, old and new, to help gather signatures, many were not interested in doing anything further. Once again, we were able to submit far more than the minimum of "good" signatures. Having already learned what was needed for a successful educational campaign, we were ready and prepared to move forward. However, Deirdre soon went off to law school, and I was essentially alone in my job as chief organizer, with a few terrific helpers.

The most important thing we did that year, in my opinion, was to update and upgrade our trifold. This time, with the work of a wonderful graphic artist and fellow fluoride fighter from Washington State, our trifold looked professionally done, was easily readable, and very convincing. We had even more wonderful benefactors who helped out with costs, thank goodness, and these trifolds were our main tool. Once again, these were handed out at public places, and we did a great job saturating the city with this basic education. I personally wrote quite a few commentaries for various local publications, but I tried to stay away from personal interviews as a result of being seriously misquoted in 1996 several times. Writing is not a problem for me, but public speaking definitely is. I had no choice but to force myself to speak publicly on occasion. Somehow, I made this work, and it made a difference.

Thinking creatively and getting the word out credibly was important in this campaign. My new PhD helped with the credibility factor. And, yes, I organized another forum of perfect professionals, again trying for a debate that didn't materialize. This time, it was well attended, including by the chief "science reporter" of the local paper, who until then either ignored us or wrote the usual media hit jobs. He told me later that he only intended to stay long enough to prove to himself that our professionals and their information were nonsense. He ended up being transfixed and converted when he heard what these people were revealing. After that, all of his articles were supportive—another key to the outcome of this battle.

So, yes, in the end, we did win, again, and by a comfortable margin. I was amused to hear that our opposition, who were waiting for a grand celebration in a rented hotel ballroom, were informed by a reporter that they lost the vote and couldn't believe it. Even our fluoride fighting friends were astounded that we won, being up against such great odds and having raised only about $8,000.

Epilogue

My health crashed that election night, and I was quite ill for several months. I also had heard that I was personally blamed by the organized opposition for their tragic loss, which frightened me. In early February, when I finally was able to work, the one foundation I had managed to apply to, giving a preliminary OK for a start-up grant for *Second Look*, let me know that they were withdrawing my grant because, post 9/11 and the following economic collapse, many foundations were tanking, and they couldn't take on new grantees. This did not bode well for my new organization, forcing me to struggle for funding ever since then.

In 2002, I started a temporary watchdog organization (*Worcester Dental Watch*) to hold accountable the dentists who had promised to improve the dental health of the poor kids whether or not they won, and we offered them some good suggestions. I think it scared them a bit, and they begrudgingly made some changes. Soon after that, I became involved with heading off a Massachusetts state fluoridation mandate, this time, mercifully, not as lead organizer. And since 2001, I have spent many hours consulting with organizers from numerous cities, states, and countries on their own fluoridation struggles.

This journey I took after fluoride captured me resulted in some significant consequences. To this day, Worcester, MA, the second largest city in New England, has fluoride-free water, a fact about which I'm very proud. Many of the cities in Massachusetts and elsewhere that followed our winning strategies were successful in their own fluoride fights. My appreciation for the concept of Environmental Health grew significantly, as did my realization that the general public's awareness of environmental toxins is minimal, something I'm trying to remedy with a new book.

And the left-over chemicals that never got used in Worcester? While gathering signatures in 2001, several signers who were water plant workers reported in whispers to our signature-gatherers that "they've been putting it in the water anyway." Researching several years of water quality reports plausibly confirmed that rumor (along with my failing thyroid...).

For many years now, having gained extensive knowledge about fluoride and fluoroquinolone toxicity through my work with *Second Look*, I've been able to guide numerous poisoned individuals–people who tracked me down in desperation after failing to find adequate medical help–to pathways enabling them to help themselves. This *pro bono* work has been aside from the help provided by *Second Look's* offshoot, the *Fluoride Toxicity Research Collaborative (FTRC)* and its separate website, FTRC WebCenter, which contains much unique information about fluoride/fluoroquinolone poisoning, with suggestions for self-help.

It is imperative that I mention with great gratitude all the many individuals who were necessary components of the successes of both Worcester battles, as well as all those who paved the way in the wider effort, for five decades prior. Some of these were doctors and scientists who bravely published the truths they ascertained, which were the basis upon which more science was built. And extremely important also were those activists who shared their collective knowledge before there was the Internet or even computers. I was very aware of these Keepers-of-the-Truth, several of whom graciously passed on to me what I needed to know to move forward in these endeavors.

I'll end here with an amusing story. A 23-year-old quote in *Worcester Magazine* answering why I thought we won in 2001 was used as major "evidence" in an April 2025 *Esquire Magazine* article by a reporter trying to denigrate the latest trajectory away from fluoridation. His efforts really didn't work, as he misinterpreted some of what I clearly said, and he chose a quote I can still stand by. Interesting how one's actions and words can reverberate for decades...

Studying the Fluoride Controversy

By: Dr Brian Martin, PhD

ABOUT: *Brian Martin is emeritus professor of social sciences at the University of Wollongong, Australia. He is the author of 24 books and hundreds of articles on scientific controversies, nonviolent action, dissent, and other topics. He is vice president of Whistleblowers Australia and hosts a large website on suppression of dissent (bmartin.cc).*

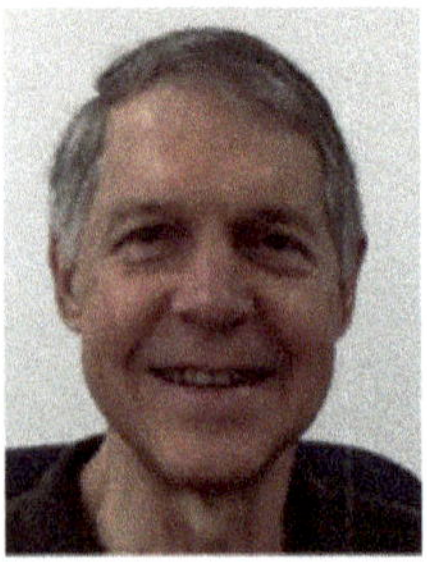

CHAPTER 24

"As soon as we abandon our own reason and are content to rely upon the authority of others, there is no end to our troubles."

—Bertrand Arthur William Russell (1872-1970)

I NEVER SET out to take a side for or against fluoridation, just to study the controversy. But proponents thought I was on the 'anti' side. Let me explain.

My background is in applied mathematics, working on astrophysics and other topics at the Australian National University. In the late 1970s, I stumbled on a quite different topic: suppression of dissent. I learned about several cases in which environmental researchers or teachers had encountered difficulties in their careers: papers censored, tenure denied, attempts at dismissal (Martin, 1981). Writing about these cases led to some publicity, and before long, I learned about ever more cases in a variety of fields.

After a decade of one-year appointments, my job in applied mathematics ran out, and I was lucky to obtain a position in science and technology studies (STS) at the University of Wollongong. STS is a social science field covering, among other things, the history of science, politics of technology, and economics of innovation. Within STS at the time, there was a small but thriving sub-field called controversy studies, looking at debates over just about any topic involving science and technology, for example, solar neutrinos, spoon-bending, intra-uterine devices, smoking, and cancer treatments.

I already knew something about some of the big controversies at the time, especially nuclear power. To cement my position at the university—to be sure to obtain tenure—I decided to make an in-depth study of a controversy. But which one? I chose fluoridation.

What Is Social Analysis?

What does a social analysis of a controversy involve? Usually, it means collecting lots of information, of one sort or another, and making sense of it. I set about my task by obtaining books and articles about the controversy, including its history, politics, economics, and psychology. That was straightforward, though tedious in pre-Internet days. I remember travelling to the Sydney University Dental School, which had a library with dental journals not available elsewhere.

I also interviewed leading figures in the Australian fluoridation debate, both proponents and opponents. Most of them were dentists, doctors, or scientists. The interviews revealed something unexpected.

At the time, the four main dimensions of the debate were benefits, risks, ethics, and decision-making. Pro-fluoridation interviewees said fluoridation was highly beneficial, had few or no risks, was ethical and that decisions should be made by governments informed by experts. Anti-fluoridation interviewees said fluoridation had dubious benefits and serious risks, was unethical and the decisions should be made by the people. Everyone lined up on one side or the other on all four dimensions. For example, no one said the benefits were enormous but fluoridation was unethical. Their views on the four dimensions were "coherent," either all pro or all anti.

What to Explain?

A common approach to studying scientific controversies is to examine just one side of the debate—the side that's wrong. The correct side doesn't need to be examined, because it accords with the evidence. The incorrect side needs explanation, to figure out why people get it wrong.

As I started collecting social analyses of the fluoridation controversy—there were lots of them, mostly from the 1960s and 1970s— this is exactly what they did. They tried to explain opposition to fluoridation, typically with some discrediting factor, like poor education or confusion. The trouble was, none of these explanations stood up to scrutiny.

Several of my colleagues used an approach to studying science called the sociology of scientific knowledge or SSK. It sounds esoteric but the basic ideas are straightforward, though perhaps hard to accept. According to SSK, as applied to controversies, the researcher—that was me—does not judge whether scientific claims are right or wrong, but instead examines explanations for beliefs on *both* sides of the debate. This was unusual.

Professions

I already knew about a body of writing about professions, most commonly medicine and law. It described techniques by which members of the profession advanced their collective interests, including via lengthy training requirements and certification by the government. In essence, professions are occupational monopolies. Entry is limited, keeping salaries high.

This helped answer a question: why would dentists support a public health measure that would reduce their income? After all, if children had fewer cavities, that meant fewer visits to dentists, so dentists seemed altruistic in their support for fluoridation. I remember one pro-fluoridation dentist telling about the old days, before fluoridation, when he had to remove all of a child's teeth, to everyone's distress and tears, including his. There was no doubt that pro-fluoridation campaigners were sincere—as were their opponents. Explaining advocacy as cynical self-interest didn't wash. But if entry to dentistry is limited, then reducing cavities in children wasn't much of a threat to dentists' incomes.

Instead, fluoridation added to the profession's prestige through its connection with scientific expertise, especially epidemiology. Dentistry, in this way, mimicked medicine with its association with science, including antibiotics, drugs, radiation, and vaccines.

Another intriguing question was why campaigning dentists pushed for fluoridation rather than other options to deal with tooth decay. It seemed simplistic to say that fluoride waste from aluminium manufacturing or uranium enrichment was a driving factor. Sure, making fluoride seem beneficial rather than toxic was helpful to industry, but was that all?

I came up with the idea of alternative trajectories for anti-cavity initiatives. One possibility was targeting sugar in children's diets, well known to cause decay. But rather than launch a major campaign to remove sugar from children's food, dentists promoted fluoridation. Why? It seemed a plausible choice when you consider who might oppose an anti-cavity campaign. In pushing for fluoridation, campaigners were mainly up against citizen opponents, who could be painted as ignorant, confused, or manipulated. In contrast, if campaigners had pushed for "desugarisation"—removing sugar from children's food via regulations or taxation—they would have come up against the powerful food industry.

The International Dimension

Since the 1970s, Australia has been highly fluoridated. However, once I started reading widely on the topic, it became clear that Australia was an anomaly on the international scene. In most countries, there was little or no fluoridation. Why not?

To find out what was happening around the world, I prepared a few questions and wrote to health departments in dozens of countries, or to their Australian embassies. As replies began coming in, they confirmed what had been reported in the few previous surveys: only a few countries had fully embraced fluoridation. Among industrialised countries, the most highly fluoridated were Australia, Ireland, New Zealand, US, and Canada, with a few outliers like Singapore, which was 100% fluoridated from a single water supply. In Europe, there wasn't much. In the Netherlands at one time, half the population drank fluoridated water but then it was all stopped. In Britain, the figure was about 10%. This raised two questions.

In most economically prosperous countries, there was little fluoridation except for the English-speaking world. How did pro-fluoridationists explain the apparently irrational dismissal of a beneficial public health measure in so many countries? After all, it was not as if the teeth of European children were so cavity-free that fluoridation wasn't needed. Or was it? I soon discovered that pro-fluoridationists didn't try to explain this discrepancy. They simply ignored that fluoridation had been rejected throughout much of the world. It seemed curious.

My other question was this: why were English-speaking countries seemingly the most enthusiastic about implementing fluoridation? What was different about them? No one was exploring this issue, so I could only speculate. One difference was the autonomy of the medical and dental professions, which was much greater in the US, Australia, New Zealand, and Canada than in most European countries, where doctors and dentists were more tied to government funding and control. It was counterintuitive. Where these professions had greater professional power in relation to the state, they pushed more strongly for fluoridation. Did this relate to the increased status associated with a "scientific" intervention? This is yet to be investigated and continues to be intriguing.

Suppression of Dissent

Whenever there's a powerful professional orthodoxy and popular opposition, dissident experts pose a special threat: they puncture the illusion of professional unanimity. Non-experts can be dismissed as uninformed and emotional, but not so individuals with credentials, publications, and prestigious institutional affiliations. These individuals become targets. They may be censored, libelled, even fired.

In such situations, prominent dissidents are like magnets. Lower-profile dissidents contact them with their stories. And so it was with fluoridation. From the mid-1950s to the mid-1970s, the most prominent fluoridation critic was George Waldbott, a US doctor and researcher. Just reading his book *A Struggle with Titans* provided enough evidence on its own of a pattern of suppression (Waldbott, 1965). Anti-fluoridation dentists were threatened, some of them deregistered. Submissions to dental journals were rejected in a suspicious pattern. Waldbott himself was subject to a sting operation in which he was listed in a dossier of anti-fluoridation activists, grouped with extreme right-wing groups and crazy-sounding health fanatics.

I didn't rely just on Waldbott's book but followed up various leads, searching for articles and writing to anyone who might know something. Albert Schatz confirmed that some of his submissions to journals had been returned unopened. Albert Burgstahler, one of Waldbott's collaborators in the comprehensive book *Fluoridation: The Great Dilemma* (Waldbott et al., 1978), sent me numerous documents, as did Waldbott's widow Edith. Before long I had a sizeable compendium of cases of suppression. I knew from experience that documented cases were the tip of an iceberg of a wider pattern of suppressing dissent.

Along the way, I wrote several articles for academic journals, and then worked on a book (Martin, 1991). This was straightforward in most ways, and there was a revealing part of the process. In my usual way, I sought comments on drafts from experts. The first three anti-fluoridation experts I approached readily agreed. However, it was difficult to find pro-fluoridation experts willing to comment. To find three, I had to approach a dozen of them. I especially appreciated the three who agreed, because they sent comments that helped me avoid mistakes and strengthen my argument. The lesson here is to seek out opponents who are open to dialogue. They are precious.

Captives of Controversy

Examining the arguments on both sides might seem like being neutral, but that's not how it worked in practice. Anti-fluoridationists welcomed my investigation because it took their concerns seriously, whereas many pro-fluoridationists were suspicious or hostile for this very reason. For ardent fluoridation supporters, anyone opposed was not just misguided but dangerous and deluded. By taking both proponents and opponents seriously, I was thereby treated as being on the side of the opponents.

This attitude of proponents was apparent in the debate itself, or rather, their refusal to debate. In dental journals, I read articles recommending that pro-fluoridationists should refuse to join public debates because this implicitly acknowledged there were legitimate reasons against fluoridation. So, to deny any such acknowledgement, they recommended declining to debate, even though this made them seem arrogant.

With this sort of rejection of the possibility of debate, much less dialogue, no wonder my investigation was seen as supporting anti-fluoridationists, because I was taking them seriously, whatever my own view.

At the time, two of my colleagues had similar experiences in studying a controversy using SSK. One was studying the debate over vitamin C and cancer, the other the debate over the Australian Animal Health Laboratory. We described our experiences as being "captives of controversy." However much we tried to be neutral, that's how we were seen (Scott et al., 1990). It wasn't the worst fate for social scientists. We learned a lot from the responses to our studies. For some sorts of insights about controversies, there is no substitute for being caught up in the clash, being seen as an ally or an opponent and treated accordingly.

Conclusion

In some ways, the controversy over adding fluoride to public water supplies isn't all that special (Martin, 2014). The same dynamics are found in numerous other controversies, including those over nuclear power, pesticides, GMOs, microwaves, and vaccination. There is the same polarisation of viewpoints, intense partisanship, involvement of vested interests, routinised rejection of contrary evidence, and suppression of dissent. Among these, the fluoridation controversy serves as an example, featuring a stable configuration of positions and techniques over many decades.

The fluoridation controversy has one significant feature not found in most others: a striking divergence of policy in different countries, with no obvious explanation. It is not easy to say why governments in English-speaking countries are so much keener on fluoridation than elsewhere.

Every long-standing controversy is maintained by campaigners on each side. For most campaigners, there is a limit to their capacity to keep going. Many campaigners have told me they are hopeful of a breakthrough, often in the next few years, when a crucial scientific study or official finding will cause the other side to call it quits. However, one of the enduring features of these controversies is that new evidence seldom makes much of a difference.

One thing I learned is the difficulty of making predictions about the trajectories of controversies, except for one thing: it is usually safe to say they won't be resolved any time soon.

Acknowledgements: For helpful comments, thanks to Mark Diesendorf, Suzzanne Gray, Julia LeMonde, Lorraine Pratley, and Karen Spencer.

When the Ivory Tower Becomes a Bull Ring

The attacks on Dr Christine Till, PhD

(*Written by:* Dr Hardy Limeback)

ABOUT: *Dr Christine Till from: tillyorkulab.com/team*

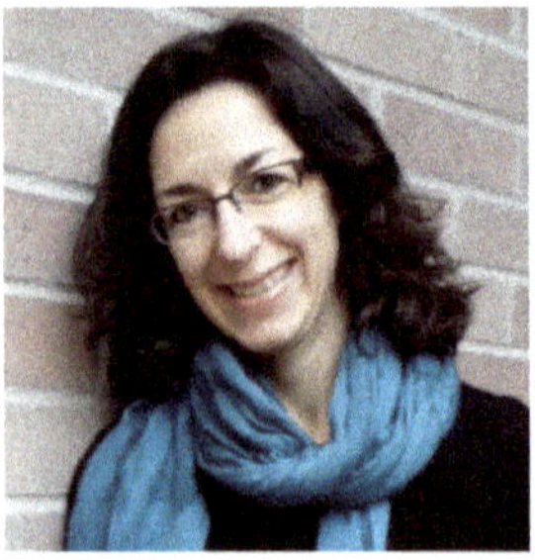

I am a clinical neuropsychologist and Professor of Psychology at York University. My lab focuses on determining how early life exposures to environmental toxicants are implicated as underlying risk factors for emerging morbidities in childhood, including ADHD. My research applies epidemiologic approaches and a biopsychosocial lens to identify risk and protective factors for children's health. My goal is to conduct research that can be used to optimize maternal-child health and the health of future generations.

Together with a highly collaborative and multi-disciplinary research team, our research aims to fill gaps in knowledge about health-related effects of environmental exposures to neurotoxicants. Our work strives to advance the measurement of environmental exposures and their potential health effects by taking into consideration factors that may increase vulnerability, such as timing of exposure, psychosocial stressors, nutrition, and sex-related differences.

I currently serve as the principal investigator for two population-based cohort studies funded by NIH and CIHR. These include the Maternal Infant Research on Environmental Chemicals (MIREC) and the New Hampshire Birth Cohort studies. This work is specifically examining how exposure to fluoride in gestation and infancy impacts learning and behaviour in children. My research is also examining mechanisms of fluoride neurotoxicity by assessing the endocrine-disrupting potential of fluoride. This work is evaluating an array of thyroid hormones and comprehensive measures of fluoride exposure, including tap water samples and dietary intake information, to better understand sources of fluoride exposure. To make informed decisions about the safety of water fluoridation, we need studies looking at sensitive endpoints in the most vulnerable populations.

CHAPTER 25

"Studies of what scientists believe have no relationship to studies of how nature behaves."

—Karl Popper (1902-1994)

DR TILL AND her research team have been at the forefront of an ambitious research initiative addressing one of the most polarized and politicized controversies in public health: the safety of fluoride. Dr Till did not set out to prove fluoride was dangerous or safe. She simply recognized the critical gap in investigating fluoride's potential as a developmental neurotoxin based on suggestive animal studies. Not a single human study had studied the impact of fetal exposure to fluoride in drinking water, despite a 2006 report by the National Research Council calling for more research in this area. This gap required scientific investigation.

Amidst prevailing skepticism and reluctance within academic circles, Dr Till set out on what was to become an earth-shaking challenge to entrenched beliefs. At the time, few scientists were willing to study or question fluoride. People who questioned the safety of fluoride were often dismissed as anti-science quacks and relegated to the so-called fringe by their peers. Questioning the health effects of fluoridation was like trying to enter a no-go zone.

Securing funding for fluoride research requires a lot of teeth gritting. In a commentary (Till & Green, 2020), she described some of the reactions her grant proposal elicited. One reviewer dismissed the proposal with the remark, "*This study is not needed. We know that fluoride is safe.*" Another reviewer commented, "*You can't look for risks of fluoride without evaluating its benefits.*" But if a researcher proposed a study on fluoride's anti-cavity benefits, it would be extremely unlikely that they would be told they must also examine potential risks!

Following numerous rejected grant applications, Dr Till and her team ultimately succeeded in securing their first R21 grant from the National Institute of Environmental Health Sciences (NIEHS) in 2016 to investigate the neurotoxicity of fluoride. Since then, Dr Till has obtained over $3 million in funding from prestigious organizations, including NIEHS and the Canadian Institutes of Health Research (CIHR), to support her ongoing fluoride research.

I first met Dr Till and heard about her research when she attended an anti-fluoridation talk hosted by an anti-fluoride activist in Toronto, Canada. She described the results of the world's largest study of urinary fluoride levels encompassing almost 2000 pregnant women living in Canada (Till et al., 2018). This work provided the necessary methodological details for informing the next phase of a series of high-quality studies examining how fluoride exposure may be linked with birth outcomes (Goodman et al., 2022a), infant neurodevelopment (Krzeczkowski et al., 2022), child IQ (Green et al., 2019; Till et al., 2020; Farmus et al., 2021; Goodman et al., 2022b), risk of ADHD (Malin & Till, 2015; Bashash et al., 2018; Riddell et al., 2019), sleep problems (Cunningham et al., 2021), and thyroid dysfunction in pregnant women (Hall et al., 2023; 2024). Dr Till formed collaborations with other highly respected environmental health researchers to test hypotheses about fluoride and child IQ in other birth cohorts from Mexico (Cantoral et al., 2021; Goodman et al., 2002c), Denmark (Grandjean et al., 2024), and more recently, the United States.

I was very impressed with her work: it was meticulous, complicated in terms of epidemiological statistics, and with results that were quite shocking, to say the least.

The Landmark Green et al. Study in 2019

Dr Till and her team's ground-breaking work used urinary biomarkers measured in pregnant women to predict cognitive outcomes in preschool-aged children. The research team studied 512 mother-child pairs from six cities in Canada and found that higher levels of fluoride in the urine of pregnant women, and in the water, they drank, were associated with a loss of 3 to 5 IQ points in boys—an effect that rivals that of lead. This study was conducted by Rivka Green, a clinical neuropsychology Master's student, who was being supervised by Dr Till.

Dr Till worked to get Rivka's Master's research published in a reputable, peer-reviewed journal. Before submitting the work for publication, the team was required to obtain approval from the Maternal-Infant Research on Environmental Contaminants (MIREC) Biobank committee. The manuscript underwent an extensive internal review by multiple experts from Health Canada and from various divisions of public health.

JAMA Pediatrics took a significant step in publishing the study, but only after subjecting it to a more than the usual peer-review process due to the controversial nature of the findings. On August 19, 2019, the study was published along with an editor's note and a podcast. The journal's editor-in-chief acknowledged that publishing the study was not an easy decision, but it was justified based on the study's methodological rigour and the strength of its tested hypotheses. He aptly observed that "it is neither the first, nor will it be the last, to test the association between prenatal fluoride exposure and cognitive development." In the accompanying podcast, the editor explained that the Green et al. (2019) study required an especially careful review because of its potentially contentious implications. He anticipated criticism for publishing it and emphasized that the journal took caution to ensure the study met the highest standards of quality. In retrospect, their caution was well-founded—this study attracted much attention and was ranked higher than 200,000 publications scored by Altmetric within two months of its publication (Altmetric "quickly collates a record of relevant online attention").

Opposition Faced by the Research Team

The pandemonium that followed after Dr Till and her team published their research was similar to the lead industry's attacks on Herbert Needleman's lead and IQ research. This was not a scholarly debate on the neurotoxicity of fluoride. Rather, this became an attack on epidemiology followed by scurrilous personal attacks on the scientists.

Those attacks were like the now banned bull fights of Spain. Picadors on horseback stab the bull with lances and banderilleros on foot use "banderillas," barbed sticks that are stabbed and anchored under the skin of the tormented bull. It is a cruel and unfair treatment meant to weaken the bull and at the same time rile it up to fight even harder, while the 'matadora' hides behind *her* red cloak waiting for an opportunity to kill the weakened beast.

What follows is a timeline of some of the academic banderillas Dr Till has had to withstand.

- In **August 2019**, major media outlets denounced the JAMA Pediatrics fluoride study. The dental profession responded swiftly and critically to the findings. Dentists and dental organizations argued that the study was flawed, pointing to methodological issues such as the reliance on urinary fluoride levels as a proxy for exposure and questioning the generalizability of the results to broader populations. Critics emphasized that "decades of research have supported the safety and effectiveness of fluoride," and some accused Till of exaggerating risks and spreading misinformation that could undermine public confidence in fluoridation. Scientists affiliated with the American Council of Science and Health publicly dismissed the findings as invalid.

- In **October 2019**, a letter signed by 30 academics and professionals from various health and dental institutions was sent to multiple organizations, including the Centers for Disease Control and national newspapers. The letter cited concerns about the replicability of scientific research and accused the team of withholding data even though anyone who asked for the data was provided with guidelines on how to access the MIREC data.

- An anonymous Rapid Response Report entitled "Community Water Fluoridation Exposure: A Review of Neurological and Cognitive Effects" was published in **October 2019** by Canada's Agency for Drugs and Technologies in Health (CADTH). This report, which narrowed in on a single study, concluded the Green et al. (2019) study was weak and had serious flaws, despite the report itself containing several factual errors. For example, the report stated that the study sample only included 369 mother-child pairs when in fact it included 512 mother-child pairs. Claims were made based on no scientific basis, such as "the fluoride-IQ association may have been driven by some outliers" (when in fact outliers were checked by the researchers) or "the decision to conduct a subgroup analysis based on sex was made post hoc" (also not true). The research team had contacted CADTH to alert them to the factual errors. They were directed to a disclaimer stating that:

  > *"CADTH is not responsible for any errors, omissions, injury loss, or damage arising from or relating to the use (or misuse) of any, statements, or conclusions contained in or implied by the contents of this document or any source of the source materials."*

  Because the authors of the CADTH report were not revealed, the public is unable to assess their qualifications and potential conflicts of interest. Without transparency about potential conflicts of interest, the report risks being biased and misleading. Regardless, the CADTH report was widely promoted by pro-fluoridation lobbyists on social media. They used the report to call the Green et al. (2019) study "fake science" and claim that the data did not support their conclusions.

  Dr Till and her team sent a formal letter to the Director of CADTH to share concerns about the accuracy of the report, the process in which the rapid review was developed, and how the report was being used by lobby groups. The report was later retracted from the CADTH website.

- In **July 2020**, a letter was sent to the York University Board of Governors by pro-fluoride lobbyists complaining about Dr Till's research and public appearances and asking for an independent review of her research. The York University President dismissed this letter and expressed support for Dr Till's academic freedom.

- In **August 2020**, pro-fluoridation activists contacted the president and executive members of the International Society for Environmental Epidemiology (ISEE) with concerns about Dr Till's research and requested that her symposium be cancelled (it wasn't).

- In **September 2020**, a second_letter to Mr. Paul Tsaparis (Appendix F) was sent to the Board of Governors at York University by the "International Group of Fluoridation Experts" and circulated to international media outlets defaming Dr Till. The letter asked the institution to establish an independent international committee to evaluate the quality of academic research conducted by Dr Till on fluoride. There is personal stress that accompanies such a complaint. Such charges can destroy a scientific career.

- An article from the *National Post*, one of Canada's national newspapers, (see Appendix G) called for an arm's-length review of Dr Till and her laboratory to determine whether 'ideology is being misrepresented as science'.

- In **May 2021**, the Calgary Rotary Club was contacted by pro-fluoride advocates asking that Dr Till not be permitted to present her research. The complaint was dismissed as members of this club wanted to hear from both sides of the fluoride debate.

- In **August 2021**, a lengthy complaint letter was sent to the President of York University, the U.S. Office of Research Integrity, editors of *JAMA Pediatrics*, and institutions of each collaborator. Allegations of research misconduct were made against Dr Till and her team, including claims of data manipulation and falsification. The letter requested that Dr Till be dismissed on "the grounds of falsification." Emails accessed through a Freedom of Information request revealed that the complaint letter was circulated to members from different dental organizations. In this email, a cautionary note is made stating that the letter "is defamatory".

- From **September 2021 to April 2022**, the Office of Research Integrity conducted investigations and determined that the allegations of research misconduct are not supported. All five universities involved in the research completely exonerate the scientists. I imagine the work of Dr Till and her team was severely disrupted by the need to defend themselves against false accusations.

- In **October 2022**, two letters were sent to the Editor of the journal *Environmental Research*, accusing Dr Till's research team of using methods that were "not scientifically proven." The letters referred to a paper examining critical windows of fluoride neurotoxicity (Farmus et al., 2021). Notably, one of the letters was sent by Ms Chris Wood on behalf of the Association of State and Territorial Dental Directors (ASTDD). She was later deposed as part of the fluoride trial (Chen, 2024) where she testified that she had never read the letter that she signed and did not understand its contents. The research team responded to each letter (Farmus et al., 2023a, 2023b).

Conversation with the Opposition

All of the *Fluoride Harm* chapter contributors regard Dr Till as an amazing bull in the academic bull ring, withstanding far more attacks than the average tenured professor. I suppose dentists and pro-fluoridation advocates thought they could 'bully' her into submission. Profluoride advocates would lie to the public and, when caught with a fact check, would simply backtrack to cover their own behinds and say "I misspoke."

Accusations that researchers are falsifying their research, covering up data, misinterpreting data, and misleading the public are serious accusations, even libelous as to warrant personal lawsuits.

But somehow, they simply thought they could get away with it.

Take, for example, this interchange between two well respected podcasters of *Undark*, Brooke Borel and Anna Rothchild, who spoke with Dr Scott Tomar (a new spokesperson for the American Dental Association) and Dr Christine Till on an episode examining whether fluoride is toxic at low levels (Is Fluoride Toxic at Low Levels? 2024). What was unique about this episode was that it focused on the "human conflict" dimension of fluoride research.

Below is the excerpt where Dr Tomar publicly admits he wanted to strip Dr Till of her tenured position at York University in Toronto. He first denies the fact and then tries to cover it up after being caught in a lie.

Brooke Borel (Undark): *So I do want to talk about a little bit about that retaliation — the potential for retaliation in this field. So, there were some letters that came out about specifically your work, Christine. And I know, Scott, you're involved in some of those letters. I was wondering if you could talk a little bit about that.*

Scott Tomar: *So, the ones that I signed — there was various attempts to access the data from the MIREC study, because there, frankly were some questions that a number of had about the data analysis. We were attempting to get the data, to do independent analysis of it. For a variety of reasons that never happened. So we've never (been) able to get it. The one that I would not sign, there was a letter and they had approached me and I flat out refused, was accusing the investigators, including Dr Till of professional misconduct. Which to this day I do not think was the case. And I would not lend my name to that. So, you know, requesting data, again, I think as part of the normal scientific process. You know, accusing people of fabrication or misrepresentation or other professional misconduct — again, I do not, I did not then and do not now feel that that is the case. And I would not lend my name to that letter.*

Brooke Borel: *A quick fact-check: Scott actually did sign some letters accusing Christine and her team of misconduct. There were many letters and this happened several years ago, but during our fact-check of this episode we found out that there were several with his signature. I followed up with him and he said that he misspoke here. He said, in part and I quote from an email: "I do not believe that there was fabrication of data, and I think that's what I had in mind when I answered your question. I was mistaken when I said that I did not sign letters alleging research misconduct." He also said that he continues to believe the paper intentionally omitted key information in its abstract and dramatically overstated its conclusion.*

Brooke Borel: *Christine, do you have any response to any of that? How, how was that and what, what do you have, what questions or comments do you have on that?*

Christine Till: *Well, what was the response? I mean, we've had a lot of letters sent, as some, by your guest here, and some more serious. Accusations of research misconduct is a serious threat to the principles of academic freedom.*

The day the paper was published in JAMA Pediatrics I said, you know, no one's going to believe this. Someone really should replicate the analyses. We did have multiple statisticians. An epidemiologist working in isolation did the analyses separate from a graduate student. Then we did hire a third analyst to replicate again. But, you know, it'd be nice to have someone outside of the group. Okay. So I was the one who originally said this should — I think all fluoride research should be done by two groups, quite honestly, because it's so polarized and nobody believes anyone. They'll say, oh, they're biased.

But, back to these letters, I received an email asking for access to the data, and I replied with here you go, there is an application, it took me almost a year to get through, it's a very lengthy and lots of forms. I went through it, I accessed the data belonging to Health Canada. It doesn't belong to me, but if you or anybody else would like to access it, you have to go through the process. So, to be accused later on — and actually I just saw it in the National Post again, just last week — that our research group are not sharing something. That's just completely false. But the media continues to — like, the damage has been done.

All of these letters that have been sent widely to media, now the media is putting those links up again. And so people naturally are confused. They don't know who to believe because they're hearing, "Oh, this group is withholding data," which is just not true. That is not the case. Anybody can write to me, ask me, can you run the analysis with this point missing or whatever. And we reply. So, you know, I should hope that people who are interested in the results can reach out to our group and ask a question and get an answer. That's, you know, how I think science should work.

***Brooke Borel:** Scott, did anyone in these letter writing campaigns try to reach out to Christine's group directly for any of this back and forth or did it go straight to the letters?*

***Scott Tomar:** I have to actually dig out the history. I don't remember where the — honestly I don't remember. I think that they did originally reach out to Christine's group.*

***Brooke Borel:** Christine's shaking her head. No, you don't remember. Yeah.*

***Christine Till:** I know who reached out and, um, definitely, well, there wasn't I can tell you.*

***Scott Tomar:** I honestly, I don't remember. I honestly don't remember the chronology of the letters.*

***Brooke Borel:** And what are your feelings about these letters now, Scott? Are you glad that you wrote them or do you have any regrets? Would you do anything — would you do things the same way or differently if you had the chance to do it again?*

***Scott Tomar:** Good question. I probably would address it in maybe a less threatening way. At the end of the day most of us on, on one side or probably in the dental world, you know we're all health care providers, most of also epidemiologists, we're parents, we're grandparents, you know. So I think at the end of the day, we all want to have some assurance of what's really going on. But I think if I were to do it again, maybe there's a less confrontational, less threatening way to have done that.*

***Brooke Borel:** I'm curious from both of you if it's harder or easier to be speaking directly about this stuff rather than these sort of confines of like the traditional sort of debate in science where it will be like a letter or a commentary or an op-ed or this sort of social media at this point, going back and forth. Like, how are you finding this conversation* *in comparison to those more formal and — informal with social media — channels?*

Christine Till: *Well. I don't engage on social media.*

Brooke Borel: *Probably wise.*

Christine Till: *It's not the forum for scientific discussion. This is a really complex topic. There's a lot of nuance. We have to bring people together, the dental community and the non-dental public health community. You know, I've come to realize that there's a differential weighting in what we value. Some value teeth more than IQ points. And it really comes down to this. I think overall, we're all invested in improving children's health. I do believe that, and it's trying to understand, can we come up with a way that we can achieve children's health with minimal harm and, you know, improve oral health and prevent any harm at the same time. So, I think, you know, we're moving in that direction. I would like to hope so. Yeah*

Brooke Borel: *I'm curious whether you have agreed or disagreed more than you were expecting during this conversation.*

Christine Till: *Well, could I ask Dr Tomar on his views on — would you recommend that a pregnant woman reduce her fluoride intake?*

Scott Tomar: *No, I don't think that I would recommend it.*

Christine Till: *OK, and if she told you she drank, you know, three cups of black tea made with fluoridated water — no problem?*

Scott Tomar: *I would say, and again I'm not the expert on the exposure to high levels of* ***caffeine*** *(??)(editor's emphasis). So, there may be other reasons that a pregnant woman might want to reduce her intake of black tea. I'm not yet convinced that this is a real effect again. Again, I may change my answer down the road. But as of today, no, I don't think so.*

Christine Till: *OK. So Brooke, to answer your question of whether we agree or disagree, I would say that on that point, I would say based on the science today it is time to at least acknowledge the evolving science, particularly for pregnant women. And knowing that there is zero benefit to the fetus of gestational exposure to fluoride, I think it is prudent to recommend reducing fluoride intake during pregnancy.*

And yeah, maybe we're all going to be — maybe the science will change. But until we see that data, I will say that I think it is prudent to reduce fluoride intake from whatever source. And black tea is one that can have very high sources of fluoride — levels of fluoride, I mean. So, that's one area I think we would disagree on.

Conclusion

Dr Christine Till's research at York University in Toronto has been both groundbreaking and contentious. Her 2019 study linking fluoride exposure during pregnancy to lower IQ scores in children challenged decades of public health orthodoxy, drawing sharp criticism and personal attacks from the dental community. Despite this opposition, her research sparked critical discussions about the safety of water fluoridation, influencing policy debates, and highlighting the need for further scientific inquiry and assessment of risks and benefits for pregnant women and young children (Till et al., 2025). Her current work continues to raise awareness about fluoride harm to the brain (neurotoxicity) and to the endocrine system (thyroid) and has contributed to an intensification of fluoride research around the world. Dr Till's resilience in the face of controversy (surviving all the banderillas) and her commitment to rigorous research exemplify her role as a leading voice in children's environmental health, even as the debate over fluoride's risks and benefits continues to unfold.

AUTHOR'S NOTE: Accusing a researcher publicly (in writing) of misconduct is libel and, in my opinion, is an attempt to destroy the good reputation of a scientist with an established track record of obtaining federal funding and publishing in well-respected international peer-reviewed journals. Given enough financial resources, I would have sued my accuser using anti-defamation laws when I had to defend myself against a frivolous complaint.

We have included in the appendix a letter sent to York University accusing Dr Till of misconduct and a news report that amplified the accusations (Appendices F and G) which includes Scott Tomar's signature contrary to his denial. These items are open access for all to read. They demonstrate the tactics of the proponents in trying to destroy the reputation of Dr Till. While we had reservations about including the letters (which might give proponents ideas on how to attack fluoride harm scientists), we decided to include them as a warning to those who think they can say anything about the anti-fluoridation researchers; your spurious actions may rebound on you. An analysis of researchers being accused of misconduct was published by Jaffe et al. (2025).

It Just So Happened...

By: Dr Kathleen M. Thiessen, PhD

ABOUT: *Dr Thiessen has worked in the field of human health risk assessment for more than 35 years, including evaluation of exposures to and health risks from chemical and radiological contaminants. She wrote two reports for the U.S. Environmental Protection Agency, including one on the health effects of hydrogen fluoride and related compounds. She has served on two National Research Council subcommittees, one charged with the review of fluoride exposure and toxicology, and one dealing with guidance levels for air contaminants in submarines, including hydrogen fluoride. Dr Thiessen was involved in the reconstruction of exposures, doses, and health risks to off-site individuals associated with historic releases of contaminants from the U.S. Department of Energy's Oak Ridge (Tennessee) facilities. She also contributed to the development of a risk-based screening approach to prioritize further investigation of contaminants and exposure situations in various assessment contexts. Dr Thiessen has led several working groups in the International Atomic Energy Agency's programs on environmental transport modeling. She has also been involved in litigation support for several cases involving chemical or radionuclide contaminants; she recently served as an expert witness for plaintiffs in a federal case involving fluoride toxicity. Dr Thiessen serves as a senior scientist and president at Oak Ridge Center for Risk Analysis, which specializes in human health and ecological risk assessments.*

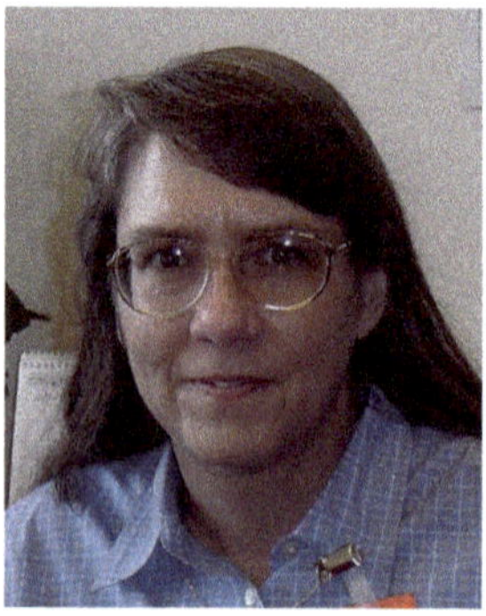

CHAPTER 26

"It is irresponsible to promote or encourage uncontrolled exposure of any population to a drug that, at best, is not appropriate for many .... and for which the risks are inadequately characterized and inappropriately disclosed to the public."

—Dr Kathleen Thiessen, PhD

IT JUST SO happened that my first professional assignment following graduate school was to prepare a draft report on fluoride toxicity for the Environmental Protection Agency (EPA). More specifically, this was to be a review of health effects associated with hydrogen fluoride, with an emphasis on airborne releases and exposures. I had joined the Chemical Hazard Evaluation Program of the Health and Safety Research Division of Oak Ridge National Laboratory (ORNL), which was contracted to provide various reports for the EPA. The scope of my review was eventually expanded, at my request, to include hydrogen fluoride and related compounds, and EPA published my report in 1988 (USEPA, 1988). This was my first significant involvement with the field of human health risk assessment, at a time when literature searches were not as easy to conduct as they are now.

As a newcomer to the field, I didn't fully appreciate all of the information that I found, and I now know that some of the information available at the time on beneficial effects was incorrect. Nevertheless, that 1988 report pointed out the dependence of chronic health effects on the total fluoride intake from all sources of fluoride, the slower clearance of fluoride and consequent higher risks for people with renal dysfunction, the likelihood that some of the decline in tooth decay attributed to fluoridated water was due to other causes, and that adverse effects as well as beneficial effects should be considered in setting fluoride levels.

At the time that I wrote the EPA report, I was only dimly aware that there was any controversy about water fluoridation. Looking back, I have wondered whether one of EPA's purposes in commissioning a review of airborne hydrogen fluoride was to provide support for the assumed safety of fluoride exposure. I vaguely remember having seen something about my hometown in South Carolina planning to fluoridate and thinking that was a good thing.

Bette Hileman's special report in *Chemical & Engineering News* was also published in 1988 (Hileman, 1988), but I didn't know about it until some years later. Some of the information on adverse effects considered as speculative in the 1980s has in recent years become much better supported, but at that time it was considered not important or not substantiated and certainly less than the benefits to be gained from water fluoridation.

Following my 1980s fluoride project, I worked on other EPA projects for a few years, while still employed with ORNL. EPA published a 1994 report on health effects associated with mercuric chloride which I drafted in the late 1980s, soon after writing the hydrogen fluoride report (USEPA, 1994). I left ORNL in 1989, did some consulting work for a while, and eventually joined SENES Oak Ridge, Inc., Center for Risk Analysis, when the company started in 1992. In 2014 we changed our name to Oak Ridge Center for Risk Analysis, Inc., of which I am now president. Our company is probably best known in the context of radiological risk assessment, but my background in chemical risk assessment at ORNL helped the company take advantage of opportunities in that area as well.

It just so happened that in 1998, a science teacher in the Lee County, Florida, school system sent a letter to the school board asking them to oppose efforts to start water fluoridation in the county. It also just so happened that my father was serving on the school board at that time. Dad sent the teacher's letter to his daughter, the scientist. I told him that water fluoridation was a done deal, everybody knows that it's a good thing. But also, for Dad's sake, I spent my Thanksgiving break looking at the issue, and I sent a letter through Dad to the school board in early December. It just so happened that by 1998, the Internet was making a large volume of literature readily available to the public, outside of university and technical libraries. Among other things, there were initial reports of increased lead levels in tap water in fluoridated areas, a finding that could have direct implications for a school board in terms of the neurological and behavioral problems already associated with lead exposure in children.

In addition, my brief review found a lack of toxicity studies of the actual fluoridation chemicals or of fluoridated tap water as consumed, the observed trend away from fluoridation in many other countries, and the failure of most studies to consider fluoride exposures in terms of individual fluoride intake rather than the fluoride concentrations in local water supplies. Given the wide range of tap water intakes in the population, considering only the fluoride concentrations in public water supplies means that a study will have significant overlap of exposure groups, potentially obscuring differences in health effects with respect to fluoride intake.

I also suggested in my letter that the Lee County School Board contact the Florida health department. At the time, my company was in the late stages of completing parts of the Oak Ridge Dose Reconstruction for the Tennessee Department of Health, assessing the effects on local populations of past chemical and radiological releases from the U.S. government facilities in and near Oak Ridge. I naïvely assumed that the Florida health officials would do a similarly responsible job with respect to questions from their constituents about water fluoridation. Later on, I came to realize that on the subject of water fluoridation, most health departments and public health agencies are not particularly objective. More than 25 years later, Florida's Surgeon General referred to community water fluoridation as "public health malpractice" and recommended against fluoridating. Florida's legislature banned fluoridation in May 2025 (Columbini, 2024; Florida DOH, 2024; Baletti, 2025b).

After my brief review of fluoridation in late 1998, my household started buying bottled water, just to try out. I had previously considered bottled water a justifiable expense mostly for beach locations where the tap water tasted pretty bad. But hey, if fluoride might cause bone and joint pain, I didn't want that. I didn't really expect to notice any difference from reducing my tap water consumption. It just so happened, however, that I was pleasantly surprised to find that some long-standing health issues disappeared in weeks. Fluoride sensitivity is real, and eminently testable, although there is relatively little recent literature about it. And it just so happened that I ended up having far more energy in my 40s and 50s than in my 20s and 30s, for which I am extremely grateful.

It also just so happened that, following my letter to the Lee County School Board, I began to hear from people around the country, both scientists and non-scientists, many of whom were concerned about possible harms from water fluoridation. One caller just so happened to be from the NRC. I had to ask her whether she meant the Nuclear Regulatory Commission, for whom I had done occasional work, or the National Research Council. It just so happened that she was organizing a committee for the National Research Council, at EPA's request, for the purpose of evaluating fluoride exposure and toxicity. The committee's efforts resulted in the 2006 NRC report (Doull et al., 2006). My work for the committee was my first major opportunity to get into the details of fluoride exposure and toxicity since my 1988 EPA report, but with the benefit of much more literature, much better search capabilities, and much more experience on my part.

Out of Scope

> *"Assessing the efficacy of fluoride in preventing dental caries is not covered in this report" (Doull et al., 2006, p. 14).*

> *"As noted earlier, this report does not evaluate nor make judgments about the benefits, safety, or efficacy of artificial water fluoridation" (Doull et al., 2006, p. 16).*

The NRC report considered community water fluoridation only with respect to its contribution to human exposures in the U.S. Specific consideration of either the safety or benefits of water fluoridation was outside the scope of the committee's assignment (Doull et al., 2006; Carton, 2006). However, we did not say or assume that fluoridation is safe or that fluoride concentrations of 0.7-1.2 mg/L (the range recommended at the time) in drinking water are safe. We specifically addressed EPA's health-based standard, the Maximum Contaminant Level Goal (MCLG), for fluoride of 4 mg/L, and we concluded unanimously that the MCLG is not protective of human health and should be lowered. This conclusion was based on the best-known (and hardest to deny) effects of dental fluorosis and skeletal fluorosis, along with increased risk of bone fracture, and should have resulted in a lowering of the MCLG by at least a factor of 10 (EPA's default minimum safety factor).

As of this writing in 2025, neither the MCLG nor the enforceable standard (the Maximum Contaminant Level, also 4 mg/L) has been lowered. Full consideration of the information now available on more sensitive endpoints such as developmental neurotoxicity and carcinogenicity should result in an MCLG of 0, corresponding to no safe level of fluoride exposure. The NRC report also noted the wide range of water consumption among members of the population; the very high water intake with respect to body mass of population subgroups such as infants, athletes, and outdoor workers; the importance of looking at individual exposures rather than average exposures of groups having different concentrations of fluoride in drinking water, given the potential for significant overlaps in exposure distributions for the groups; the importance of including all sources of fluoride exposure, not just the contribution from drinking water; and the need for further study of the actual fluoride chemicals used in water fluoridation, particularly the silicofluorides. The report considers fluoride to be an endocrine disrupter, and did not rule out a carcinogenic effect of fluoride. Research since the 2006 NRC report has consistently supported the NRC's findings with regard to the toxicity of fluoride.

It just so happened that the NRC contacted me again in 2008, to help with a report on potential health effects of selected air contaminants in

U.S. Navy submarines. One of those contaminants was hydrogen fluoride. The 2009 NRC report, which has largely escaped widespread notice, dealt only with healthy young adult men. Among other things, the report summarizes estimated average exposures associated with a variety of adverse health effects, based largely on the 2006 NRC report and within the range expected in populations served with fluoridated drinking water (NRC, 2009).

Although the NRC's 2006 report was prepared at the request of the EPA, and EPA "accepted the NRC (2006) findings as the summary of hazard for inorganic fluoride" (USEPA, 2010a, p. i), it appeared that EPA either did not fully read the report or hoped that no one else would read it. The 2006 NRC report concluded that EPA's drinking water standards are not protective against several adverse health effects, and, supported by the 2009 NRC report, it demonstrates that exposures from fluoridated water overlap with estimated average exposures of groups in which adverse health effects occurred. By their usual risk assessment procedures at the time, EPA should have identified a "safe" level of exposure and then applied appropriate safety factors to set the drinking water standards; properly done, this would have meant an end to water fluoridation. Instead, however, EPA inappropriately included an assumption of benefit in its assessment of adverse effects, left some of the most important subgroups out of their exposure assessment, allowed no margin of safety whatsoever (USEPA, 2010a; USEPA, 2010b), and to this date has not revised the drinking water standards that the NRC concluded were not protective.

Eventually, the U.S. Department of Health and Human Services (DHHS) changed its recommended concentration of fluoride in drinking water to 0.7 mg/L, instead of the former temperature-dependent range of 0.7-1.2 mg/L. This was an admission that the previous recommended levels of fluoride in drinking water were too high. The revised recommendation, which was proposed several years earlier (Federal Register, 2011), simply used the lower end of the previous range, but without demonstrating that the change would in fact bring about a reduction in dental fluorosis, the only adverse effect considered (USDHHS, 2015).

Expert Opinion v. Misinformation

In 2010, it just so happened that the Association of State and Territorial Dental Directors (ASTDD) wrote to the head of my company, suggesting that I was communicating misinformation about water fluoridation and otherwise being unscholarly and unethical in my research. Several years later, we were provided evidence of the involvement of the Centers for Disease Control and Prevention (CDC), the New York State Department of Health, and others in the sending of that letter. Ironically, a paper that ASTDD said I should use with respect to fluoride effectiveness contained essentially the same data as the paper that ASTDD objected to my using. Both papers used data from a 1986-1987 survey which, in fact, show essentially no difference in caries experience with respect to fluoride concentration in drinking water, but a very clear dose response for both prevalence and severity of dental fluorosis (Heller et al., 1997; Iida and Kumar, 2009). I just wasn't supposed to point this out.

It also just so happened that for several years, including the time period in which the NRC reports were prepared, I did a considerable amount of contract work for the Radiation Studies Branch of the CDC, representing them in projects at the International Atomic Energy Agency. Naturally, I felt a certain amount of gratification that while the CDC's Oral Health Division and others were hoping to derail my career, the Radiation Studies Branch of the CDC was sending me to Europe twice a year.

In 2015, it just so happened that I co-authored a paper that examined the significant financial benefit commonly attributed to water fluoridation, along with several key papers underlying the estimates of caries reduction attributed to water fluoridation (Ko and Thiessen, 2015). In fact, benefits are minimal at best, and many costs of fluoridating are typically not included.

A few years later, it just so happened that I was asked to serve as an expert witness for plaintiffs in a lawsuit against the EPA regarding the risk of developmental neurotoxicity from use of fluoridation chemicals in drinking water, a use that potentially exposes 200+ million people in the United States. After several rounds of reports and depositions and two trials, the judge's ruling in September 2024 concluded that water fluoridation poses an unreasonable risk of injury, and EPA is obligated to regulate it (Chen, 2024). This case would not have been necessary had EPA followed its own risk assessment procedures any time from the 1980s on. EPA's actual response to the court ruling is still to be seen.

Conclusion

I could not have planned my professional career in the way it turned out, even if I could have imagined it in advance. Providentially, it just so happened that I had the qualifications and experience necessary to contribute to the NRC reports, and later to testify against the EPA. I have simply tried to do a responsible job with the opportunities and challenges in front of me, especially where my efforts could improve the lives and health of others.

> *"Whatsoever thy hand findeth to do, do it with thy might."*
> *(Ecclesiastes 9:10a)*

"And who knoweth, whether thou art come to the kingdom for such a time as this?" (Esther 4:14b)

"The sixth commandment requireth all lawful endeavors to preserve our own life, and the life of others." (Westminster Shorter Catechism 68. A.)

Retired Before Fired

By: John Mueller, BSc, PE

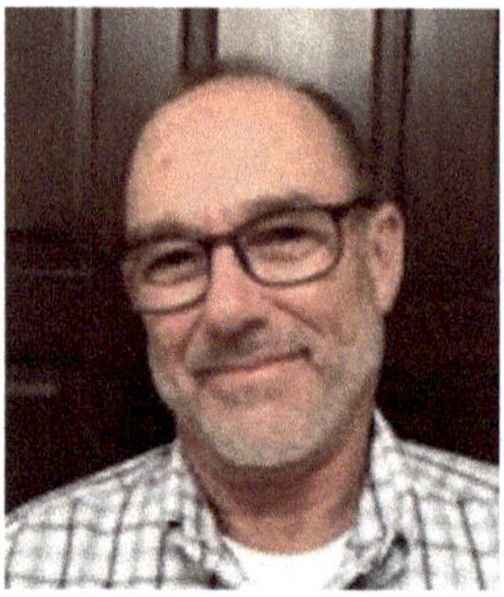

ABOUT: *John Mueller PE (Civil and Control Systems) is a 1984 graduate of the Colorado School of Mines in Golden, Colorado, with a BSc in Geophysical Engineering. He retired from his employment with the City of Tulsa, Oklahoma, and his Senior Engineer position in the city's Water and Sewer Department, effective January 1, 2016. He enjoyed a 25-year career in public works, mainly in water resources engineering, which began as an assistant engineer with the Santa Clara Valley Water District in San Jose, California, in 1990. During his 11 years with the Water District, he obtained his Professional Engineer license as a Civil Engineer, in addition to a Grade 4 Water Treatment Plant Operator certificate from the California Department of Health Services. That certification is authorization "TO OPERATE OR SUPERVISE THE OPERATION OF A WATER TREATMENT FACILITY FOR PRODUCTION OF WATER FOR DOMESTIC USE." He and his wife Sally reside in Edmond, Oklahoma near their family with growing young grandchildren. John's interest in fluoridation began around Earth Day in 2009. He started experiencing professional difficulties for that interest after authoring an article published in the Tulsa World newspaper in July 2014, titled "Water fluoridation needs a second look." What follows is part of his story.*

CHAPTER 27

"A people that values its privileges above
its principles soon loses both."

—U.S. President Dwight D. Eisenhower (1890-1969)

Arsenic—the Trigger

I HAD RECENTLY filled the vacancy for the Senior Engineer position in the Water Supply Section of the Tulsa Water and Sewer (W&S) Department when I received the assignment that started me on a path to get Tulsa to stop adding fluoridating chemicals to its drinking water. Little did I anticipate where it would lead, and the mission continues as of this writing.

It was April 2009 and only a couple months after I had transferred from the Water Design Section, I was given the assignment by Bob Brownwood PE, my boss, and Water Supply Section Manager. In the chain of command, Bob reported to the Director of W&S, who in turn reported to the Tulsa Metropolitan Utility Authority (TMUA, aka Utility Board). TMUA consists of six members appointed by the Tulsa City Council (nine councillors for nine council districts) and the mayor.

My new task was to review and update as needed the Technical Specifications for the Purchase Agreement for fluorosilicic acid (FSA) (chemical formula H2SiF6). That's when the arsenic contaminant caught my eye.

Significant at that time was the fact that fluoridation and its underlying conflicts in controversy were all new territory for me. The Water District in California did not start fluoridating San Jose's water until December 2016, more than 15 years after our move to Tulsa. My first seven years with the City of Tulsa, 2002 to 2009, focused mainly on providing engineering, technical and administrative support in offices where there was no direct connection with the fluoride being added at the city's two large drinking water treatment plants.

Launching into my assigned task, I perused the Purchase Agreement in effect at that time, along with a number of related historical files. It was a well-established requirement that a copy of the Certificate of Analysis (CofA) be provided with each FSA shipment upon delivery. The CofA listed the chemical analysis of that tanker truckload of FSA solution being delivered. That's when I learned—discovered, realized, and got somewhat concerned—that we were knowingly adding not just fluoride but also arsenic, a strictly regulated contaminant, to the public water supply.

The images in the Appendix E are copies of a Certificate of Analysis and a tabulation of periodic analytical results from the FSA supplier validating variable arsenic contamination in the fluoridation additive. A recent study states, "These findings suggest that public water arsenic exposure is associated with adverse birth outcomes, even at levels below the current US Environmental Protection Agency maximum contaminant level" (Nigra et al., 2025).

That was in the early days of a steep and challenging learning curve about the history and science of fluoridation. I became somewhat of an amateur lobbyist, approaching elected and appointed officials, arguing and advocating for the end of the fluoridation practice. With unbridled optimism, I tried cultivating relationships and sharing informative materials that I had gleaned from respected sources. But instead of educating them, I received an education in the decision-making process and resistance to change. It was a formidable obstacle that would inherently but ultimately manipulate the end of my cherished career; way too soon for this healthy and active person driven by a sense of purpose to make a difference for the public good. It became clearly evident that resistance to change and affinity for confirmation bias prevail among entrenched TMUA members and public health officials, some of whom have held their privileged appointments for decades.

The Learning Curve

Learning that the FSA added to drinking water was the washdown solution collected from air pollution control systems—the smokestack scrubbers—at phosphate mining and fertilizer production facilities in Florida, preyed on my mind. My passion for ending the practice of fluoridation was crystallizing. I was being forced to come to terms with the fact that the FSA added to Tulsa's tap water was a highly toxic, regulated, environmental pollutant, and if not sold for drinking water or for a select few other industrial uses, it would require costly disposal as industrial hazardous waste.

This chemical is a highly corrosive liquid with a pH of 1.2, a strong acid since it dissociates almost completely in water, releasing H+ ions. That chemistry is not important in this essay, but what is highly relevant is what I have labeled as the "regulatory compliance mindset," that prevails among water utility owners and managers and committed workers on down the line. It is the mindset that as long as we are not in violation of any water quality regulations, then we are doing our jobs and doing them well, on the premise that we were being completely effective at protecting public health by all federal, state and local regulatory standards.

My initial resolve, as such, was that even though we were knowingly adding carcinogenic arsenic to all the treated drinking water, we were legal because after dilution into the finished water, the arsenic's reportable concentrations in the water leaving the treatment plant were below the enforceable Maximum Contaminant Level (MCL) of 10 parts per billion (ppb; EPA's MCL and MCLG are explained below).

After setting aside my regulatory compliance mindset that everything was okay because we were legal, my major concern and argument soon became the overarching and nagging fact that we were knowingly adding for public consumption a carcinogenic contaminant with an MCLG of zero. I saw that as a serious violation of the spirit and intent of the federal Safe Drinking Water Act (SDWA) administered by the EPA, and more importantly a violation of the public trust. FSA contaminated with arsenic was consistently added to the drinking water at concentrations exceeding the EPA's MCLG of zero. Yes, it gets diluted to below the enforceable MCL, so we were legal, but legal does not equal safe, and that realization was clawing at my conscience.

For moral support I relied on prayer and McGraw-Hill's *Standard Handbook for Civil Engineers, Third Edition, Frederick S. Merritt, Editor,* a favorite in my personal library. In the first section on the very first page of narrative text and under the subtitle is a list of four canons to be embraced by the practicing engineer. The first states the engineer shall "Hold paramount the safety, health and welfare of the public . . . ." Practicing fluoridation, as I was learning, fundamentally contradicted that moral and ethical code of conduct.

Challenging my employer's deeply entrenched practice and pushing to repeal a city ordinance and an enshrined policy that had been in place for more than fifty years, was not in my published job description. If I persisted in my contrarian ways to some point of crossing a line, I could face disciplinary action for insubordination, even termination if they so desired, with my end of the deal having no plausible recourse; and there goes my pension to which the city and I had contributed during my 13+ years of productive employment as a civil servant for the City of Tulsa.

Back to the 'Regs'

The enforceable limit, or Maximum Contaminant Level (MCL) for arsenic was and is 10 parts per billion (ppb), or micrograms per liter (µg/L). MCLs are enforceable for regulated contaminants and are established by first determining a maximum safe level, or the unenforceable Maximum Contaminant Level Goal (MCLG). EPA's definition on its website states:

"The MCLG is the maximum level of a contaminant in drinking water at which no known or anticipated adverse effect on the health of persons would occur, allowing an adequate margin of safety." That margin of safety in EPA's standard practice is typically a factor of not less than ten, by their standards for establishing a safest level. So for a math example only, if we were to say fluoride's safe concentration level in water was scientifically determined to be 1.5 parts per million (ppm), then applying a safety factor of 10 would divide the safe level by 10, resulting in an MCLG of 0.15 ppm. The EPA's safety margin for the *unenforceable* MCLG is supposed to ensure the safety of the most vulnerable population groups. The *enforceable* MCL is established after considering the economic and technological feasibility of treatment processes required to remove the contaminant; it is supposed to be as close to the MCLG as possible.

A Bold Move on My Part

In the summer of 2014, I had written an opinion piece for the city's major newspaper, the *Tulsa World*, with the title "Water fluoridation getting a second look" which went to print in the July 30, 2014 edition. The editor of the opinion section thoughtfully and generously coached me through several drafts before accepting it for publication, and it was published as a "Readers Forum" column in the Opinion section, with face photo and a biographical byline.

My article was mainly based on industry standard fluoridation practices, but I did not reveal to the editor that I was a city employee, and I excluded that tidbit from the byline I provided. Soon after its publication, I was told by a coworker that after learning that the article's author was a city employee, one of the TMUA members had voiced his reaction with, ". . . *maybe we need to let him go*." I got nervous. What made it more difficult for the W&S director was the fact that I was no longer in the Water Supply Section but had transferred to a Senior Engineer vacancy at one of the largest wastewater treatment facilities, so anything to do with the drinking water side of W&S was no longer within my responsibilities or job description.

The second incident that put my future employment at risk involved the attached photos of the eyewash station, part of the emergency shower and eyewash station in the bulk FSA storage room at one of the treatment plants. The room is in the chemical building and is only for housing the FSA and associated mechanical infrastructure.

Should the need arise, in this toxic, corrosive ambient air in the bulk FSA storage room, how safely could an accident victim place their eyes directly over water spraying through the crusty deposits on the two nozzles of the emergency eyewash station? FSA vaporizes to hydrogen fluoride (HF), which makes hydrofluoric acid when combined with water moisture in air; it etches the glass in the building's windows. Plant operators had commented that FSA spilled on the floor can make the concrete look like Swiss cheese.

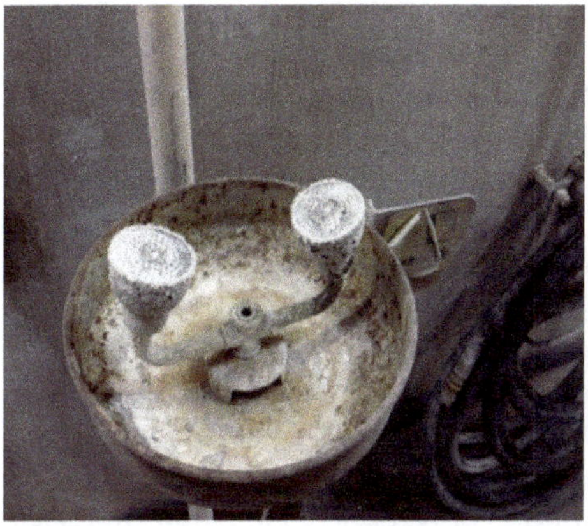

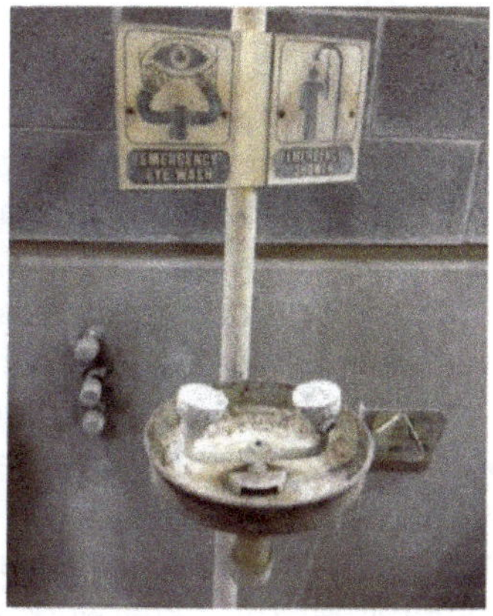

At a city health fair for employees, hosted by Human Resources, one of the information tables was manned by staff from the mayor's office representing a new committee created to collect employee suggestions for saving money during a budget crisis at the time. I shared these photos with the committee suggesting, as a conscientious employee, that ending fluoridation would save maintenance costs incurred from the damage to plant infrastructure due to the chemical's high corrosivity as seen in the bulk FSA storage room where these photos were taken. Then when I got on my soapbox with one of the mayor's staffers, it caused a bit of a stir. That's when I first heard words of warning about insubordination. I was getting close to crossing the line.

My suggestion for saving money was dismissed, and interestingly, not long afterwards the City entered into a construction contract for about $400,000, including the expense for a consulting engineering firm to design and oversee the work of completely refurbishing that bulk storage room and all associated equipment housed in it, including a completely new ventilation system, all due to FSA's extreme corrosivity.

After the situation with the photos of the emergency shower and eyewash station, the director of the Water and Sewer Department, Clayton Edwards, called me at my office at the wastewater plant and said he was coming out to talk to me. And he did the next day. We had a friendly visit, and he told me I really had to stop my activism about fluoridation because it was not in my area of responsibility. It was a friendly meeting, as we had known each other for years, including watching youth sporting events as our families were growing up.

The photos of the eye-wash station were taken in March of 2015. By that time, my interest in ending fluoridation had become somewhat of a crusade. I was fueled by a passion that would not let up. I had been studying the science and history of fluoridation since Spring of 2009, for about six years, continually discovering more reasons to stop adding this toxic hazardous waste to everyone's drinking water. Among other literature, I read Christopher Bryson's book, *The Fluoride Deception*, and juxtaposed it to the American Dental Association's *"Fluoridation Facts,"* a defining example of apologetics and seemingly riddled with misleading propaganda or falsifications to promote the practice.

I had a nice office at the wastewater treatment plant. I enjoyed and got along well with coworkers and contractors for plant maintenance projects I managed. My initiatives in areas of need were appreciated; I was productive and conscientious, did good work and I received positive performance reviews. But I could not, with a clear conscience, get off my soapbox about fluoridation.

I submitted the paperwork for my retirement soon after that visit from Clayton because I knew that if I was terminated, I would lose my pension, a future source of retirement income guaranteed for life. I arranged my effective retirement date for January 1, 2016. Clayton came out to the wastewater plant for my retirement party, and his quiet comment off to the side as he was leaving, and a compliment I later realized, was that he envied me.

But he was at the mercy of the Utility Board; he reported directly to them and the mayor. And I got to the point of knowing full well that they could direct him at any time to have me terminated if they got the notion. Continuing in my position for any more productive years would be doing so under a stressful dark cloud and at considerable risk. The Utility Board even had a financial incentive; my termination would separate me from my pension, and they could replace me with a lesser burden on the payroll. I value and depend on that monthly bank deposit from the City of Tulsa and still feel an allegiance to the city where we still do certain business and have lasting friendships.

Conclusion

Even today, I continue sharing facts and figures with Tulsa's leadership, keeping them apprised of current fluoridation-related activity at federal, state, and local levels, all of it informing a most responsible decision to end the practice.

I remain optimistic, the tide is turning. The message is getting through. People in my community go out of their way to thank me for my efforts to make our drinking water safer.

Most importantly, I can sleep at night knowing I have been doing the right thing.

The Struggles and Satisfactions of Being Editor of the Journal *Fluoride*

By: Dr Bruce Spittle, MB, ChB, ECFMG, DPM

ABOUT: *I was born in Oamaru, New Zealand, in 1945, graduated from Otago University with distinction in medicine (1969) and a Diploma of Psychological Medicine (1974), and became a fellow of the Royal Australian and New Zealand College of Psychiatrists. After some research experience, I was a Post-Doctoral Fellow and Physician in Psychiatry, University of Missouri and Mid-Missouri Mental Health Centre, Columbia, Missouri, USA, while in receipt of a Fulbright Hayes Research Scholarship and a Travelling Scholarship in Medicine. I then worked as a senior lecturer in the Department of Psychological Medicine, University of Otago, and as a consultant psychiatrist to the hospital board, 1978–2004.*

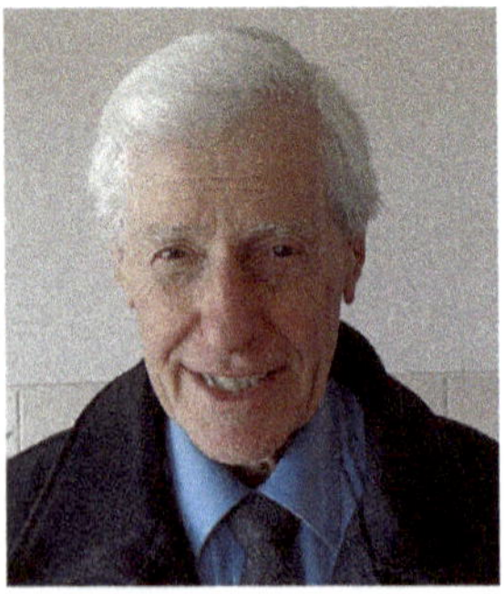

My interest in fluoride was sparked while on sabbatical leave in London in 1988 after reading Hans Moolenburgh's book, Fluoride: The Freedom Fight (Moolenburgh, 1987) and subsequently listening to John Colquhoun, a dentist who famously changed his mind about fluoridation (Colquhoun, 1997). After John became editor of Fluoride, 1991–1998, I helped him and became a co-editor, 1994–1998. Following John's death in 1999, Albert Burgstahler became editor and I helped Albert as managing editor, 1999–2013. Following Albert's death in 2013, I became the editor-in-chief, 2013–2024, and then a rotating editor-in-chief, 2024 to the present.

CHAPTER 28

"All truth passes through three stages: first it is ridiculed, second it is violently opposed, third it is accepted as being self-evident."

—Arthur Schopenhauer (1788-1860)

FLUORIDE, QUARTERLY JOURNAL of the International Society for Fluoride Research Inc. (ISFR) commenced publication in 1968. The previous editors were George Waldbott, 1968–1982; Albert Burgstahler, acting editor 1982–1991, editor 1999–2013; Edith Waldbott, interim editor 1982–1991; and John Colquhoun, 1991–1998. The position of rotating editor-in-chief was created in 2024 to make future transitions in the editor-in-chief role smoother.

For George Waldbott the struggles with fluoride began before he became editor. He said he had a good wife, Edith, who had a searching mind and drew his attention to the whys and wherefores of water fluoridation (Waldbott, 1965). He said initially his interest in the matter was lukewarm. However, his interest became aroused because of his experience with a patient drinking fluoridated water and his interest in drug sensitivity and drug intolerance.

He commented that in the past he had been credited with several basic contributions to knowledge in allergy and did not anticipate the repercussions involved in carrying out research on fluoridation. This was totally different from engaging in research on allergy. He said that he was not aware that it might wreck a man's career. He said that when he began questioning the safety of water fluoridation, a large segment of Detroit dentistry began questioning his competence and representatives of the Detroit District Dental Society requested that the Council of his medical society censure him.

Dr Wadbott wondered if he should drop what would be an extremely challenging study but asked himself if he was a coward and could be intimidated. He considered that he could withstand the campaign of disparagement and slander which had begun and decided to go on. He spent many months at the library searching the literature, consulted biochemists and dentists, studied microscopic sections of teeth and bones and took up the study of Italian and Spanish in order to acquire at least a reading knowledge of these sources. He had already covered the French and German literature. He documented his findings in a review article, "Medical evidence against fluoridation of public water supplies." After contacting the American Medical Association (AMA) *Journal and the New England Journal of Medicine* he realized that the subject had already become such a political issue with the medical profession that it would be impossible to have the article published in any American medical journal. He therefore printed the paper at his own expense and sent it to members of his medical society and to some Detroit dentists. Eventually it reached dental groups outside the USA and *The Australian Journal of Dentistry* requested the privilege of publishing his paper (Waldbott, 1955a).

In response to the paper's publication two proponents of fluoridation, Professor Philip Jay and Dr Fred Wertheimer, requested critiques of the paper from Dr Gerald J. Cox, Dr F.J. McClure and Dr A.L. Russell. The critiques were used to prepare a dossier on Dr Waldbott which became part of a brochure, "Comments on opponents of fluoridation," which was disseminated by the Bureau of Public Information of the American Dental Association (ADA) and by the United States Public Health Service (USPHS).

The dossier accused him of intellectual dishonesty and incompetence. Subsequently, wherever he raised his voice against fluoridation, the dossier always showed up like a steady companion. It was widely distributed to fluoridation committees of district dental societies, officials of medical societies, key lay persons, and leaders of clubs and organizations, whenever and wherever there was a need for countering his data. It reached hundreds of communities in the USA. It was received in Germany; Holland; the Svenska Dagbladet, Stockholm, Sweden; the Berner Bund, Switzerland; and the New Zealand Fluoridation Commission of Inquiry.

The report of the 1957 New Zealand Commission of Inquiry on the fluoridation of public water supplies (Stilwell et al., 1962) did not refer to receiving a dossier on Dr. Waldbott but reviewed three of his papers (Waldbott, 1955a; Waldbott, 1955b; Waldbott, 1956) and formed the opinion that the individual signs and symptoms of the alleged syndrome might be due to any number of unrecognized causes and that there was no causal relationship between any of these signs and symptoms and the ingestion of water containing 1 ppm of fluoride and food cooked in this water.

Dr. Waldbott said that in spite of the efforts of the ADA and the USPHS to eliminate him from the fluoridation battleground, his article gained him the reputation of being a conscientious and thorough student of the subject among many of his colleagues and certainly among those in the habit of arriving at their own conclusions without relying upon so-called "authorities" to do their thinking for them.

Waldbott commented that by 1960, many physicians and scientists in both the USA and abroad recognized the need for meetings and free discussion on fluoride research. Following a successful conference in Bern, Switzerland, in 1962, the newly formed *American Society for Fluoride Research* held a similar conference in Detroit in 1966 and Waldbott then formed the ISFR which held its first conference in Frankfurt am Main, Germany in 1967. Through its conferences, and its official journal, *Fluoride*, the ISFR has contributed materially to the advancement of research on fluoride, especially on matters biological and medical (Waldbott et al, 1978). He noted that at no time has the Society been involved with the politics of fluoridation and that its members hold widely differing views on the subject and on the role of fluoride in air and water pollution. Biochemists, physicians, dentists, veterinary scientists, botanists, physicists, and engineers from many parts of the globe have participated in its meetings. Thirty-six conferences have been held with the other hosting countries being Spain, Austria, the Netherlands, England, the United States of America, Switzerland, India, Japan, Hungary, the People's Republic of China, Poland, New Zealand, Canada, Iran, and Thailand.

Waldbott observed that, nevertheless, the promoters of fluoridation had interfered with this worthwhile congregation of researchers with a conference planned for Rome in 1962 being cancelled at short notice with no reason given and the publisher of the proceedings of the 1963 Bern conference being threatened with a boycott of future business if he went ahead with the publication. Another publisher did the job (Gordonoff, 1964).

Waldbott noted that several US scientists who had at one time contributed papers to the conferences or to the *Fluoride* journal suddenly withdrew their involvement without giving any reasons, despite strong previous interest. One scientist, who had been engaged in basic research on fluoride at his institution, informed him that he was no longer permitted to pursue research on fluoride at his institution, which relied on USPHS research grants. Another, who was scheduled to participate in the program at one of the conferences, candidly acknowledged that USPHS, which was supporting his research, would not give him permission to attend.

Waldbott described *Fluoride* as a veritable encyclopedia covering all aspects of fluoride research. Nevertheless, Index Medicus, published by the USPHS's National Library of Medicine (NLM) and a major source of references to fluoride-related health topics, has repeatedly declined to include *Fluoride* in its list of journals indexed. Since this journal was the only one in the world devoted exclusively to fluoride research, he wondered why the NLM consistently decided "not to include *Fluoride* in *Index Medicus*" although other journals far less important to human health such as purely chemical journals were included. He was concerned that the foremost effect of banning *Fluoride* was that various public health figures, such as doctors and dentists, were deprived of access to information about the numerous effects of fluorides on humans, animals, and plants. Waldbott asked in 1978 why most scientists and laymen remained ignorant of the dangers of fluoridation? He reflected that no single reason by itself sufficiently explained the general state of mind regarding fluoridation but that one point was clear: scientists and the public were not ignorant because the many opponents of fluoridation had been silent. Quite the contrary, from the very beginning they had cried out with loud voices, enumerating the scientific, logical and moral reasons for not adding an unnecessary cumulative toxic substance to public water supplies. Their reward was harassment, intimidation, and persecution, as well as loss of previous reputation, research grants, and employment. His sad conclusion was that had the USPHS taken another posture, fluoridation would, in 1978, have been on the historian's shelves with the other mistakes of the past (Waldbott et al., 1978).

Waldbott concluded that no other procedure in the history of medicine had been praised so highly and condemned so thoroughly at the same time. He saw that few other examples existed where health-bringers had ignored so much unequivocal scientific evidence of human harm—actual as well as potential—in order to implement a controversial health measure. Fluoridation, a program of almost inescapable mass medication, had no parallel in the experience of man.

Waldbott, born in Speyer, Germany, on 14 January 1898 was aged 80 when he wrote about his struggles as editor of *Fluoride* in 1978. However, he also described satisfactions. He wrote, "As I enter the twilight of my long and active medical career, I know that the path I chose long ago, though strewn with many obstacles, is the only one I could have taken. No more satisfying or humane goal can be attained than the truth which alleviates the suffering of mankind. When medical practitioners everywhere also recognize the severity of the problems of chronic fluoride toxicosis, and laws mandating truly safe drinking water are sincerely enforced, the health of millions will dramatically improve. Only then will fluoridation cease to be *The Great Dilemma*." George Waldbott died on 17 July 1982.

In 2008, a new application made to the NLM for inclusion of *Fluoride* in MEDLINE was again rejected (Burgstahler et al., 2009). In declining it, Sheldon Kotzin, MLS, Associate Director, Library Operations, NLM, reported that *Fluoride* did not receive a high enough score for inclusion in MEDLINE at a journal selection panel meeting. A number of examples of shortcomings in the journal were noted including the insufficient development of animal models, vague end points in some human studies, lack of ethical clearance for some fetal studies, references to other articles in *Fluoride*, lack of information on conflict of interests and informed consent, and a predominance of articles on fluoride toxicity.

To many, these concerns would appear to be comparatively innocuous and even specious but they were answered (Burgstahler, 2009):

- The collateral review panel cited no examples of animal models being insufficiently developed. In fact, the effects of fluoride in rats, for example, have been extensively studied.

- In the human studies published in *Fluoride*, there were no vague end points; in every case, the adverse effects were consistent with those expected from fluoride.

- The fetal studies were performed outside the USA where the IRB standard would not be applicable. *Fluoride* is an international journal and reports the research done in many countries. In the general information section, each issue of *Fluoride* noted that authors must indicate whether their institutional and national guidelines for the care and use of laboratory animals were followed. When reporting experiments on human subjects, authors should indicate whether the procedures followed were in accordance with the ethical standards of the responsible committee on human experimentation (institutional and national) and with the Helsinki Declaration of 1975, as revised in 2000 (World Medical Association, 2000).

- Citing articles published in *Fluoride* can hardly be construed as a scientific shortcoming when those articles are relevant to the report at hand. Since it is devoted to publishing reports of fluoride research, *Fluoride* can hardly be faulted for self-citation, which occurs as expected in virtually all research journals.

- In regard to conflict-of-interest or informed consent issues, these matters are usually dealt with by authors in their covering letters of submission and/or in the acknowledgements section of their papers

- As for "balance" between pro- and anti-fluoride articles, a list of pro-fluoride items published in *Fluoride* was in fact sent to Mr. Kotzin and acknowledged by him. Why, however, should there even have to be any kind of "balance," since no exclusively pro-fluoride dental and medical research journals are excluded from MEDLINE? By taking this position of excluding *Fluoride* because it is deemed as having "insufficient balance" between pro- and anti-

> F research reports, the collateral review panel revealed its own conflict-of-interest in standing by the official dental health policy endorsement of water fluoridation by the National Institutes of Health under which the NLM operated as part of the US Department of Health & Human Services. In making this decision not to index *Fluoride* in MEDLINE, the NLM clearly appeared to be out of step with the National Research Council of the US National Academies (NRC) whose 2006 report on Fluoride in drinking water: a scientific review of EPA's standards (Doull et al., 2006) contained far more citations (57) of research published in *Fluoride* than in any other journal among its 1077 references.

This non-indexing of *Fluoride* in MEDLINE obviously makes citing relevant research published in *Fluoride* less likely. For example, a report on the genetic susceptibility to dental fluorosis in mice (Carvalho et al. 2009) did not cite a highly relevant study in *Fluoride* on prior related work in humans (Liu et al., 2006).

Although Mr. Kotzin stated that *Fluoride* was rejected for inclusion in MEDLINE because of professional shortcomings and insufficient scientific quality, the rejection really appeared to stem from the fact that peer-reviewed reports in *Fluoride* by well-qualified researchers dealt with toxic effects of fluoride that called into question the credibility of the unwavering endorsement of water fluoridation and dental fluoride use as completely safe by the US Department of Health & Human Services.

A further application for inclusion of *Fluoride* in MEDLINE in 2013 was again rejected by the NLM (Spittle, 2014). The negative decision appeared to stem from the unyielding endorsement of water fluoridation and dental fluoride as being completely safe.

Again in 2021, *Fluoride* was not recommended for MEDLINE. The overall comments and basis for the recommendation by the Literature Selection Technical Review Committee (LSTRC) were: "There is no one element by itself that tends to disqualify a journal from being recommended. The overall appraisal of a journal's scope and coverage, editorial policies and processes, scientific rigor of article content, production and administration, and impact determine the LSTRC recommendation."

The reviewer comments noted that most of the previously identified defects had not been corrected, that the journal's impact could be increased by increasing the scientific quality of the articles and reducing the acceptance rate, speeding up the time to publication, improving production and administration, reducing spelling errors, improving the figures, enforcing ethical policies better, and making the website more user friendly

After taking these comments on board with a website upgrade, clearer ethical policies, and the use of a template to speed up publication, a further application for listing *Fluoride* in MEDLINE was made in 2025. This time the Journal passed the initial assessment including the editorial policies and the policies on the peer-review process, conflicts of interest, human and animal rights, and informed consent.

However, NLM determined that the journal was not currently suitable for the NLM Collection, due to significant concerns over the scientific and editorial quality. In the future, NLM would like to see evidence of more rigorous evaluation methods and improved clarity of the reporting across articles. No other details of the concerns were given. A further application can be made after 24 months.

At present, community drinking water continues to face choppy waters (Spittle, 2025) with a United States District Court ruling that community water fluoridation at 0.7 mg/L presents an unreasonable risk of injury to health (Chen, 2024) and a Cochrane Library report (Iheozor-Ejiofor et al., 2024) finding the benefits of community water fluoridation are slight and less than previously. Florida and Utah have now passed legislation prohibiting community water fluoridation. While the goal of having excellence in journals is laudable, the flip side of excluding from MEDLINE journals still to reach this high standard is the risk that papers reporting toxicity, such as developmental neurotoxicity from low levels of fluoride, may receive less attention than is ideal. This is detrimental to public health. For example, a paper published in *Fluoride* showing that fluoride, in doses comparable to those often being consumed by some individuals, can adversely affect male fertility (Long et al., 2009) was not listed in MEDLINE.

My Tenure

Being an editor of *Fluoride* has had both struggles and satisfactions. My life may have been easier by avoiding taking up the challenge presented by fluoride. My affiliation with *Fluoride* was regarded with disfavour rather than being a source of pride by the local university which has a School of Dentistry that continues to strongly support fluoridation. One of the papers presented at the Otago Medical School's 150th celebrations on May 31, 2025 was by a strong supporter of the safety of community water fluoridation and the lack of any associated developmental neurotoxicity, Professor Jonathan Broadbent (Department of Oral Sciences, Faculty of Dentistry), whose topic was "Are we communicating with facts on community water fluoridation?"

My involvement with fluoride research was also seen adversely and as supportive evidence of my being eccentric in a court case resulting a conviction on two charges of indecent assault. The case involved a seriously mentally disordered inpatient of mine in a psychiatric hospital who alleged, 14 years later, that I had repeatedly indecently assaulted her. The alleged offences existed only in her mind and not in reality. No evidence that the offences had actually occurred was presented in court and it was a situation of she said/he said. An 11:1 majority jury guilty verdict was accepted by the judge from a jury of 11 women and 1 man. This gross miscarriage of justice resulted in my medical registration being removed. Appeals to the Court of Appeal, the Supreme Court, Te Kāhui Tātari Ture, and the Criminal Cases Review Commission were unsuccessful. A second application to the Commission is currently being considered.

The National Library of Medicine takes very seriously the need to ensure that the material included in its collection is scrupulously correct in every aspect. However, it is not the only approach that can be productive. *The Annals of Improbable Research*, a six-issues-a-year magazine, is unlikely to ever be granted MEDLINE coverage but plays a useful role spotlighting genuine, improbable research culled from the entire world as well as original improbable research. They publish real improbable research about anything and everything, from everywhere that makes people LAUGH, then THINK. The company, Improbable Research (https://improbable.com/), and a much larger volunteer community of improbable researchers gather all this stuff, write about it, and produce events such as the presentation of the Ig Nobel prizes. They are an international group of scientists, journalists, teachers, artists, musicians, indescribables, introverts, extroverts, short people and tall people and also medium size people, each and every one of whom is somewhat delightfully quirky. Examples of their papers are: "Is Anything That's Alive Kind of Complicated?", "Does Health Insurance Make You Fat?", and "Calculating the guano-equivalent output of NYC residents". In publishing papers that make people laugh and think, the editors of *Improbable Research* "hope to spur people's curiosity, and to raise the question: How do you decide what's important and what's not, and what's real and what's not—in science and everywhere else?" They quote Isaac Asimov who noted that "The most exciting phrase to hear in science, the one that heralds new discoveries, is not 'Eureka!' but, 'That's funny...'" and Sherlock Holmes, a creation of Sir Arthur Conan Doyle, who credited for his inspiration, Joseph Bell, a surgeon at the Royal Infirmary of Edinburgh, said "Once you eliminate the impossible, whatever remains, no matter how improbable, must be the truth."

It is perhaps improbable that a journal such as *Fluoride,* a diamond open access journal which is free for both readers and authors, has continued to be published for 58 years with the lack of recognition from established institutions such as the National Library of Medicine. Like Improbable Research, it has many international volunteers doing most of the work and quirky persons have not been entirely absent from its ranks. In addition to his concerns about fluoride, Albert Burgstahler was also passionate about the authorship of Shakespeare and spent many hours researching cryptological evidence to support the case that the 17th Earl of Oxford, Edward de Vere, was the true author.

However, two realities remain. One, which encourages promoting knowledge to reduce fluoride-induced harm once its reality is recognized, is inscribed on the wall near the entrance to the Hercus Building of the Otago Medical School, Dunedin, New Zealand: "Where the love of man is, there also is the love of healing" (Hippocrates). Another, which encourages persistence in the face of adversity, is: "All truth passes through three stages: first it is ridiculed, second it is violently opposed, third it is accepted as being self-evident" (Arthur Schopenhauer).

An Oregon Story

By: Lynne Campbell, BA, MA

ABOUT: *My unusual parents, Malcolm and Mary Ellen, researched the things they cared about most, so that my sisters and I were raised with unconventional perspectives, mostly on health and nutrition, that are fairly widely accepted today. We grew up attending silent Quaker Meeting, and I still resonate with Quakers 'belief in listening to "the still, small voice" within and following one's conscience. Maybe it's why I feel compelled to speak out—often quaking inside—against what I see as injustice or deception. My eclectic education includes a Bachelor's in Music Composition, a Canadian Secondary Teaching Certificate, and a Master's in Organization Systems Renewal. Over the years, I have had a varied career, holding various positions in offices, teaching High School English and Music Theory, and buying media for advertising clients. The skills I acquired served me well in managing the nonprofit I would found in 2001 and in doing what I consider my most important work, educating people about fluoridation. My father died in 1993, but I will always be grateful to my sisters and my late mom for their support. During legislative sessions, Mom would come from Montana to winter with me, taking over cooking and housekeeping chores, and even collating documents, so that I could keep working. To oppose fluoridation is to be challenged, and my family always had my back.*

CHAPTER 29

"The controversy about fluoridation was inevitable because fluoridation was, in a real sense, conceived in sin. Fluoride is a major waste product of industry and one of the most devastating pollutants of the aluminum industry. The government not only dismissed the danger and left industry free to pollute, but it has promoted the intentional addition of fluoride - most of which is recycled industrial waste - to the nation's drinking water."

—Professor Albert Schatz, PhD (1995)

THE YEAR I WAS BORN, 1950, was the year the US Public Health Service endorsed community water fluoridation. It was a time when DuPont's tagline "Better Things for Better Living Through Chemistry" conveyed a sense of optimism about what was possible in the seemingly modern 20th century.

While growing up, conversation about fluoride and fluoridation was fairly common around our house. My dad Malcolm and granddad Julian Campbell, both Yale graduates with degrees in engineering, had concerns. As engineers, they questioned a water utility's ability to maintain a consistent concentration of fluoride throughout its system. They were aware of fluoride's extreme toxicity and its source as an industrial waste product and worried about adverse health effects. As a child, I could understand their frustrations both with a policy that was ridiculously wasteful—less than one percent of treated water is ever consumed by people—and with proponents 'emphasis on the so-called safety of the *concentration* added to water, rather than the actual *dose* each person would ingest.

Granddaddy Campbell, a self-made man with over 50 patents to his name, was a colorful character. On one of his rare visits, he embarrassed Mom in a restaurant by twirling paper napkins and sticking them in his ears as a signal to management that he didn't care for their music. He liked big cars—I remember a Chrysler Imperial and a Lincoln Continental—on which he affixed a large, professionally-rendered sign featuring a monkey holding a sack of poison over a pool of water. It read, "Don't Let Them Monkey With Our Pure Water. No On Fluoridization."

Years later, when I became involved in the issue full-time, I inherited a collection of documents from an elderly activist. Among them I found one of Granddaddy's 23-page pamphlets, "Fluoridization; 'The Crime of the Century.'" (The word "fluoridation," he explains—"a perfectly good geological term"—was "purloined" by promoters, making it easy to confuse with "chlorination." The correct word, he insisted, is "Fluoridization.") I don't know how his pamphlets were distributed, but this particular one is from a 1965 tenth edition of 25,000.

Although I was born in California, at age nine, our family settled in Newberg, Oregon, a small town 25 miles southwest of Portland. The year was 1960, and in '62, a second attempt was made to fluoridate Oregon's "Rose City." Those are years I particularly associate with the names Drs George Waldbott, Fred Exner, and Albert Burgstahler, names that would be familiar to anyone who has ever delved seriously into the science of fluoride's effect on health. Dad knew Dr. Exner personally and considered him a friend; his connection with Burgstahler is less clear to me now, though I'm sure they were in touch at least by mail or telephone.

Despite numerous attempts made over decades to fluoridate Portland's water, strong opposition has always prevailed, and the city remains the largest in the U.S. never to have adopted the practice. And, so, fluoridation was something that faded from my attention until the 1990's when I learned of repeated efforts to mandate fluoridation throughout the state by way of bills in the Oregon legislature.

Oregon Trail

While the idea of mandatory legislation was gaining ground at the state level, a local effort emerged in Lake Oswego, a suburb of Portland and my hometown at the time. Somewhere along the line, I had connected with the late Jeff Green, founder of Citizens for Safe Drinking Water based in San Diego. I came to rely on Jeff and his website as sources of accurate, science-based and well-documented information which I used extensively to bring myself up to date on the issue. I joined with other Lake Oswegans in opposing the fluoridation effort, and, perhaps due to the significant public outcry, the matter was dropped.

But as we approached the end of the year 2000, promoters of the statewide mandate seemed poised for victory in the upcoming legislative session. They had garnered even more support than I'd been aware of. From a *Willamette Week* article (Budnick, 2001), I learned:

- The Oregon Health Division had been given an $88,000 grant to "promote public acceptance" of water fluoridation.

- Dr. H. Whitney Payne, a Public Health Service employee, had been hired as Oregon's new dental director. In an email sent to prominent fluoridation promoter Michael Easley, Payne exudes confidence in their success. He writes, "...the entire Oregon Health Division is behind water fluoridation... I will be able to take Portland off the Surgeon General's list."

- Support for a mandatory bill had continued to grow at the legislature with key committee members on board as well as the senate president and the minority leader who claimed "the entire health community [is] behind us," and that the governor, physician John Kitzhaber, was ready to sign the bill.

Then, on December 20, Portland's *Oregonian* profiled Dr. Martin Wasserman, Oregon's new chief health administrator and reported that fluoridation was one of his top priorities (Koglin, 2000). That was the tipping point for me; I knew then that without a massive, well-organized counter effort, mandatory fluoridation would become our reality. At the time, undertaking that effort felt like a calling. I closed my advertising buying business and began building the nonprofit I would direct pro bono for the next five and a half years—Oregon Citizens for Safe Drinking Water (OCSDW), loosely affiliated with Jeff Green's national organization.

On January 9, 2001, the Oregon legislative session began, and SB99, seen as "the keystone of the Oregon Health Division's plan for improving the dental health of Oregonians," was introduced. The bill required all communities of 10,000 or more to fluoridate their drinking water.

As I look back, I am amazed at what we accomplished between the opening of the session and the hearing that was held in committee on April 11. Jeff became an invaluable mentor over those months; he traveled to Oregon twice, and we stayed in frequent contact. Without the benefit of his strategy and wise counsel, I doubt we would have been successful.

First of all, we were not anti-fluoridationists; we were safe water advocates. Jeff strongly believed that people were more attracted to efforts that were for, rather than against, something.

Next, instead of going head-to-head with dentists and physicians by engaging in their arguments about children and teeth, we would change the conversation (much as one redirects an opponent's energy in the practice of Aikido). It isn't that we would never talk about teeth or health, but that we wouldn't start there. We would focus primarily on the product by suggesting to a legislator, "If you choose to enact this policy, at some point, a truck loaded with fluoridation chemicals is going to show up in your community. Let's talk about what's on that truck, where it came from, and how poorly it is regulated." These were conversations legislators had never had. Even the promoting dentists at the time were unaware of the source of the chemicals.

Jeff recommended introducing his draft of counter legislation that later came to be known as the "Water Quality Assurance Act." Our bill would help neutralize a promoter' bill while serving as an educational tool. The Act 1) prevented the addition of any drug to drinking water that had not been FDA-approved for its intended purpose, and 2) made it illegal to add something to public water laced with contaminants at levels above their EPA-established Maximum Contaminant Level Goals (MCLGs).

Finally, throughout my tenure as director of OCSDW, I carefully followed another one of Jeff's maxims, one that served me well: To never make a statement publicly I couldn't support with documentation that would stand in a court of law.

And so, that January, I began the work of doing whatever was required: getting my Board of Directors in place; developing a body of supporters I would update regularly; preparing documentation for legislators and the public; getting media attention and interviews; finding credible people who would testify on our behalf at the hearing; lobbying legislators, something I had never done; and securing a sponsor for our bill (SB744 was never heard in committee but served to help legislators better understand the issue).

Jeff's strategy seemed a perfect fit for me. Talking about fluoridation products didn't put legislators already favoring the mandate on the defensive. I was presenting new information that opened up conversation. Because appointments were typically short—I could count on about 15 minutes unless a legislator had questions—focusing on the product allowed me to be effective in dealing with the complicated, multi-faceted issue that fluoridation is. And, as a lay person, it lent me credibility I would have lacked, in spite of authoritative documentation, had I concentrated on teeth and health.

Focusing on the product gave me another advantage. In those first few months, I aggressively sought and was successful in gathering environmental support. Not only was the product—hydrofluorosilicic acid (FSA) and its salt derivatives—the untreated waste of phosphate fertilizer production, contaminated with heavy metals and other toxins, but classic studies done on the Columbia River and at Hood Canal in Washington had found that very low levels of fluoride in fresh water—as low as one-fifth of the one part per million level recommended for drinking water—were toxic to salmon, an important Oregon industry.

I remember on more than one occasion thanking my lucky stars for some of the breaks that came my way. Salmon was one; another came in the form of Nick Budnick, a reporter with Portland's alternative paper *Willamette Week.* Nick had recently moved to Oregon from California where Jeff had known him and trusted his work. In Nick's big February story on the fluoridation push, rather than characterizing me as a "crazy," I'm described as "a soft-spoken woman with graying dark hair...[who] was until recently a successful ad buyer..."

"Today, however," he goes on, "she is the volunteer head of Oregon Citizens for Safe Drinking Water. In the '50s and '60s, extreme conservatives considered fluoridation a communist plot. Campbell's views bear little resemblance to theirs; her opposition is based on science and individual rights." Under a photo, it reads, "Lynne Campbell, fluoridation's worst nightmare, isn't talking conspiracy theories..." (Budnick, 2001)

By the time of the April 11 hearing, we had secured an impressive line-up of people who would testify. Key presenters included:

- Hardy Limeback PhD DDS, (another one of my lucky breaks) a practicing dentist, former president of the Canadian Association for Dental Research, and Head of Preventive Dentistry at the University of Toronto, Ontario, Canada;
- Eric Dover MD, a family physician and member of Physicians for Social Responsibility representing himself;
- Ann Durrant DC, vice president of Oregon Doctors of Chiropractic;
- Paul Engelking PhD, professor of chemistry at the University of Oregon, an ion expert knowledgeable about fluoride's effect on fish;
- Travis Williams, executive director of Willamette Riverkeeper;
- Mary O'Brien of the Science and Environmental Health Network; and
- Rhett Lawrence, Environmental Advocate for the Oregon Student Public Interest Group (OSPIRG). Because the national organization USPIRG had not taken a position on the issue, Mr. Lawrence was unable to officially oppose fluoridation, but he supported us by invoking the precautionary principle.

The hearing was long. Held in the Senate Committee on Health and Human Services, we knew that the chair, Senator Bill Fisher, was in favor of the bill, but, to his credit, he gave everyone an opportunity to speak. Numerous representatives of water utilities from around the state shared their opposition based mostly on the issues of local decision-making and choice.

But the most memorable testimony came from one of the legislators' own. Representative Alan Bates, a physician from southern Oregon, was expected to fully support the bill. After thanking the committee for their invitation to speak, he began, "If you'd asked me six to eight weeks ago what I thought of fluoridation, I'd have told you that it's a good health policy, should be done without question..." (Bates, 2001a).

Proponents and opponents alike sat in stunned silence as Bates continued. He explained that he'd been talking to and doing research with colleagues and had been unable to locate "good outcome data" showing that fluoridation works and doesn't have "unexpected side effects." His "two queries to CDC," a reliable source of outcome data in the past, had gone unanswered. In the end, he urged caution saying, "I've not seen really good, long-term, large studies on whether fluoridation is safe or unsafe" and advised the committee, for the moment, to "put this debate aside."

Bate's reversal was likely our luckiest break of all. Unraveling the backstory, credit for this turn of events falls to Michael Framson of Medford, Oregon. While doing some carpentry work for local cardiologist Nick Dienel, he and the doctor became friends. And when the Jackson County Public Health Advisory Committee began pushing to fluoridate Medford, Michael started attending their meetings. After one of these meetings, he wrote up a lengthy paper about fluoridation and asked Dr. Dienel for his review. After several weeks, Dienel got back to Michael saying, "You're absolutely right," and subsequently arranged a meeting in which he shared information with other physicians in the area. According to Michael, it was likely Dr. Dienel and a local gastroenterologist, both highly respected in the community, who went to Bates with the information and their concerns.

In the end, SB99 never moved out of the committee. A Master's thesis written by public health student Kendra Wise at Oregon State University helped me better understand key reasons why: Protonernts'. claim of a consensus in medicine and dentistry on the safety and effectiveness of fluoridation had been effectively challenged by the testimony of Drs Limeback, Dover, and Bates. While acknowledging their good intentions, Dr. Dover created doubt about their understanding of the issue, saying, "In medical school and residency training, we were never told anything except that it [fluoride] supposedly helped prevent dental caries, no more information than that." And finally, importantly, we had secured the support of environmental organizations typically aligned with the medical community, yet they were raising concerns promoters knew nothing about and had no answers for (Bates 2001b).

In her thesis, Wise writes, "With politically influential groups such as the OMA [Oregon Medical Association], ODA [Oregon Dental Association] and OSPIRG on opposite sides of the table and faced off on the issue, legislative caution may have been heightened. The opponents of SB 99 successfully portrayed the bill as a controversial issue with unanswered questions, perhaps making it difficult for the committee members to support the bill. Terminating the bill in committee was probably the easiest route for the committee members to take, reducing their risk of ostracizing any of the groups involved by having a vote on the bill." (Bates 2001c)

It must be said, too, that the public had been vocal on the issue. In a congratulatory message I sent thanking supporters on the demise of SB 99, I wrote:

"Many of you personally, and numerous organizations with which you are affiliated, participated in this critical effort: Forwarding our updates, testifying at the hearing, writing newsletters, position papers and letters to the editor, or endorsing our own SB744... Thousands of letters, postcards, and emails were sent to legislators–Senator Fisher's aide reported 1,200 letters received by their office alone. Countless phone calls were made."

In subsequent years, we continued to grow our support—especially environmental—and helped locally in opposing fluoridation efforts in Sutherlin, Hillsboro, Willamina, and Hood River, Oregon (though we lost Beaverton), and in White Salmon and Goldendale, Washington. We would go on to defeat another mandatory bill in the 2005 legislative session.

But I've always seen our defeat of SB99 as the most critical to our ongoing successes. It established OCSDW as a fact- and science-based force to be reckoned with. Dr Bates continued to be an ally and, over time, his opposition deepened. His ongoing influence in the legislature until his death in 2016 cannot be overestimated.

Frames

I'm now looking back nearly a quarter of a century. I had so much good information and documentation at my disposal during those years—and more kept coming forward—that it felt as if fluoridation would surely soon come to an end. So many of us who've engaged with this issue have naïvely assumed that just by sharing our information, people would see and embrace the truth, as in the rare case of Dr. Dienel. How wrong I was.

I don't remember when I first read neural linguist George Lakoff's work, but it gave me real insight into how the human mind "thinks" and why, in spite of the voluminous scientific evidence showing harm, fluoridation persists. Lakoff explains that rather than thinking rationally, most of human thought is actually unconscious, and that we really "think" in terms of frames, metaphors and narratives. When the frames are strong and reinforced by repetition, such as the frame that fluoridation is "safe and effective" —something we've been told now by trusted medical, dental, and public health officials for 75 years—it doesn't matter how many facts are presented showing the framing to be false, our brains find a way to dismiss the facts in order to keep the frame.

Nevertheless, based on all that is happening now, my hope is renewed. There are so many people to whom I am deeply grateful: those who are active today (particularly Paul, Ellen, and Michael Connett), those who worked with me in Oregon and carried on after I resigned (especially Kim Kaminski and Brent Foster), and those from years past upon whose shoulders we've been standing. I wish I could name them all. These friends and colleagues, like my parents and sisters, provided me with a frame, a scaffolding for my life.

Conclusion

There were significant personal costs to the work involved–physical, emotional, and financial. But to stand in the truth, in the company of the extraordinary people of courage and integrity across this continent who I've come to know–if I had it to do over, I would do it all again.

Eliminating Fluoridation

Quebec's long, painful, but successful story

By: Dr Gilles Parent, ND

ABOUT: *Dr Parent has been a naturopath since 1972. He is a member of the Association des naturopathes agréés du QuébecNaturopaths of Quebec (ANAQ), where he served as its long-time vice-president. Since 1970, he has closely examined the scientific, environmental, and legal aspects of fluoridation. He was the editor of the journal La fluoration en Question from 1976 to 1977. He has authored and co-authored many works on fluoridation since 1975. His most recent work, "La fluoridation: autopsie d'une erreur scientifique" with Dr Pierre Jean Morin, PhD and Maître John Remington Graham was translated into English as "Fluoridation: autopsy of a scientific error" by the Éditions Berger. He is a scientific spokesperson for "le Front Commun pour une Eau Saine", and "Eau Secours".*

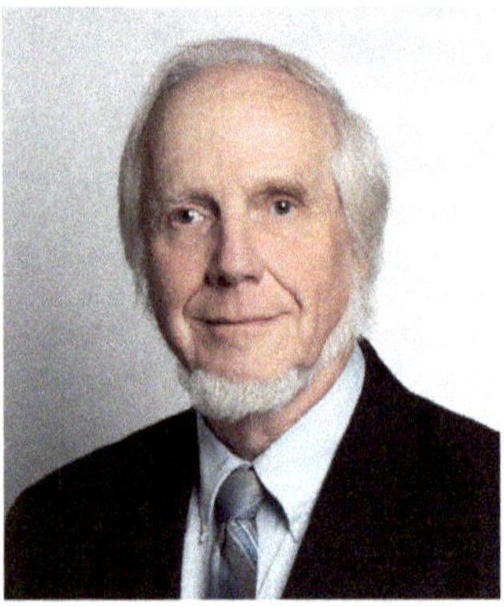

Dr Parent has been involved in the cessation or rejection of fluoridation in a number of municipalities including: Montreal, Quebec City, Gatineau, Longueuil, the Ville du Lac Etchemin, Mont-Joli, Saguenay, Ste-Marie-de-Beauce, Verchères, Richmond, La Prairie, Chateauguay, Trois-Rivières, Pointe-Claire, Dorval, Quebec, Waterloo, ON, Moncton, NB, and Prince George, BC. He has prepared and presented the largest and most documented brief on fluoridation for "le Front Commun pour une Eau Saine" to the "National Assembly Parliamentary Health Committee on Fluoridation" in April 2013, in collaboration with several scientific experts.

CHAPTER 30

"Ironically, the 'antis,' who are usually portrayed as unscientific, often act more scientifically in the debate. By contrast, the political pro fluoridation stance has evolved into a dogmatic, authoritarian, essentially anti-scientific posture, one that discourages open debate of scientific issues."

—Professor Edward Groth, III (1991)

Background: Quebec's Social, Political, and Economic Context

TO UNDERSTAND THE phenomenon of the fight against fluoridation in Quebec, one must understand the historical, socio-economic, linguistic, and political context of Quebec.

French is the dominant language in Quebec. Until 1960, the province was under the influence of the omnipresent Catholic religion and under the economic domination of the English-speaking minority, which held a significant portion of the economic and political levers and kept the management positions of companies and banks for itself. Quebec society underwent a profound transformation starting in 1960, called the "Quiet Revolution." This was a turning point that led the health system to become socialized. In this social awakening, old institutions were called into question and fluoridation didn't escape this questioning.

Against the status quo, groups for environmental protection, organic farming, and natural health products emerged, as well as alternative medicine professions. These emerging professions were frowned upon by the Quebec medical establishment which tried to curb them. In this ecological and alternative medicine movement, a more or less underground network was created among environmental associations, alternative medicine, the natural food industry and more open conventional medicine professionals, including in dentistry. They have all played a role in the history of opposition to fluoridation in Quebec.

In 1969, the Quebec government established the Régie de l'assurance maladie du Québec (Quebec Health Insurance Board), which administers the health system. The government aimed to reduce dental health costs. At that time water fluoridation was being promoted as an effective and completely safe panacea for reducing tooth decay.

Already, some twenty municipalities in Quebec, some since 1958, had introduced fluoridation of their drinking water.

Since 1971, the Ordre des dentistes du Québec, supported by the Collège des médecins du Québec, has been increasing pressure and lobbying both the government and municipalities to promote fluoridation.

Chance Thrust Me into the Center of the Fight Against Fluoridation

It was in this social context that I found myself playing a decisive role in ending fluoridation in Quebec. By luck, I met with renowned researchers, leaders of environmental organizations, and determined citizens, often just at the right times.

Opposing fluoridation was consistent with my awareness of the importance of a healthy diet, nutrition, organic farming, and naturopathy. It was meant to be.

Scientific Logic Awakens Me to Fluoridation Absurdity

In 1966, I worked in one of the first natural health food stores in Quebec where I discovered *Rodale Books* and the magazine *Prevention*, which published on organic farming, nutrition, and prevention. I discovered there was a dissonance between fluoride-as-a-nutrient, which might be beneficial but was also toxic, and fluoride, the environmental pollutant. The subject of fluoridation concerned me because I did not find this public health measure logical, scientific, or ethical.

In 1968, my textbooks in biochemistry and in toxicology explained that fluoride inhibits several enzymatic systems and that no enzyme in animal physiology depends on fluoride for its function unlike other trace elements. As part of my course on environment and health, forced to choose a topic for a research project, I selected fluoridation. However, in my naïveté, I did not realize that I was about to open a Pandora's box where the myths and beliefs of health authorities go against the most fundamental principles of science. I was even less aware that I would soon become a central architect of the blocking of the implementation of the Quebec Fluoridation Program. At that time, I was only writing a research paper for a course, without thinking that it would later become a book... a book that would change the history of fluoridation in Quebec.

Instigated Meetings with Renowned Researchers

During my research for my book, I discovered the 1966 article by Marier and Rose from the National Research Council of Canada, "The Fluoride Content of Some Foods and Beverages: A Brief Survey Using a Modified Zr-Spands Method," which discussed the significant fluoride content of foods. Fluoride deficiency was therefore unlikely. I requested a meeting with Dr Marier, PhD, in Ottawa, which he granted me, but only if it took place in the evening, at his home, and surreptitiously through the back door. His bosses mustn't find out. It was then that I began to understand that the highest health authorities exercised control over anyone who might question the dogma of fluoridation.

Genesis of a Law to Make Fluoridation Mandatory in Quebec

In 1973, the year I graduated as a naturopath, one of my colleagues, Jean-Marc Brunet, published a short book on fluoridation, *Dossier Fluor*, to counter this public health idea. It was rather brief and aimed at the general public. Convinced that a more comprehensive and better-argued work, covering scientific, nutritional, and environmental aspects, could make health authorities realize the stupidity of fluoridation, I decided to publish my work under the title of *L'Inconsequence de la Fluoration* (Parent, 1975).

Two erroneous assumptions on my part were: first, not realizing that the fluoridation project of the Ministry of Health and Social Affairs was already forging ahead and secondly, thinking that scientific arguments on the ineffectiveness and toxicity of fluoridation could bring down a dogma advocated by prestigious health organizations.

In September 1974, the Minister of Health and Social Affairs, Mr. Claude Forget, announced that Bill 88 would make fluoridation mandatory, supported by "Dossier technique sur la fluoration 1974" which presents fluoridation as a panacea against dental caries capable of reducing dental caries by 60 to 75% without any health risk.

The *Front commun contre la fluoration* (Common Front Against Fluoridation) emerged to oppose Bill 88.

On January 27, 1975, we received unexpected help from Dr Pierre Jean Morin, PhD, the director of medical research at the Laval Hospital affiliated with the Faculty of Medicine of Laval University, in Quebec City. He and two medical doctors, Dr Roy and Dr Boutet, published an article in the newspaper *Le Devoir*, a daily newspaper renowned for its journalistic rigor. Without taking a position against fluoridation, these authors raised some concerns about the risks of fluorides on dental health (dental fluorosis) and bones (osseous or skeletal fluorosis) and addressed the problems of fluoride pollution around the fairly numerous aluminum smelters in Quebec.

I attended the Parliamentary Commission on Bill 88 that took place on February 27, 1975, in Quebec City. I was amazed by the rhetoric and ignorance of that body which unreservedly endorsed the document on fluoridation from the Ministry of Health?

Fluoridation law for all municipalities of 5,000 inhabitants was passed on June 27, 1975 requiring mandatory compliance January 1, 1977.

Elements of a Fight Against Fluoridation Take Shape

I published my book, *L'Inconsequence de la Fluoration*, in March 1975. At the same time, I took over the leadership of the *Front commun contre la fluoration*, which I organized as an association with dues-paying members. With the funds raised, I published in the newspapers several promotional advertisements for the *Front commun contre la fluoration* and its mandate. I managed to get several op-eds published, too.

Two environmental groups, the Society to Stop Pollution (STOP) on the English side and the *Société pour vaincre la pollution* (SVP) on the French side, joined our group and Montreal Mayor Jean Drapeau announced that Montreal would never be fluoridated as long as he would be mayor. It goes without saying that the *"Front Commun"* supported Mr. Drapeau.

When I met with Dr Pierre Morin, PhD, who was research director at Laval Hospital, he agreed with our premise. He told me, "We need to analyze the fluoridation file deeper; the toxicity and environmental aspects seem troubling to me," and then led me into a room where enormous computers were set up. These were new acquisitions from the Research Center that allowed them to obtain all the references with a short summary on a given subject within a few hours. Shortly after, Dr Morin launched a search that retrieved more than 700 publications relevant to fluorides and health and environment.

It was during this meeting that Dr Morin revealed a secret to me: two weeks before the Parliamentary Commission, he received a long-distance call from Dr Augustin Roy, the president of the Collège des médecins du Québec, asking for his opinion on fluoridation because, despite his advocacy, he had no idea about the effectiveness and safety of this dental health measure.

Opposition to Fluoridation Extends to the Government

Three weeks later, I met again with Dr Morin. With all the recently gathered scientific studies in hand, he joined the government's Advisory Council on the Environment (ACE), then chaired by one of his acquaintances, Dr J. Benoît Bundock, MD, a physician and former Deputy Minister at Health Canada who was a leading authority. The Advisory Council on the Environment would later become the Bureau d'audiences publiques sur l'environnement (BAPE). Soon after, in August 1975, it published an article in *Le Devoir,* expressing its concerns about the increase of fluoride in the environment through fluoridation.

On November 15, 1976, against all odds, the Parti Québécois took power in Quebec. In 1977, faced with growing opposition to fluoridation, including from the Advisory Council on the Environment and several municipalities besides Montreal, the compulsory requirement of the Bill 88 to fluoridate water was suspended but did not subside.

In the Trenches

Right from the start, I consulted with learned experts from around the world to discuss fluoridation policy and their findings. I shared those findings with our audience in Quebec. Dr Morin became the second reviewer of our popular level science journal, renamed *La fluoridation en question.* Our objectives were:

- to disseminate information in French to members of the *"Front Commun contre la fluoration"*, a membership benefit;
- to inform ministers and government officials and the media about the dangers of fluoridation;
- to enable the publication of scientific articles in French;
- to give scientific credibility to opponents of fluoridation.

We published the Chilean study by Dr Albert Schatz, PhD, on higher mortality rates among newborns in a fluoridated city compared to those in a non-fluoridated city.

We connected with the Safe Water Foundation led by Dr John Yiamouyiannis, PhD. Yiamouyiannis' PhD was in biochemistry and he served as the editor of *Chemical Abstract Services*. Dr Yiamouyiannis was working closely with Dr Dean Burk, one of the founders of the National Cancer Institute. I facilitated a meeting between Drs Morin and Yiamouyiannis. Together they conducted a study documenting a nearly 10% increase in cancer incidence in ten large fluoridated American cities with over a million inhabitants compared to ten equivalent large non-fluoridated cities. *La fluoridation en question* published an interim version of their study in French in 1977.

I also published in journals for water workers and engineers not only about the risks to consumers, but also the risks to worker health and environment. Beginning in 1980, Dr Pierre Morin became the scientific advisor to the association of technicians and engineers in water works in Quebec.

Political Shifts

A significant trial took place in Pennsylvania in 1978 on the link between cancer and fluoridation involving attorney John Remington Graham. Drs Dean Burk, John Yiamouyiannis, Pierre Morin, and George Waldbott were expert witnesses. Justice Flaherty concluded that, according to a preponderance of evidence, fluoridation of drinking water could be carcinogenic. This judgment supports the credibility of Quebec's opponents of fluoridation (Graham & Morin, 2018).

However, evidence of harm was trumped by jurisdictional issues. Judge Flaherty commented in 1988: "Nothing I have seen changes my view of the serious hazards occasioned by public fluoridation. To the contrary, what I have read convinces me all the more that in depth, serious, scientific effort should be undertaken before further expanding a questionable practice. Those who belittle critics of fluoridation do the public a mis-service, yet it seems in the face of strong, uncontradicted prima facie evidence, that is the tactic most often employed."

The Parti Québécois had made the environment one of its priorities, and in November 1979, it officially created the Ministry of the Environment under the leadership of Mr. Marcel Léger, one of the party's big guns. Dr J. Benoît Bundock, MD, previously president of the Advisory Council on the Environment, was appointed deputy minister. Together, Dr Morin and Dr Bundock, who headed the Advisory Committee on Water Fluoridation team within the Advisory Council on the Environment, produced an official 210-page report for the Ministry of the Environment, entitled *Les fluorures, Fluoration et la qualité de l'environnement* (with a red cover) (English version in 1980). It recommended suspending water fluoridation at least until studies could fully assess and evaluate the impact on public health and the environment.

However, we were not working in a vacuum. Dr Denis Lazure MD, the Minister of Health and Social Affairs, took a very dim view of the "*Red Book*". He ordered the Environment Ministry's report shelved in order to protect policy. Since the Ministry of Health is more powerful than the new Ministry of the Environment, and since this report is far too incriminating for the policy of water fluoridation, he won his case. The report was made public. Still under embargo, there are only a few copies of the report.

Coincidentally, I had a meeting with Dr Morin that day and I stole, with complicity, a copy of the *Red Book* which I handed over to the environmental journalist of *Le Devoir*, Mr Louis-Gilles Francoeur, who published a two-page article summarizing the report on the front page the very next day. *Le Devoir* is considered to be a reputable media source in Quebec. This was explosive!

The Ministry of Health tried to put out the fire. It forbade Dr Morin, under penalty of immediate dismissal, from speaking to any journalist. He obeyed the order, except that luck was still on our side: the Laval Hospital Research Center had just achieved a major world-first in medicine—the successful simultaneous transplantation of a liver and a lung in a patient. As director of experimental research, Dr Morin was the architect of the procedure, and it was essential for the international prestige of the Laval Hospital Research Center and the Quebec Ministry of Health that the news of the transplant made the headlines. Dr Lazure, the Minister of Health and Social Services, asked him to hold a press conference immediately. Dr Morin replied that he could not because he had been ordered not to speak to journalists. Dr Lazure lifted the ban and Dr Morin gave his press conference on this first liver-lung transplant. Obviously, it was impossible for him to avoid questions about fluoridation and the *Red Book* which was still front-page news.

Because it covered so many troublesome aspects of fluoridation, the *Red Book* could kill the Quebec Fluoridation Program. We, the opponents, were then convinced that the fluoridation file was dead, really dead, stabbed in the heart by the *Red Book.* It was wounded and it never fully recovered. And there was an unofficial 1980 moratorium, but fluoridation had many resurgences in Quebec.

Second Court Case Against Fluoridation Involving Quebec

In 1982, another legal case against fluoridation involving Quebec opponents was held in the United States. This one generated considerable publicity. It was presided over by the Honorable Anthony Farris, Judge of the District Court of Texas in Houston (Safe Water Foundation of Texas v City of Houston, 1982). Naturally, the prosecution's experts included Dr Dean Burk, Dr John Yiamouyiannis, and Dr Pierre J Morin. The fact that Dr Morin—author of the *Red Book,* produced by a government ministry—was one of the key expert witness in the trial, that the lead lawyer was Mr Graham, a Quebec resident, and that the judgment was in favor of the prosecution further lent credibility to the anti-fluoridation movement in Quebec. Several excerpts from the trial minutes would appear in the book *La fluoration: autopsie d'une erreur scientifique*, which was published in 2005.

Political U-turn and Attempt to Fluoridate Montreal

In 1985, the Parti Québécois lost power to the Liberal Party, which came back with a majority. As expected, in 1988, the Public Health Department relaunched the promotion of fluoridation.

At the Municipal Commission on Fluoridation, professional organizations marshaled by their political leaders repeated exactly the same refrain: "Water fluoridation is essential, effective and safe." On the other hand, truly without financial means but organized, the *Front commun contre la fluoration* ensured that a dozen organizations came to present briefs, each in depth on only a specific aspect of fluoridation. Thus, the opponents demonstrated that they had much more detailed knowledge about fluoridation than the professional associations.

Our big coup at the Commission was the contribution of Dr John Yiamouyiannis PhD, whom I had invited. He arrived with a pile of more than 600 studies illustrating the toxicity of fluoride or fluoridation. Surprised by the existence of so many studies, one of the commission's advisors asked him how he had all these studies in hand when the authorities claimed that there were no such studies on the harmful effects of fluoridation? Dr Yiamouyannis replied:

"Gentlemen, you have before you more than six hundred studies published in credible and recognized scientific journals, so go ask these professionals why they were unable to find them. Yet, you have proof that they do indeed exist!"

Given the evidence presented and following the precautionary principle, the Montreal municipal commission recommended against fluoridating Montreal's water. It called on the Quebec government to impose fluoridation if it was so keen on it.

In 1994, Bill 88 was repealed.

In 2000, the City of Laval, the third largest city in Quebec after Montreal and Quebec City, stopped fluoridation following a damning report by water technicians regarding the costs incurred by pipe corrosion related to fluoridation.

New Fluoridation Promotion Act

In 2001, the Parti Québécois' position shifted. It voted on a huge omnibus, catch-all public health bill that included four articles related to water fluoridation on December 20, 2001. It prescribed an active promotion of fluoridation and was accompanied by a grant program that covered all construction costs for fluoridation facilities, equipment, and products. However, the decision to fluoridate was left to municipalities. Consequently, the fight would have to be waged municipality by municipality.

New Allies in the Fight

An association of holistic dentists was formed during this period and after a presentation that I had given, it joined the anti-fluoridation movement. Some members got involved in the fight, but not without facing reprisals.

So, starting in 2002, the front commun contre la fluoration, which later became "Le Front Commun pour une Eau Saine," led the fight against fluoridation municipality by municipality. Later the Coalition Eau Secours joined in as another pivotal organization. As experience grew, a *modus operandi* was created to be able to act at the municipal level.

I found myself in the role of manager, resource person for establishing links with experts, organizer, and captain. I wore the hat of scientific advisor and spokesperson for both organizations.

Modus Operandi

Citizens or citizens' associations of a community who wanted to end fluoridation or prevent its introduction eventually reached out to me, often through a member of a group of one of the coalitions.

Meetings were held with these activists to study the local situation, structure the group, ensure their training on fluoridation and how to conduct the debate respectfully, reach out to local media, find local allies, plan actions, meet with municipal officials and make representations, inform the population with leaflets, and organize public lectures or debates or make a presentation directly to the municipal council, often with our experts.

Sometimes the struggles were long and bitter, sometimes easy and cordial; sometimes the invitation came from municipal councils, occasionally, it was the citizens themselves who decided to end fluoridation on their own. Since 2002, nineteen communities in Quebec have ended or rejected fluoridation.

Fluoridation: Autopsy of a Scientific Error

We had the trial transcripts in hand, and no one was more knowledgeable about the link between cancer and the cytotoxic, genotoxic, mutagenic, and carcinogenic effects of fluoride than our experts, Dr Morin and Mr Graham. We decided to write another book.

In October 2005, we published, *La fluoration: autopsie d'une erreur scientifique* (Morin, Graham & Parent, 2005; Morin, Graham & Parent, 2010). It received good media coverage, at least in Quebec. With the help of Dr Pierre Larose DDS, who was then a member of the governing council of the International Academy of Oral Medicine and Toxicology (IAOMT), I contacted Dr David Kennedy DDS, its president, who introduced me to Dr Hardy Limeback, DDS PhD. As Dr Limeback was one of the twelve experts on the upcoming US National Research Council report, *Fluoride in Drinking Water—A Scientific Review of EPA Standards*. He graciously agreed to write a foreword for our book.

Multiple Fronts

Also in 2005, the Quebec Public Health Department published the *2005-2012 Public Dental Health Action Plan*, whose objective was to fluoridate 50% of the Quebec population while at that point the rate had dropped from 17.5% to 7.5%.

The Ministry of Health tried to convince large municipalities to join the Quebec Fluoridation Program. In the fall of 2005, fluoridation became an issue in Montreal for the November 2, 2005, elections. Our book, *La fluoration: autopsie d'une erreur scientifique* became part of the electoral debate. Mayor Gérald Tremblay, well informed about the dangers of fluoridation, won the election. The City of Montreal would not be fluoridated.

More pro-fluoridation alliances developed, as the rhetoric heated up with accusations of eco-terrorism and un-democratic tactics, adding additional spice to our efforts. This was abetted by a pro-fluoride cartel of primarily dental scientists.

In 2007: The Institut national de santé publique du Québec (National Institute of Public Health of Quebec) launched a major promotional document for the measure: *Fluoration de l'eau : analyse des bénéfices et des risques pour la santé – un Avis scientifique*. For years afterward, opponents to fluoridation would clash with the authors, Dr Michel Lévy, DDS and Dr Christian Fortin, DDS, in public debates, on radio and television, and during presentations to municipal councils.

Also in 2007, I met with the Coalition Eau Secours, a coalition of environmental and educational organizations, unions, committed artists, and citizens. It added the opposition to fluoridation as one of its mandates. With considerable social credibility in the environmental field, the Coalition Eau Secours has played an important role in the fight against fluoridation in Quebec.

Legal Tools

We started to use Freedom of Information requests to obtain information that was not openly available in 2008. We searched for the review of toxicology tests attesting to the safety of fluoridation chemicals which was the responsibility of the government.

In 2010, Pierre J. Morin and I sent three petitions under the aegis of the Commissioner of the Environment of the Office of the Auditor General of Canada and addressed to Health Canada, the Ministry of Justice and Environment Canada. These petitions are a form of Freedom of Information requests, but instead of seeking to obtain documents, they request answers.

We learned that Health Canada does not approve, does not regulate, and does not exercise any oversight over the sanitary quality of fluoridation products despite its assertion that fluoridation is safe. Health Canada relegates fluoridation products to simple "water treatment products," whose legal classification falls under the jurisdiction of provinces. Health Canada establishes fluoridation standards in collaboration with the provinces and territories, which are actually responsible for fluoridation in their province. Health Canada is the only government agency with constitutional jurisdiction over all products having a therapeutic function and a therapeutic claim, and despite attributing a therapeutic function to fluoridation, it refuses to take responsibility for it.

Health Canada was unable to provide a review of the toxicology tests on fluoridation products and claims that the National Sanitation Foundation (NSF) conducted them, but the NSF does not certify safety, only compliance with a limited protocol. Fluoridation products are not approved by Health Canada which has no documentation of safety—facts that are ignored by the provinces and municipalities.

In 2010, the *Protecteur du citoyen du Québec* (Quebec Ombudsman) advised that since it is the municipalities that decide whether or not to fluoridate, they bear full legal accountability of fluoridation in case of injuries. In 2013, we double-checked it.

Contracts

In 2009, as more and more Quebec municipalities were withdrawing from fluoridation programs, the Ministry of Health and Social Services established a standard contract defining the commitments between the Ministry and the cities that decided to fluoridate. This contract included a stipulation that, in the event of cessation, the cities would have to repay the generous subsidies allocated to them for the design, construction, equipment, and development related to fluoridation. By 2025, only the City of Trois-Rivières, had signed the said contract, which it would later tear up because the Ministry had been unable to adequately defend fluoridation against opponents.

From 2010 to 2017, a fluoridation reinstallation project was relaunched in Trois-Rivières following the obsolescence and failure of fluoridation equipment. Trois-Rivières is one of the major cities in Quebec with a population of 144,500.

Having obtained a copy of the contract, thanks to the Freedom of Information Act, we discovered that all the planned piping and some of the piping already installed was made of stainless steel, incompatible with hydrofluorosilicic acid and capable of releasing toxic fumes of hydrogen fluoride. It would have to be completely replaced; this made the headlines and the mayor's credibility was affected: his first setback. Then the City was unable to provide the toxicology tests requested by the Freedom of information Act: his second problem.

On February 17, 2016, *Le Nouvelliste* published an article: "Are Trois-Rivières residents threatened with lead poisoning?" The article was signed by Christian Linard, a clinical biochemist and full professor, and Joan Hamel, lecturer, both at the University of Quebec in Trois-Rivières (UQTR). Other signatories included Mireille Guay, PhD, whose doct-orate is in organic chemistry and spokespersons for the *Coalition trifluvienne pour une eau très saine* (CTETS).

The medical officer from the Public Health Regional Directorate, Dr Isabelle Goupil Sormany MD, responded that this is not a problem because there is a government program in place to replace the lead pipes in the water inlets in Trois-Rivières, where a significant portion of the built heritage predates 1970, the period when these types of pipes were used. The full lead pipe replacement will take 20 years.

At that time, the issue of lead poisoning in children from drinking fountains with lead solder in schools was also making headlines. Shortly after her gaffe on lead poisoning, Dr Goupil Sormany resigned. This left Mayor Lévesque to defend himself against the respectful and scientific attacks of the Trois-Rivières Coalition without the support of Public Health.

On February 20, 2017, in protest against Public Health and the Ministry of Health, and against all expectations, Mayor Lévesque threw in the towel and the project to reinstate fluoridation in Trois-Rivières was abandoned. This six-year fight against fluoridation in Trois-Rivières was the longest and most difficult in Quebec and a major victory.

In 2009, my neighboring community of Richmond faced a fluoridation mandate. Because of community resistance supported by experts of my acquaintance, a popular consultation was held on Sunday, October 20, 2014. Fluoridation was rejected by 75%.

In December 2014, the fluoridation project was abandoned and the Richmond citizens were forced to reimburse the government $127,000 for its installation subsidies, resulting in substantial tax increases for the next two years. Yet, the City had never signed such a contract.

On September 12, 2011, the *Comité d'éthique de santé publique de l'institut national de la santé publique du Québec* published its "Avis sur un projet de fluoration de l'eau potable." This Ethics Committee never considered that the chemicals used for fluoridation were not approved by Health Canada and that they were merely "water treatment chemicals." Using "water treatment chemicals" to treat a population without informed consent should raise serious questions about the ethics of fluoridation.

In September 2011, faced with the failure to make progress with the fluoridation program, the Ministry of Health and Social Services (MSSS) postponed its 50% implementation target for the program until 2015. At that time, the rate of the population receiving fluoridated water in Quebec had fallen by nearly 200%, to 2.6%.

In 2013, our alliance of professional organizations opposed to fluoridation launched a petition on the website of the National Assembly of Quebec to demand that a parliamentary commission shed light on fluoridation. The list can be found in the Appendix C of this book.

As part of the petition to the National Assembly, 80 Quebec municipalities each passed a motion at their municipal council meeting rejecting fluoridation of their drinking water.

In its final report, the Parliamentary Commission confirmed that fluoridation **lacks social acceptability in Quebec** and that, consequently, it will be necessary to better sell the effectiveness and safety of fluoridation to the public, maintain the fluoridation program, and monitor the positive and negative effects of the measure. The government's efforts to promote fluoridation were in vain, and it continued to decline thereafter as the people realized with increasing clarity that the government had neither evidence of safety nor effectiveness to back up their policy.

Last Resistance in the Province

Ending fluoridation in the West End of Montreal was unique. Per usual, councils of the municipalities served were committed to water fluoridation, fearing a dental health disaster if fluoridation ended.

Since Montreal is responsible for the filtration plants and, therefore, for drinking water, we approached the city councillor responsible for water at the City of Montreal. Without a clear response on safety and accountability, Councillor Coehlo, with the help of a lawyer, sent two formal notices to the City of Montreal demanding that fluoridation cease, since fluoridation products are not approved and not regulated by Health Canada, and, therefore, present a health risk. The petition, two formal notices, concerns over the fact that 99% of the fluoride added to drinking water would eventually reach the environment—not to mention that trucking hexafluorosilicic acid on the highways of densely-populated areas to reach two filtration plants presented a civil security risk—these were tools Montreal used to end fluoridation.

Saint-Georges-de-Beauce is the last fluoridating municipality in Quebec. It serves approximately 25,000 citizens, equal to 0.25% of Quebec population. A group, Saint-George sans fluor, began to pressure the municipal council in 2019 with interventions at council meetings, a press conference, and a public PowerPoint presentation by Mrs Mireille Guay and myself on May second, 2025. A petition is currently circulating.

Conclusion

My allies and I have fought the good fight against water fluoridation policy for over fifty years. None of us could have done it alone, and none of us intended for fluoridation to take up so much of our time and our lives. I, for one, do not regret a single minute of it.

Infant Formula Fluoride Risks

Dental fluorosis risks from infant formula prepared with fluoridated tap water

By: Douglas Cragoe

ABOUT: *Doug Cragoe works in video and film production in Hollywood.*

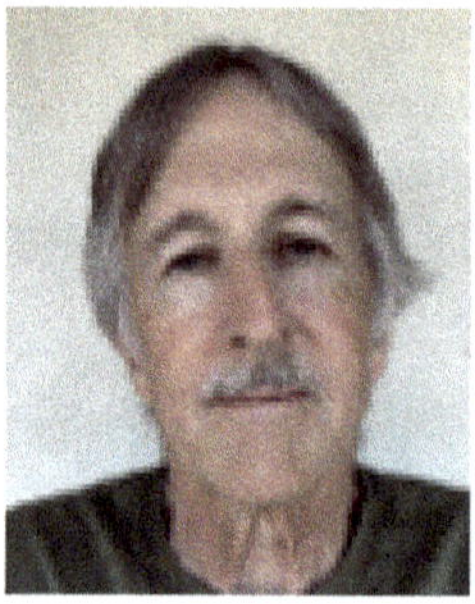

His YouTube channel is @DougCragoe. Doug joined an activist group when Los Angeles, California, was considering starting up water fluoridation. Despite the group's best efforts, the city council approved fluoridation in a split vote. Doug sent a legal duty to warn letter that was acknowledged, but ignored. The L.A. activist group subsequently filed a lawsuit. The judge ruled in favor of the city but noted that the city had violated the state open meeting law regarding the planning for fluoridation. That one cause of action should have allowed the trial to proceed, but a new judge dismissed the open meeting violations. An appeal was unsuccessful, and Doug found his mission: forcing authorities to follow the law and to remove false information from websites.

Doug's wins include: The Los Angeles Department of Water and Power removed a webpage that claimed fluoride was essential; the American Dental Association (ADA) stopped claiming it was a "fact" that 60 nations fluoridated their drinking water (there were only 23); the federal National Institute of Dental and Cranial Research (NIDCR) removed their claim from its website that H. Trendley Dean found no increase in fluorosis with water fluoridation; the CDC eliminated an entire webpage that claimed a National Academy of Sciences report said fluoride was essential.

CHAPTER 31

"It is particularly worrying that statements which mislead the public about the review's findings have been made in press releases.... The review did not show water fluoridation to be safe. The quality of the research was too poor to establish with confidence whether or not there are potentially important adverse effects in addition to the high levels of fluorosis."

—*Professor Trevor Sheldon, MSc, DSc (2003)*

I LEARNED THAT water systems with over 2 mg/L fluoride were required by EPA regulations to issue public notifications. Seven states had water systems with violations for not informing their customers about high fluoride levels. The notifications advise parents to not give this water to their children as it puts them at risk for severe dental fluorosis. In 2016, I wanted to learn how the notifications were distributed. I quickly discovered that most water systems in Texas were failing to send the required notifications. This problem was rectified after Texas got an EPA grant to fix its water quality report generator system which automatically adds the proper advisory when needed.

After digging into more public records, I discovered that 95% of the Texas water systems were in violation of the law. The EPA's own system for creating water quality reports had the same deficiency as the one in Texas. I found that EPA deficiency led to water systems violations in New Mexico, with the state regulatory agency unaware of the violations. But the EPA refused to fix their water quality report system. I eventually documented a total of seven states with violations which are regulatory failures.

The Los Angeles Fluoridation Battle

In the 1960s, the city water department was going ahead with plans to fluoridate the water when the city council stepped in and said 'wait, you need to get permission from us first. Then, over the course of many years fluoridation was debated in front of the city council. The top experts on both sides of the issue spoke in front of the council. In 1975, the city council voted to start up fluoridation in a split vote. Environment activists then threatened to gather petitions and force the issue onto the ballot for voters to decide.

Since San Diego activists had done exactly that resulting in city law forbidding the city council from fluoridating San Diego, a law that lasted for decades, the L.A. City Council decided in 1975 to put the issue on the ballot themselves as an advisory vote and pledged to abide by that vote.

Despite virtually all major media, medical, and dental groups advocating for fluoridation, the voters turned them down; fluoridation lost in the election. The city council respected the will of the voters for 20 years, but a city council split vote again decided that fluoridation would commence in 1995.

Fluoridation started in L.A. in 1999, but so far there is no evidence of any direct benefit. On the other hand, a recent L.A. study using the MADRES cohort of mother-child pairs suggests neurotoxic harm from pre- and post-natal exposure (Malin et al., 2024).

Babies Don't Like Fluoridated Water

I learned about Dr. Hans Moolenburgh who led the successful effort to stop fluoridation in the Netherlands in 1976. I produced a video interview of him (. Hans Moolenburgh, 2014).

In that video, Moolenburgh explains how he and his doctor group saw the adverse effects of fluoridation first hand when it started up in the Netherlands. Babies who had their powdered infant formula made with fluoridated tap water experienced colic; they cried and yelled around the clock. Switching to non-fluoridated water eliminated their distress.

Dr. Moolenburg also spoke about how children and adults were plagued by stomach aches and reoccurrences of rashes and other conditions that had previously been under control—all of which were eliminated with a switch back to non-fluoridated water. It was this clinical experience and subsequent investigation (Grimbergen, 1974) that led to the banning of fluoridation in the Netherlands.

Fluorosis Risk from Powdered Infant Formula

Infants 0-6 months of age have no erupted teeth and their ideal food is breast milk, which is extremely low in fluoride. But many infants are fed powdered infant formula reconstituted with fluoridated tap water.

In 1980, infant formula makers in the U.S. voluntarily stopped using fluoridated water in the manufacturing of ready-to-feed products but, at that time, infants were still being prescribed fluoride supplements from birth. It wasn't until 1994 that the schedule was changed, so that infants 0-6 months of age were no longer prescribed fluoride supplements. Dentists realized that powdered infant formula combined with tap water still posed a potential fluorosis risk, but thought it would only affect primary teeth and considered it unimportant. Moreover, they gave no consideration to other potential problems such as colic and rashes.

By 2004 and 2005, there were a substantial number of studies showing that infants and toddlers getting a large dose of fluoride every day early in life experienced increased fluorosis in their permanent teeth.

By 2006, the evidence for fluorosis risk in permanent teeth was strong. Because of a press release concerning the 2006 National Research Council (NRC) review on fluoride in drinking water (Doull et al., 2006), the American Dental Association (ADA) and the Centers for Disease Control and Prevention (CDC) issued lukewarm advisories for parents about fluorosis risk from early life exposure. They suggested parents consider using non-fluoridated water to prepare infant formula in order to reduce the risk of "mild fluorosis." The story made national news in the U.S., but it did not lead to any substantial changes in public policy. The CDC had a small webpage on this risk with a sentence saying parents should consider the potential for a systemic fluoride benefit before making a decision to use non-fluoridated water when preparing infant formula. I wrote to the CDC challenging them for data showing toothless infants benefited from fluoridated water. That sentence was removed from the CDC webpage not long afterwards.

A systematic review by Philippe Hujoel clearly showed that infant formula made with fluoridated tap water increased the prevalence of dental fluorosis (Hujoel et al., 2009). Breast milk typically contains essentially no fluoride at 0.006 mg fluoride/L (Sener et al., 2007).

Using ready-to-feed formula does not solve the fluoride/fluorosis problem as the fluoride content is quite variable in those milk and soy products—0.01 to 1.3 ppm—which is much higher than breast milk fluoride content; and reconstituted formula made with tap water that has low levels of naturally-occurring fluoride, such as at 0.3 ppm, exposes babies to 40 times more fluoride than received by breast-fed babies (Velez-León et al., 2023).

Another issue relevant to dosage was first revealed in a 1975 study that showed 6-month-old infants received fluoride at 0.16 mg/kg/day when they consumed formula prepared with artificially fluoridated tap water (Wiatrowski et al., 1975). If that high daily dosage was extrapolated based on weight, an adult weighing 198 pounds (90 kg) would consume 14.4 mg of fluoride per day, enough to cause crippling skeletal fluorosis. Consequently, as weight increases with age, the fluoride dosage (by weight) decreases, but the variations in exposures based on multiple factors makes it impossible to suggest any dose that does not pose a risk to the developing teeth of the infant or young child.

Even with warnings not to use fluoridated water, there remains a risk for dental fluorosis in babies fed infant formula in communities without artificial fluoridation programs, which is ignored by government and health authorities upon whom the public relies.

The WIC in California

In the U.S., there is a program called "Women, Infants, and Children" or WIC which provides free powdered infant formula to low-income parents. I did an informal survey of all the state WIC programs in 2009 to see if the parents were being informed about this fluorosis risk. Very few WIC state programs did anything with this advice.

In California, I obtained WIC documents that trained the WIC advisors how to address the fluorosis risk, but at the same time, the WIC advisors were only supposed to talk about it if the parents brought up the subject first. Parents were deliberately being left in the dark. Some WIC programs might provide ready-to-feed infant formula. But since that is more expensive the parents would get less product. WIC will not provide non-fluoridated water to prepare infant formula.

I sent some questions to the CDC about fluoride and infants. The CDC did not respond. So, I requested California Senator Barbara Boxer submit my questions. The Director of the CDC replied to her. The CDC director said they had no data showing any additional fluoride intake above the adequate intake level of 0.01mg per day for infants 0-6 months of age provided any additional benefit. Fluoridation policy, like fluoride supplements, pose only risks for this age group, and the CDC and other fluoridationist organizations knew it. Using fluoridated water to prepare infant formula creates risk with no potential benefit for infants 0-6 months of age.

Oral Health Conferences

A few years later, I attended a high-level Oral Health Conference. The Surgeon General was there, along with public health dentists and top fluoridationists. I talked to many of them, and one of them was aware of the "Senator Boxer letter." At this conference I asked many people a simple question: "Should parents be informed about the fluorosis risk from preparing infant formula with fluoridated tap water?" All but one of the many experts there refused to answer that question. The one who answered the question said parents should be informed. At the end of the conference, one of the organizers said to me "we did not answer your question" before proceeding to tell me what she knew about the fluorosis risk with a non-responsive monologue, which did not answer my question as to whether parents should be informed.

During a study session on fluoridation at another conference where no recording was allowed, Oregon fluoridationists discussed their recent (2013) referendum defeat in Portland. I brought up the infant formula fluorosis advisories that were being proposed for water quality reports. The speaker then complained that anti-fluoridationists were going too far in their proposed wording of the advisories. He never said if those advisories were a good or bad idea, or if they should or should not be on the water quality reports. In 2010, a book titled "Infant Feedings: Guidelines for Preparation of Formula and Breastmilk in Health Care Facilities" was being written by the American Dietetic Association's Pediatric Nutrient Practice Group. I sent them a three-minute video (Use Nonfluoridated Water, 2009)

None of the authors replied to my e-mail. There was no mention of fluoridated water in the "Infant Feedings" book. All I could conclude was that these authors had no problem with infants being overdosed with fluoride for no benefit.

Recently, I've suggested the Los Angeles Department of Water and Power add an infant formula fluorosis advisory to their water quality report. Since I wanted to see if there would be resistance from local fluoridation supporters, I sent an identical e-mail to the deans of the public health schools at USC and UCLA, and the top leadership of the L.A. Dental Society which is associated with the ADA, referencing an advisory recommendation proposed in New Hampshire. None of them sent me a reply.

Just a few years after the 2006 admission of a fluorosis risk, the political implications of this advice to parents prompted even more extreme statements and recommendations from leading fluoridationists trying to justify, dismiss, or ignore that risk. In 2010, U.S. fluoride scientist Steven Levy, who is funded by the government, said no formula advisories were needed because the fluorosis might not be disfiguring. He is essentially saying let infants be heavily overdosed with fluoride and that parents and doctors should be kept in ignorance about the risk. Levy and his co-authors claimed that:

> *"Nearly all of the fluorosis in our study participants was mild. A recent review of the effects of mild dental fluorosis on oral health-related quality of life concluded that the effect of mild fluorosis was not adverse and could even be favorable."*

The ADA broadcast excerpts of that article included:

> *"This suggests that concerns about mild dental fluorosis may be exaggerated. Therefore, no general recommendations to avoid use of fluoridated water in reconstituting infant formula are warranted." (Levy et al., 2010)*

That kind of reasoning justifies letting children swallow toothpaste, and exposing them to more than "mild dental fluorosis" risks. The ADA has flip-flopped over the years, trying to find the right spin that won't discourage fluoride use.

Water Notifications about Infants and Dental Fluorosis Risk

I am not the only one campaigning for parental warnings regarding the fluorosis risk to infants and young children. When the Irish government considered issuing a warning to parents, political factions feared this advice could lead to the end of fluoridation in Ireland. So, all the plans to inform parents were canceled (FAN, 2012).

Stuart Cooper of FAN lobbied for a law in New Hampshire that would place the CDC advice on water quality reports. This is the required wording:

> *"Your public water supply is fluoridated. According to the Centers for Disease Control and Prevention, if your child under the age of 6 months is exclusively consuming infant formula reconstituted with fluoridated water, there may be an increased chance of dental fluorosis. Consult your child's health care provider for more information."*

While the law that mandated this advisory made its way through the New Hampshire legislature, it was opposed by the local chapter of the ADA. The law passed anyway with a huge majority in the New Hampshire house of representatives, despite the campaigning against the advisory by the New Hampshire ADA chapter. They claimed that the advice should be given in a doctor's office. The American Academy of Pediatrics (AAP) and the American Academy of Pediatric Dentistry (AAPD) are strong supporters of fluoridation that choose not to inform their membership about the risk of dental fluorosis and instead continue to advise pediatric fluoride supplements be prescribed in non-fluoridated communities.

The national water fluoridation level was lowered to 0.7 mg/L fluoride for the entire country in 2015. This reduced the fluoride exposure from water by 30% in New Hampshire. The CDC fluoridation engineer, using that news, told a top state water system official in New Hampshire that the CDC advisory about infant formula should no longer appear on water quality reports. She unilaterally ordered the advisories removed. She was quite embarrassed to later find out what she did was illegal. The advisories then reappeared on New Hampshire water quality reports.

Just a few years after the 2006 admission of a fluorosis risk the political implications of this advice to parents prompted even more extreme statements and recommendations from leading fluoridationists trying to justify ignoring the overdose risk.

Back in California, the L.A. County dental director admitted to me that he lied when he wrote in a pamphlet distributed to doctors and dentists stating that water fluoridation did not cause fluorosis. It certainly has been confusing.

In 2006 the ADA's initial advice was to have parents avoid fluoridated water to prepare infant formula, but in 2011 the ADA changed its advice on this fluorosis risk, saying fluoridated water *could* be recommended for infant formula preparation (Berg et al., 2011).

At my suggestion, the very large Los Angeles water system recently added a new section to their water quality report, pointing out that the use of their fluoridated tap water to prepare infant formula creates a fluorosis risk that can lead to discolored teeth. No one opposed adding this section to the water quality report, and internal discussion at the L.A. Water department showed they were aware of the new attention on fluoride and thought it was a good idea to add this section. Things are slowly changing for the better, slowly but surely.

Conclusion

The activities of the CDC, ADA and other organizations who suppress the facts about dental fluorosis and other risks posed to infants and young children by fluoridated water and supplements can have only one justification—any advice that casts doubt on using fluoridated water to feed babies casts doubt on water fluoridation in general. Since the public can still vote on fluoridation in some states, that doubt poses a political difficulty. The public perception of water fluoridation as good is more important to stakeholders than saving infants from any damage, whether to their brains, their guts, their thyroids, or their teeth.

Why Do We Have High Levels of Fluoride in Our Food?

The Background to EPA's Approval of Sulfuryl Fluoride

By: Ellen Connett

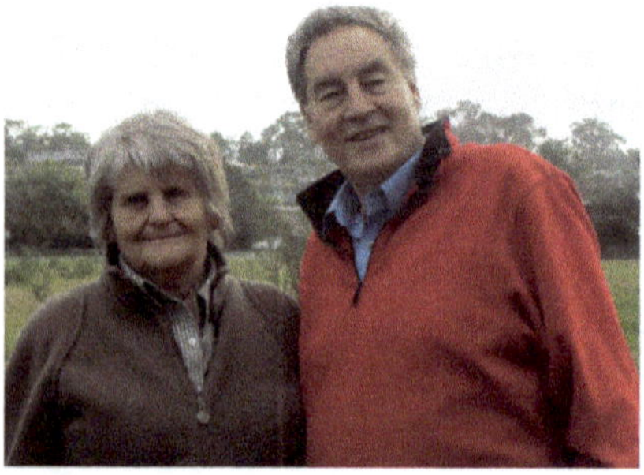

ABOUT: *I worked at an ad agency in NYC and met Paul while volunteering at the American Committee to Keep Biafra Alive. We married and moved to London where I became a pacifist and worked at Peace News, a weekly newspaper. I co-founded Operation Omega, an effort to get supplies to those in need in East Pakistan (now Bangladesh) who were too weak to cross the border into India during the 1971 Indo-Pakistan war. My colleague and I were sentenced to two years in prison for "illegally" crossing the border, but were freed by the Indian army as they advanced into Bangladesh.*

We had three beautiful babies in London, then moved back to the states to help my brother who sustained a catastrophic injury. In 1986, Paul and I became deeply involved in fighting municipal waste incinerators after one was proposed in our upstate NY county. The last 29 years have been spent fighting fluoridation and two years fighting the genocide in Gaza.

CHAPTER 32

"The prime purpose in this life is to help others.
And if you can't help them, at least don't hurt them."

—Dalai Lama XIV

ON JANUARY 19, 2011, my phone rang and it was Jonathan Fleuchaus, the General Counsel for the Environmental Protection Agency's Pesticides Division (EPA). He rang to "give us a heads-up" that the Federal Register, the official journal of the federal government, would be publishing a "Proposed Order Granting Objections to Tolerances" for Sulfuryl Fluoride. He told me that, as far as he knew, **"this was the first time in EPA's history that they granted an Objection." Translation: the EPA agreed with our Objections to their approval of the use of the post-harvest food fumigant Sulfuryl Fluoride, that leaves high fluoride residues on food, and that it was going to be phased out.** According to protocol, EPA simultaneously solicited public comments on the phase-out. And then...

Well, let's start at the beginning.

In the summer of 1996, my friend Georgena Hull called to ask me to speak out against the fluoridation of our drinking water at an upcoming village meeting in upstate Canton, NY. She told me it was dangerous for our health. She was a bright and well-read woman, and I thought she went off the deep end on this. I told her NO as I knew nothing about the issue, and I didn't even know that our water was fluoridated. We had our three sons in the UK and there was no discussion of this issue there.

Then for the next week she called me each day asking the same question. I got so angry that the last time she asked, I yelled into the phone "YES" and slammed the phone down. Belated apologies, dear friend. This was a gut reaction to the fact that I would have to put a ton of effort into understanding fluoridation and fluoride and that I would likely disappoint her.

As editor of *Waste Not*, a small weekly newsletter fighting incineration proposals across the country, I was in an unusual position, as I had lots of information on toxic substances. I had a part-time helper, Pat Perry, who meticulously filed everything into a huge number of four-drawer file cupboards in our basement. I first looked through the 'Tox Profiles' the government had recently begun issuing and found the 1993 "Toxicological Profile for Fluorides, Hydrogen Fluoride, and Fluorine" article by the Agency for Toxic Substances and Disease Registry (Clement International Corporation, 1993). My husband Paul, a chemistry professor, was away for three weeks fighting incinerator pollution somewhere overseas. I was on my own, with no email at that time. So, I went to my desk and read the report straight through. I found this on page 112:

> *"Existing data indicate that subsets of the population may be unusually susceptible to the toxic effects of fluoride and its compounds. These populations include the elderly, people with deficiencies of calcium, magnesium, and/or vitamin C, and people with cardiovascular and kidney problems."*

This was helpful. If the elderly (people over 50!) could possibly be harmed, then this would be an argument I would use for discontinuing fluoridation.

I also rang several environmental groups that we worked with in fighting incineration. I thought for sure Clean Water Action in D.C. would have some good info. I asked them to send me everything they had on fluoridation, and I would pay for all costs. They rang me back with, "We don't have anything." That was the refrain I heard from every national group I asked.

I found several unread items sent to Paul in our files on fluoride. I began reading them and found the story of William Marcus, the EPA's senior toxicologist, who stated that there were serious errors in a 1990 report on fluoride that the U.S. Congress requested EPA provide. And for that, he was fired. The information in my files didn't have the updated story, so I rang the EPA and asked for the office of their professional's union. Someone answered, and I blurted out, "What happened to Marcus?" I was told that Secretary of Labor Robert Reich "ordered" the EPA to reinstate him. According to Labor Secretary Robet Reich:

> *"... Labor found the EPA guilty of falsifying employment records, discrimination, and retaliation against an employee whistleblower. It also granted Marcus the largest compensatory damage award ever upheld under the federal environmental employee protection statutes. ...Reich disputed the EPA's position, stating, 'I agree with the ALJ that this rationale is pretextual and that the true reason for the discharge was retaliation'.* ***Both Reich and the ALJ found that Marcus was actually fired for publicly criticizing and opposing***

EPA's policy on fluoride in drinking water..." *(National Whistleblower Center)*

While on the phone with the EPA's Union office, I mentioned that I couldn't find any groups concerned about the fluoride issue. He recommended that I speak to Eleanor Krinsky on Long Island and gave me her telephone number. I called her straight away, and we spoke for a few hours. She explained the issue to me, and I believed her. She told me their group (which included Carol Kopf) stopped all fluoridation on Long Island, with a population of 7 million, by 1996. She said she would have activists send me studies. And they did! And I read them.

When Paul came home, I bribed him with a sandwich and cup of tea to read the studies. I trusted his opinion. If he didn't agree that I and the other women were on the right track, I would have dropped it. He agreed, and so it began.

I remember the night Paul and I walked to the village meeting with our son Michael to address fluoridation for the first time. Paul declared that this would be the easiest issue we would ever be involved in! He couldn't have been more wrong.

I was stunned at the huge turnout for our village of 6,000 at that meeting. Nearly every dentist in St. Lawrence County was there, including my dentist. I went up to him and told him what I learned. His response was, "Be careful; the anti-fluoridation people lie." I then learned that he was the president of the county's dental association! When I had a dental emergency a year later, his office told me I was no longer their patient.

It took our little community seven years to end fluoridation, even though the long-time head of our water department, William Hamilton, was opposed to fluoridating the water. His job was always in jeopardy because of that, but he was so good they never fired him.

It took a petition signed by 130 professors and the Dean of Students from St. Lawrence University to end fluoridation in Canton.

It was during this period that a group of us set up the Fluoride Action Network (FAN) in 2000. During this past quarter of a century, we had a front-row seat to the hubris and corruption that protects fluoride use, destroys careers, and irreparably damages human and environmental health.

Federal Hubris

We got our first real taste of the hubris of those promoting fluoride in 1997 when the Food and Nutrition Board at the Institute of Medicine (IOM) made the decision to include fluoride as a "beneficial" non-nutrient element as part of its Dietary Reference Intakes (DRI) recommendations for health. The DRI recommended "adequate intakes" with no special considerations up to an assumed safe upper limit (UL) of 10 mg a day for children and adults (IOM, 1997). This report led people to believe, mistakenly, that fluoride is an essential nutrient.

Paul and Bill Hirzy, a risk scientist for EPA, attended the public comment meeting that discussed that decision. Paul videotaped the proceedings. He phoned me immediately after the meeting. It was the only time he told me that he "needed a drink!" The meeting was terrible. Herschel Horowitz, DDS stood up and said that fluoride doesn't accumulate in the body and everyone clapped. Horowitz was the chief of community programs and clinical trials for the caries prevention and research branch at the National Institute of Dental and Craniofacial Research. He was a major promoter of fluoridation. He and his dental associates accused Paul of making money on his videos, an accusation that riled Paul and provoked much yelling.

Ian Munro was the chair of the IOM meeting. He was also the head of CanTox, a Canadian consultancy group with which I had been involved. In the late 1990s, his group approved a risk assessment for an incinerator scheme, slightly more advanced than a barbecue pit, to burn PCBs in Cornwall, Ontario. Anyone who knows the health statistics of Ontario knows that Cornwall stands out as being one of its sickest communities. I got party status as an opponent of the incinerator project, as did the Mohawks from Akwesasne who lived nearby on Cornwall Island. I read all the health reports available at that time. Past industrial practices in Cornwall resulted in significant mercury contamination. divides Cornwall in Ontario, Canada, from Massena in New York. Cornwall was a mile or two downwind of the two aluminum smelters in Massena and had major fluoride contamination. It was impossible to understand why this pro-industry consultant was selected to referee a public comment meeting under the aegis of the Institute of Medicine.

Ironically, the CDC said in 1999, and repeated in 2001, that its assumption of the need for ingestion for reducing cavities was flawed and that the negligible fluoride in saliva was similarly non-effective (CDC 1999; Adair et al., 2001). There is little doubt in my mind that many of the staunchest fluoride advocates at that meeting were aware of the science disproving their aggressive promotion.

We thought that when the CDC said the benefit was "predominantly" or "primarily" from topical use of toothpastes, that fluoridation would be phased out and the IOM would reverse itself. We were mistaken. The stakeholders in the fluoride mythology doubled down—and they used the controversial IOM decision as a talking point.

Fluoride in Food

Up until 2004, the major source of fluoride in U.S. food came from the use of the pesticide Cryolite (Sodium hexafluoroaluminate). Cryolite was the pesticide used on nearly all vegetables and fruits, grains, and more.

Cryolite

Sodium hexafluoroaluminate (its molecular structure, from Wikipedia, is shown here).

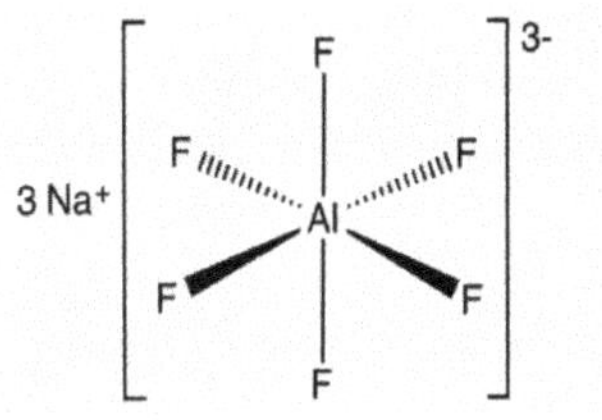

Cryolite was the pesticide used on nearly all vegetables and fruits, grains, flour, and more. No other country used it as the US did. Notice that it contains aluminum, another neurotoxicant that we want to keep out of our food.

EPA set tolerances (levels of residues) of fluoride from the use of Cryolite at 7 parts per million (ppm) "in" and/or "on", blueberries, broccoli, Brussel sprouts, cauliflower, cucumber, citrus fruits, eggplant, grapes, kale, lettuce, raspberries, strawberries, tomatoes, and many, many more foods.

Sulfuryl Fluoride

From 2004 onwards, an added source for contaminating U.S. food with fluoride was sulfuryl fluoride. This is its molecular formula:

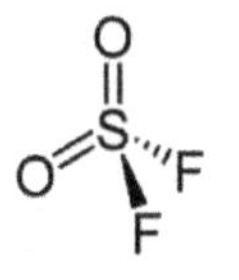

Also in 2004, EPA made its first-time approval of the use of sulfuryl fluoride as a post-harvest fumigant on a wide variety of foods such as dried fruits like raisins and legumes like lentils, and again in 2005 approved more high tolerances for foods, including 900 ppm residues for "dried eggs." At the time one-third of all eggs in the U.S. were dried and used in all food making facilities.

In 2004, Jay Feldman's group Beyond Pesticides joined with us as Objectors, and in 2005, the Environmental Working Group joined as Objectors due to the concerns of its co-founder, Richard Wiles. And we had a masterful pro bono lawyer, Perry E. Wallace, who worked to reverse EPA's approval through a series of substantive submissions to the EPA—which were incredibly demanding to write. Each person brought something to the table. We also went through obtuse mediations with Dow Chemical that went nowhere.

According to the EPA, sulfuryl fluoride breaks down rapidly in the human body to fluoride. And because of that, EPA approved two "tolerances": one for fluoride and the other for sulfuryl fluoride. They were the highest tolerances ever set by the government for fluoride.

Our team submitted copious well-documented and scientifically-referenced comments to the EPA regarding the risk to health, only to be repeatedly ignored.

More information on the fluoride exposure from food due fumigants can be found in the Appendix J.

Farm Bill

We continued to reach out to the EPA. What follows are a few of the comments we submitted:

- EPA failed to consider the potential for unexpectedly high fluoride accumulation in certain, unforeseen processed foods that had been granted tolerances for an incalculable large number of food items under the catch-all heading: "all processed foods will contain 70 ppm fluoride"

- Only a small fraction of current "processed foods" had any actual residue tests conducted on them

- Considering that the composition of each food item, particularly its protein and fat content, is a major determining factor for how much fluoride it will retain, the absence of any test data on most processed foods raises the distinct possibility that— as with dried eggs— some processed foods may concentrate fluoride to higher-than-expected levels. The following statement from EPA underscores the basis for this possibility:

  > "*For a number of finished products; the residues of sulfuryl fluoride in the packaged configuration were greater than in the open configuration... Method performance leaves a high degree of uncertainty surrounding residues of sulfuryl fluoride in Oreo® cookies, powdered eggs, and baking soda; and for residues of fluoride in white cake mix, pet foods, parsley, and baking powder.*"

- When we identified children's aggregate or cumulative exposure to fluoride from other sources as high, particularly from swallowing toothpaste, EPA misrepresented published data on toothpaste ingestion and assumed that ingestion of toothpaste would not be a problem due to the presence of instructions in fine print

- We found regulations that determine whether a pesticide residue is safe: the Federal Food Drug and Cosmetic Act (FFDCA), as amended by the Food Quality Protection Act (FQPA):

- *"[T]he term 'safe' with respect to a tolerance for a pesticide chemical residue, means that the Administrator has determined that there is a reasonable certainty that no harm will result from aggregate exposure to the pesticide chemical residue, including all anticipated dietary exposures and all other exposures for which there is reliable information." 7 U.S.C. § 346a(b)(2)(A)(ii)*

- The Reference Dose (RfD) used by EPA is the maximum acceptable oral dose of a toxic substance "below which no adverse noncancer health effects should result from a lifetime of exposure." The EPA changed the fluoride RfD for a 7-kilogram infant twice over four years, each time increasing the RfD and thus allowing for higher levels of fluoride for infants. These increases resulted in the highest allowable dosage of fluoride ever sanctioned by a government agency in the nation's history and were based on changing interpretations of the twenty-year old standard: the Maximum Contaminant Level Goal (MCLG). This makes sulfuryl fluoride the only pesticide ever registered where the allowed safe dosage for infants and children is higher than it is for adults. It is an unprecedented decision that warranted a high burden of proof that was not met.

- We objected to the substantive lack of adequate factual and scientific support underpinning critical assumptions and choices made in evaluating the tolerance petitions. Notable among these was EPA's choice, now thoroughly rejected by a National Research Council (NRC) report in 2006, to use the MCLG for fluoride of 4 ppm as the foundation of a safe exposure level for setting tolerances for Sulfuryl Fluoride under FQPA. The NRC study concluded that serious adverse health effects would occur at exposure to 4 ppm, a finding that undermines the notion that the tolerances meet the legal requirement of a reasonable certainly of no harm for infants and children in FQPA. EPA's reliance on an unsafe MCLG as the foundation of food tolerances for Sulfuryl Fluoride made it impossible for the process that established these tolerances to meet the legal requirements of the FFDCA, which mandate a careful, logical and sound assessment of the health risks associated with fluoride exposure. This failure pervaded and flawed the entire decisional process.

- Study after study of Dow's animal experiments with Sulfuryl Fluoride had the same outcome: severe and significant damage to the brains of all animals tested.

- Animals (rabbits, rats, and dogs) exposed to Sulfuryl Fluoride developed "malacia (necrosis)" of the brain. This is a very rare effect defined by Dow scientists as "liquefaction necrosis" (Quast et al., 1993). A more explanatory definition of liquefactive necrosis (from Uppsala University) is:
    - Necrosis characterized by dissolution of tissue
    - Necrotic area is soft and filled with fluid
    - No cell architecture remains
    - Results from enzymatic degradation of tissue.

- Sulfuryl Fluoride is the only pesticide with food tolerances in EPA's pesticides database that produces liquefactive necrosis. The only other non-pesticide chemical that we could find that produces liquefactive necrosis in the brain is soman (Armed Forces Institute of Pathology, 2002). Soman is an organofluorine warfare nerve agent.

- Vacuolation of the brain is a rare effect that is seldom found in animal experiments with pesticides. Dow reported vacuolation in the cerebrum, thalamus/hypothalamus, medulla, caudate-putamen nucleus and white fiber tracts of the internal capsule of the brain, white matter of the brain for females only, putamen, globus pallidus and internal and external capsules in the brain, and choroid plexus ependymal cells. There are only seven current pesticides used in the U.S. that are known to produce vacuolation in the brain of experimental animals. Of these seven:

    - One is Sulfuryl Fluoride
    - Two are fluorinated (Fluazinam and Indoxacarb)
    - Two are fluorinated and brominated (Bromethalin and Chlorfenapyr)
    - Two are non-fluorinated (Propamocarb hydrochloride and Propetamphos)

- According to a July 2006, California EPA Health Risk Assessment: "The cause of the vacuolation and malacia in the brain after sulfuryl fluoride exposure is unknown... In neural diseases, the formation of intracellular vacuoles in the brain is a marker for the diagnosis of a group of neural degenerative diseases called spongiform encephalopathies (De Girolami et al., 1999). Vacuolation of the neurons in the cerebrum, cerebellum, and other nuclei is also a finding in aging rats..."

- Due to the finding in animal studies of vacuolation of the white matter in the brain, we sent several copies of *The Behavioral Neurology of White Matter* (Oxford University Press, 2001) by Christopher Filley to EPA with our first submission objecting to Dow's request for an Experimental Use Permit. Filley wrote:

  "Early clinical features of cerebral white matter involvement typically include confusion, inattention, memory dysfunction, and personality change."

- We requested that a Developmental Neurotoxicity test (DNT) on animals be performed for fluoride before consideration of setting tolerances. EPA's action in waiving the DNT study was based on faulty reasoning and flawed science.

- Independent animal studies—investigating the effect of oral fluoride intake from water—have also reported elevated levels of fluoride ion in the brain (Zhai et al. 2003; Inkielewicz & Krechniak 2003; Vani and Reddy 2000; Long 2002; Guan et al 1998; Mullenix et al. 1995)

- Fluoride crosses the placenta (WHO 2002) and has been found in the brains of aborted human fetuses. Du (1992) examined the brains from 15 aborted human fetuses from an endemic fluorosis area and 16 aborted brains from a non-endemic area in China. He found:

  -the fluoride levels in fetal brains from the endemic fluorosis area were higher than the levels in the non-endemic area

  -fluoride passes through the placenta of chronic fluorosis mothers and accumulation within the fetus brain impacts the developing central nervous system and stunts neuron development".

- EPA only considered individuals with "average consumption" of fumigated foods.

The points above are some of the arguments in our Objections which resulted in the EPA granting our Objections.

And that's when the Dow Chemical Company, the proprietary owner of sulfuryl fluoride, did everything a powerful corporation can do to dissuade EPA from enacting the phase-out of "their" product. They lobbied the U.S. Congress. In January 2014, the Agricultural Act of 2014 (the "Farm Bill") was released with language inserted at the eleventh hour that reversed EPA's proposed phase-out of sulfuryl fluoride (and erased 9 years of hard work). Here's the language Dow wanted and got:

Agricultural Act of 2014 – Sec. 10015 Regulation of sulfuryl fluoride.

> *"Notwithstanding any other provision of law, the Administrator of the Environmental Protection Agency shall exclude non-pesticidal sources of fluoride from any aggregate exposure assessment required under section 408 of the Federal Food, Drug, and Cosmetic Act (21 U.S.C. 346a) when assessing tolerances associated with residues from the pesticide."*

By getting rid of the "aggregate exposure assessment," they nullified concerns of overexposure to infants and children, which was the basis of our objections.

But there's more. Having salvaged their post-harvest food fumigant from the phase-out, Dow Chemical sold sulfuryl fluoride in 2015 to Douglas Products. Congress allowed Dow to enrich itself on a chemical that is so extremely toxic to the brain that it should be forever banned, certainly not used on the foods we eat.

It didn't matter which political party was in power when the EPA made its decisions. Both parties and our regulatory agencies let down the American people and left our children unprotected.

FAN's team worked thousands of hours on this issue. When the U.S. Congress gave Dow what it wanted, I felt like I was literally run over by a train. It took me five years to pick myself up and write the end to this American tragedy on FAN's website.

Protect Yourself

I was told that Dow AgroSciences campaigned hard to get the EPA to accept sulfuryl fluoride as the replacement fumigant for methyl bromide. Because methyl bromide is an ozone destroyer, western countries were obligated under the UN Montreal Agreement to end all uses. Dow was the producer of both methyl bromide and sulfuryl fluoride, so they profited either way. In all their animal studies, Dow never looked for effects on bone.

Sulfuryl fluoride is exceptionally toxic, and workers who use it are at risk. A 1998 study by Calvert et al. compared the effects on fumigation workers who used either methyl bromide or sulfuryl fluoride. The study found that sulfuryl fluoride workers suffered 'subclinical effects on the central nervous system" as well as observable "cognitive deficits."

In addition to its use on foods, sulfuryl fluoride is also used as a structural fumigant to rid structures, libraries, ship containers, etc. of pests. Its trade name is Vikane. A 2024 study by Gaeta et al. noted that California uses ~85% of sulfuryl fluoride use (by mass) for structural fumigation, while ~15% is for agricultural and commodity fumigation. California emits 60-85% of U.S. sulfuryl fluoride emissions, with the highest from Los Angeles, Orange, and San Diego counties.

The good news:

- People buying organic and growing their own food avoided fluoride intake from pesticides.

- Homeowners now have alternatives to ridding their property of pest infestations. One alternative is heat-treatment: "a non-toxic method that involves gradually heating a structure or space to temperatures high enough to kill all bed bugs or other insects that have invaded that area..." See also online advice from "Beyond Pesticides."

Conclusion

Paul and I were accidental activists. We have three wonderful sons, albeit one is in heaven. We had fun together and can still laugh about embarrassing moments. We made wonderful friends and were inspired by people we wouldn't have otherwise met.

EDITORS' NOTE: We found a cancellation order registered in the United States, which forbids the distribution, sale, or use of cryolite and propazine, published in the U.S. Federal Register with a June 8, 2021 effective date.

From Light Posts to Litigation

By: Derrick Broze

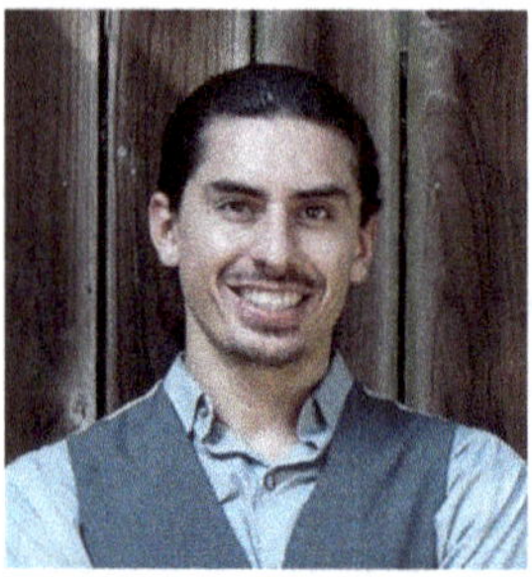

ABOUT: *Derrick Broze is an author, journalist, documentary filmmaker, and activist originally from Houston, now based in Mexico. In 2010, Derrick founded the activist alliance The Houston Free Thinkers, organizing protests, music festivals, community gardens, skill shares, and other community events. He also co-founded Fluoride Free Houston, an effort to end water fluoridation in the fourth largest city in the United States. Derrick has been producing videos, essays, and articles since 2011. In 2013, he founded The Conscious Resistance Network, a site dedicated to multimedia journalism that exposes corporate and governmental corruption while also highlighting solutions and exploring spirituality. Since 2015, Derrick has also published several books, including The Conscious Resistance Trilogy, The Holistic Self-Assessment, and his latest work, How To Opt Out of the Technocratic State. Derrick has also produced numerous documentaries, including Bringing Down Jeffrey Epstein, The 5g Trojan Horse, and the 17-part series, The Pyramid of Power. Since 2013, he has given presentations in the United States, Europe, and Central America.*

CHAPTER 33

"Unnecessary, unproven, and unsafe!"

—Dr Bruce Lanphear, MD, PhD (2023)

THE FIRST FORM of activism I ever participated in was putting flyers on the light poles in my neighborhood. They were simple enough—a picture of a running faucet, with big block letters flowing down, and the subtle phrase "There's Poison in the Tap Water!" Within 24 hours several of the posters had been torn down. I still remember the excitement I felt when I realized someone went to the effort to rip them down. It was the first time I felt like I had a voice. It was also the first time I felt like someone wanted to silence me.

I had only recently read Christopher Bryson's brilliant book *The Fluoride Deception* and shortly after discovered the Fluoride Action Network. I quickly went from completely ignorant about the dangers posed by water fluoridation to being overwhelmed by all of the data confirming that fluoride was causing harm to human health. I learned as much as I could, as quickly as I could, stopped drinking and cooking with tap water, and made it my mission to tell anyone who would listen.

In the years that followed I founded an activist group called Fluoride Free Houston, taking inspiration from other "Fluoride Free" groups I'd seen taking action across the world. We began visiting Houston City Council to share our concerns during the public speaking session. We also started meeting with council members, and quickly learned how difficult a fight it was going to be to convince the Mayor and the Health Department to take us seriously.

By 2014 I was a correspondent for the local news on Houston's Pacifica station, 90.1 KPFT. Since I was keenly aware of the stigma around the fluoride conversation—I'd heard my fair share of Dr Strangelove references by this point— I sought to normalize discussion of the dangers involved in water fluoridation. I used every opportunity I could to report on fluoride as a correspondent, and when I was eventually given the opportunity to co-host my own show, fluoride was a regular topic.

Around this same time, I also scored my first paid writing gig in independent media and regularly wrote about various studies relating to water fluoridation, as well as efforts to ban fluoridation chemicals. Headlines included *U.S. Government to Lower Amount of Fluoride in Water*; *STUDY: Infants at Risk from Hidden Fluoride Exposure in Commercial Foods*; *New Studies Indicate Exposure to Fluoride Affects IQ of Infants, Sleep Patterns*; *New Study Confirms Negative Impact of Fluoride on Thyroid Gland;* and *New Study Provides Further Evidence of Low IQ in Children Due to Fluoride Exposure.*

By 2018 I had learned about the Fluoride Action Network's back and forth with the U.S. Environmental Protection Agency. I kept my eyes on the situation and shared any updates I could with my audience. By February 2020, I interviewed Dr. Paul Connett, one of the founders of the Fluoride Action Network, regarding the developments in the legal battle with the EPA (Dr. Paul Connett on the Historic Trial, 2020). Connett informed me that the issue was finally headed to court later that year. In June 2020, during the height of COVID19 lockdowns, the San Francisco trial began online via Zoom. I tuned in to the court proceedings over the next two weeks and live blogged/tweeted what was happening.

While I was busy tweeting and writing articles on the developments, I immediately noticed a complete lack of interest in the lawsuit from the corporate press. The only reporting other than my own, and one or two other reporters in independent media, were from legal blogs with paywalls. The average person was hearing exactly zero about this historic trial which would impact all Americans. After the judge decided to put the trial on hold until the U.S. National Toxicology Program released their final report on water fluoridation and neurodevelopment in children, I did my best to write articles, record video reports, and keep attention on the issue.

Four years after the online hearings, the case was finally going to proceed in person in Judge Edward Chen's federal courtroom in San Francisco, California. Once the dates were set, I ensured I could be there in person for the entire two-week process.

On January 31st, the lawsuit proceeded with the star attorney Michael Connett representing the plaintiffs which included the Fluoride Action Network against the EPA et al. In the first week, I had the opportunity to interview Michael, as well as three of the expert witnesses - Dr. Howard Hu, Dr. Bruce Lanphear, and Dr. Phillipe Grandjean.

Dr. Howard Hu was the principal investigator in the Mexican ELEMENT study; a pregnancy and birth cohort focused on fluoride's impact on neurobehavioral development. The research was funded by the EPA and the National Institutes of Health. Hu had previously been involved in research on lead toxicity and antisocial behavior.

Following his testimony to the court, Dr. Howard Hu confirmed to me that he believes fluoride is a neurotoxin:

> *"Yes. I would say that, in my view, the evidence is quite persuasive that there is a negative impact of fluoride exposure on the neuro-development of children, particularly the research that's been coming out in prenatal exposure."*

Dr. Bruce Lanphear is a public health physician & pediatric epidemiologist who specializes in environmental exposures including lead & other toxic chemicals. Dr. Lanphear has an MD from the University of Missouri at Kansas City and an MPH from the Tulane School of Public Health. He is an expert on lead toxicity whose own work has been used by the EPA to develop their standards on lead.

Lanphear told me he also concurs with the NTP's conclusion on lower IQ in children exposed to higher amounts of fluoride. He also shared about his own studies on IQ:

> *"Well, what we found, whether we looked at urinary fluoride from the mom as a measure of exposure, or water fluoride, or an estimate of fluoride intake during pregnancy, in every case, we saw IQ deficits in the children."*

As to why it was only the boys who showed signs of deficits, Lanphear said the researchers "can't explain everything at this point." He acknowledged that this "raises more questions," however, he reiterated that the data has "really raised questions about practices like community fluoridation."

Dr. Philippe Grandjean is a Danish scientist working in environmental medicine. He is the head of the Environmental Medicine Research Unit at the University of Southern Denmark and adjunct professor of environmental health at the Harvard School of Public Health. Grandjean has an extensive history of researching mercury.

Following his testimony, I asked Dr. Grandjean about statements he made in the 1st phase of this lawsuit in 2020 regarding threats made against him at Harvard, and the "fluoride lobby" exerting influence over the World Health Organization (Broze, 2020).

Grandjean told me that after he began researching fluoride and its impacts on IQ, members of the Harvard University staff became concerned.

> *"A professor from Harvard University came to my office and asked me to sign a statement that my work on fluoride had nothing to do with fluoridation. He actually wrote this draft,"* Grandjean stated. *"And since I didn't sign this immediately, he instead went to my dean*

and had the dean sign a statement that he supported water fluoridation in accordance with the policy of the CDC."

Grandjean would later be told by "the leadership at Harvard" that his research on fluoride was "unwanted" and had never been approved by Harvard.

"Because we couldn't agree on my....what I would consider academic freedom, I left Harvard."

Grandjean also discussed what he meant by the "fluoride lobby" influencing the WHO. He said he had been invited by the WHO to help develop an "environmental health criteria" document on fluoride. Once he began gathering data, including animal data and epidemiological studies, changes were made to his draft.

"They inserted changes in my draft indicating that fluoride could perhaps be toxic, but only at immense concentrations," Grandjean said. *"I protested and said that in accordance with the scientific documentation, it would be wrong to insert the word immense."*

"And so, WHO published a document, without my name, because I'd asked to have my name stricken, but then they inserted some other colleague's name as the author of the draft, which is, of course, erroneous. But that was what WHO felt was necessary in order to protect the interests of water fluoridation."

I was astounded to learn these details from Dr. Grandjean. Of course, that's not to say that I was surprised. I had long ago learned that there does indeed exist a lobby of organizations like the American Dental Association and the American Fluoridation Society. While those groups, and the fluoride lobby Dr. Grandjean exposed at the WHO, play a powerful role in maintaining the public's ignorance regarding the dangers of water fluoridation, they are not alone.

The compliant and silent corporate media do their best to keep the general population in a matrix of false fact checks and slogans about "trusting the science." Other than myself, there was not another single journalist in the courtroom for the entire two-week proceedings. Thankfully, Brenda Baletti of Children's Health Defense came in person for the first week.

I was honored to be in this position— to be live tweeting, interviewing the expert witnesses, giving interviews about the happenings, and reconnecting to my activism roots. Fourteen years after my "poison in the tap water" flyers were torn down; I had the privilege of holding that space for all of the fluoride-free warriors who'd fought for decades to bring the truth about water fluoridation to a court of law.

Thankfully, in the end, Judge Chen saw the evidence against fluoride and ruled in favor of the plaintiffs on September 24, 2024. However, the EPA decided to appeal Judge Chen's ruling.

Wherever the fight goes next, I will be there reporting.

> **EDITORS' NOTE**: The EPA, through the Department of Justice (DOJ), began the process of appealing the verdict on July 18, 2025. The action was approved by Attorney General Pam Bondi and supported by an amicus brief from the American Chemistry Council (ACC). The ACC membership includes corporate polluters and fluoridation chemical distributors. The appeal is not questioning the findings of fact in the verdict, but rests its case on claims of legal technicalities. As promised, Derrick Broze is reporting on the continuing saga at:
> https://www.thelastamericanvagabond.com/category/health/fluoride-trial/

From San Francisco Union Square to the Federal Courts

How a Promise to End Water Fluoridation
Took Me Everywhere I Never Expected

By: Clint Griess

ABOUT: *Clint Griess spent five years interviewing the world's leading experts and advocates in the fight against water fluoridation and has gained extensive knowledge of the history, science, and politics of this misguided policy. He is a professional campaign consultant with 20 years of experience as a coach and trainer helping companies and political campaigns build effective, purpose-driven teams. An archive of the fluoride teleconferences he hosted and other related information can be found at* InternationalFluorideFreeTeleconference.org.

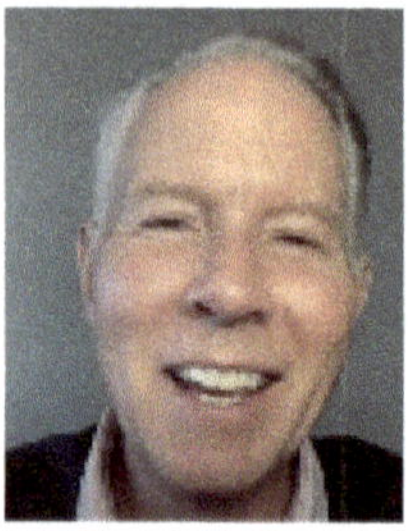

CHAPTER 34

"Fluoridation must be stopped.
Politics, not science, keeps it afloat. Let's sink it."

—Paul Beeber, JD (2018)

IN 2011, AT 46-years-old, I made myself a promise: I would find one cause, go all in, and stick with it until the very end—no matter how long it took, no matter where it led me.

I didn't know then that this promise would take me from organizing a marching band down Market Street to testifying before the NAACP, from running an international teleconference series to sitting in a federal courtroom watching scientists spar over the future of America's water. I didn't know it would pull me into the strange backrooms of politics, forge unlikely alliances, or demand a kind of perseverance I didn't know I had.

Choosing My Cause

By 2011, I'd dabbled in plenty of causes—cleaner air, healthier food, fairer elections, and even sound money. I'd donated to many organizations, but I'd never planted my flag and said: This is it. I'm staying until it's done.

I wanted a cause where success would be tangible, immediate, and undeniable. I spent more than a year weighing options. Then I landed on fluoridation.

It matched my deepest values:

- **Health:** Stop adding a known neurotoxin to public water, and everyone benefits instantly.
- **Personal choice:** When a government adds a biologically active substance to the water supply, it robs people of consent.
- **Practicality:** The Fluoride Action Network had already built a world-class library of science, politics, and news—a heavy lift done.

The moment it became real was a late-night conversation with my best friend Jonathan. We were both looking for something worth our full commitment. When fluoridation came up, the connection was instant—a shared outrage, a shared purpose. We promised to take it on together and, together, we traveled many unexpected roads.

The First Big Step: San Francisco

Jonathan and I moved fast. Our circles were full of artists and musicians, many already fluoride-aware. Soon my living room was a hub of spirited debate over whether to launch with an expert lecture or a marching band parade. We chose both.

When I arrived at Union Square that morning, my heart soared: a crowd of fresh-faced, eager people from all walks of life, holding signs, smiling, ready to move. The band struck up, brass echoing off the buildings as we marched down Market Street. People stopped, stared, asked questions.

We ended at the San Francisco Main Library, where an eccentric East Bay dentist opened with a lively talk linking oral health to overall health. Then Dr. Paul Connett took the stage, delivering a masterclass in science and policy. We'd promoted for weeks—flyers in cafés, laundromats, posts online—and we left with something even more valuable than applause: a list of people ready to stay involved.

Then came the game-changer: a middle-aged couple with a charitable fund offered us $75,000. We formed Clean Water California, a 501(c)(3), and began strategizing.

I wanted to run a San Francisco campaign—take the risk, make the splash. Others argued the city was too entrenched, too expensive, too risky if we lost at the ballot box.

There was no formal vote. It was a slow, quiet drift toward a decision I resisted for weeks. Eventually, I accepted what I'd fought to deny: San Francisco wasn't ready. The money went instead to the Fluoride Action Network to hire a communications director: our own Jay, a gifted musician turned natural professional advocate.

Portland: A Masterclass in Campaigning

With our local push stalled, I visited Portland, Oregon, for the final week of a special election to overturn the city council's surprise vote to fluoridate. Portland was the largest unfluoridated city in the country, and the backlash was fierce.

At campaign HQ, about ten of us crowded into a rented room. We were trained together, handed professional phone scripts, and put to work calling voters. The discipline, the focus, the efficiency—this was what a winning grassroots campaign looked like.

I brought those lessons home, hoping to ignite a local effort. Instead, I only underscored how far we were from that standard. If my city wouldn't run a campaign, maybe I could help *everyone else* run better ones.

The International Fluoride-Free Teleconference

That realization became one of my proudest creations: the International Fluoride-Free Teleconference.

Long before Zoom was routine, I hosted monthly calls linking activists, scientists, dentists, and lawyers from Ireland to Canada, Colorado ranches to federal courtrooms.

Over 48 sessions—two hours each—we built a library of more than 100 hours of testimony, strategy, and solidarity. Guests included:

- An Irish activist in a pink superhero costume rallying crowds with flair
- A Canadian water-system trainer who, after decades of adding fluoride, reversed course to expose its dangers
- A mother who discovered her autistic son's violent outbursts were triggered by fluoridated water.

We learned together, grew stronger, and connected across borders. But we also saw the sobering truth: where fluoridation existed, it was almost impossible to remove; where it didn't, it was nearly impossible to add.

From Teleconferences to a Book

By 2022, I had years of stories, strategies, and hard-won lessons. Activists worldwide were still reinventing the wheel in their towns. I wanted to hand them a map.

In October 2022, I published *Something in the Water: 12 Steps to Ending Fluoridation in Your Town*.

It's part manual, part rallying cry—distilling the best advice from campaigns worldwide into a clear, actionable path for any resident ready to take on their local water system. It's rooted in the belief that health, consent, and community choice are worth defending, and it carries the voices of those who've lived this fight, so others can avoid the pitfalls.

Although I wanted to devote my energies to an achievable worthy cause consistent with my values, I did not set out to become an "activist," much less an author. But the book was the natural next step in keeping my promise: if I could give new campaigners a head start, the whole movement could advance.

The Lawsuit: A Slow-Motion Silver Bullet

Then came the EPA lawsuit—a legal strategy with the potential to force the agency to regulate fluoride levels to protect the brain.

I attended every early hearing in San Francisco's federal courthouse, convinced we'd met the burden of proof. The judge delayed a ruling, waiting for a massive National Toxicology Program (NTP) meta-study.

When top HHS officials blocked its release, FOIA requests forced it into daylight.

Seven years after the case began, we won. I read the news from the Fluoride Action Network's bulletin and felt both satisfaction and caution. We'd had other moments in 70+ years when fluoridation should have ended. Instead, renewed propaganda kept it alive. This time, I knew the verdict had to reach the public—and force policymakers to act.

Politics: The Detours I Never Expected

Activism pulled me into politics more directly than I'd planned. A civics course from the Center for Self-Governance required meeting an elected official. That led to an internship at City Hall, then a staff role on a mayoral campaign.

The lesson came fast: politics is tribal. Personal alliances often trump sound public policy.

I learned this the hard way when I was fired a week before Election Day over false claims I'd sought a Republican endorsement—political suicide in San Francisco. I was persona non grata with Democrats and wary of Republicans, too. It was a bitter education in how quickly allegiances shift, and how often truth is irrelevant when power is on the line.

Why I'm Still Here

I began this journey thinking I'd chosen a health policy issue. I now know it's about far more than fluoride. It's about informed consent. It's about the role of government in personal health decisions. And it's about whether determined citizens can force entrenched systems to change.

This fight has taken me to parades, libraries, federal courtrooms, NAACP boardrooms, campaign war rooms, and conference calls spanning continents. I've been inspired, discouraged, surprised, and blindsided.

And I'm still here—because I promised myself, I would be.

As of now, the EPA has appealed our hard-won verdict—an appeal that could be withdrawn. The propaganda machine still spins. The opposition is as entrenched as ever. But we have momentum, truth, and each other. Every conversation, every flyer, every alliance—no matter how unlikely—chips away at the wall.

The end of tap water fluoridation may not come quickly, but it will come. And when it does, I will know I stood the whole way, through every detour, until the last tap runs clean.

Drinking Deception
Injury and Intrigue

By: Karen Favazza Spencer, BS, MA

ABOUT: *Karen Favazza Spencer began her career in education before transitioning to Corporate America. Her interests include social psychology and learning disabilities. Her Master's thesis was on the learning processes of children, adults, and organizations. A good Italian-American parochial schoolgirl, she never swore until she read the studies in PubMed on the effects of fluoridation, in particular the early studies by Feltman and Kosel (1956, 1961) and Grimbergen (1974), who determined that a percentage of the allergic population had immediate, acute, and debilitating adverse reactions to low-dose exposures from fluoridated water and supplements. These studies are supported by the testimonies of Dr Hans Moolenburgh and Dr George Waldbott who documented that many more people developed persistent illness over time due to chronic low-dose fluoride exposure. Karen was also motivated by the writings of Dr Philip R.N. Sutton and Dr John Colquhoun who found that the proclaimed reduction in cavities was a scientific fraud from the start. She not only followed their example of speaking truth to power, Karen co-authored a peer-reviewed study with Dr Hardy Limeback demonstrating how organizational bias can result in studies designed to fail (Spencer & Limeback, 2018).*

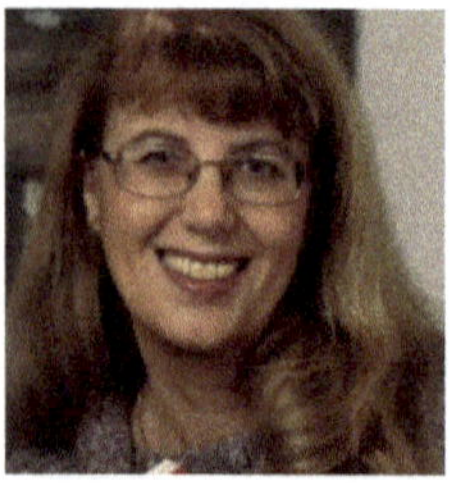

CHAPTER 35

"When injustice becomes law, resistance becomes duty."

—U.S. President Thomas Jefferson (1743-1826)

IT NEVER WOULD have occurred to me in a million years that someone would hire a virtual hitman in order to silence my voice. A free-lance software developer from Romania, no less! But that is exactly what happened.

It all started when I realized that not only were my thirty-plus years of arthritis, chronic fatigue, and irritable bowel syndrome caused by the fluoride my city added to our water supply, but that my emerging kidney and liver issues were also the result of fluoride-induced inflammation.

In the beginning

I didn't use fluoridated dental products because they irritated my mouth, neither did I drink green or black tea or consume any grape products, potatoes, or soft drinks, which are also often high in fluoride. They didn't agree with me, something I euphemistically called an allergy.

When I first realized in 2014 that my low-allergenic diet and high-quality water filter were essentially useless when it came to protecting me from fluoride poisoning and that I needed to strictly adhere to a no-fluoride diet that involved using bottled water even to brush my teeth, I began my investigation into fluoride science.

Since I am an analyst with a passion for research, this was not a problem. After a couple of months of study, I wrote my first letter to my local paper on this topic. It was a calm and professional letter stating that, whether they knew it or not, a significant portion of the community was having its health compromised by our fluoridation program. You would have thought I had committed a capital crime!

A flurry of vicious social media comments was posted on my local Massachusetts paper calling me "unintelligent," a "conspiracy theorist," and a shill for national players. Since I was a free-lance consultant with a good reputation in my residential and professional communities, I found this virtual assault very upsetting. I didn't know any of the people attacking me. But as I said, I was good at research.

I was amazed when I discovered this small group of social media trolls were posting the same vitriolic comments on local papers across the United States, as well as in Canada, Australia, New Zealand, and the UK. When I called them out as an organized troop of globe-trotting trolls whose members lived in North Carolina, Michigan, Colorado, Canada, and New Zealand, they denied it.

When a group of them from Australia to Florida tag-teamed me on Easter Sunday afternoon in 2015 within minutes of one of their number taking offense to my outing him as an out-of-towner who had "made the papers" in his Oregon hometown for his questionable fluoridation promotion behavior, I knew I had to speak out. Since I knew someone who knew someone who knew environmental health activist Erin Brockovich, I succeeded in getting Erin and five credentialed professionals to sign a letter to the Institute of Medicine in April demanding an update to its controversial 1997 categorization of fluoride as a beneficial non-nutrient. We included 100 hyperlinked science references. To my surprise, that letter was reprinted many times, internationally (Spencer, 2015).

Naming Names

However, it was my personal September 2016 letter with a much smaller reach that resulted in the paid hit. When a young woman at a nearby college wrote a dissertation misrepresenting the Cape Ann fluoridation battle, I wrote a rebuttal that was published by the Fluoride Action Network (Spencer, 2016c). A few weeks later, I realized that all of my social media comments on Facebook, Disqus, and elsewhere were muted; I could see them when I was logged in, but not when I was logged out. More importantly, no one else could see my comments, ever.

The letter that apparently prompted this attack named names. It included an appendix with copies of full-page advertisements paid for by two dentists. The advertisement ran every day the week before our non-binding referendum. It called those of us who protested fluoridation "anti-public health conspiracy theorists" and "fear-mongers" who were making "bogus attacks" that would cost the community hundreds of thousands of dollars in dental bills—all in large or bolded type.

Also included in the appendix was an opinion piece by one of the dentists who paid for the advertisements. He claimed that voting to end fluoridation up to a concentration of between 1 and 1.4 ppm per our annual water quality report would cost the community millions of dollars, implying that our effort included removing the natural calcium fluoride from our waters, a concentration below 0.2 ppm.

Our local editor should never have published the libelous advertisements or the dishonest opinion piece, but he was pro-fluoridation. He often censored or unfairly edited our letters.

The appendix to the September 2016 "Salem State letter" additionally featured a poster for a Gloucester event inviting interested parties to an "Interactive Speaker Training" sponsored by the Better Oral Health Massachusetts Coalition. The topic was "framing" the community fluoridation conversation. It was the young director of the sponsoring coalition who wrote the dissertation to which I had responded. The poster listed the names of the presenters. I understand from attendees that one of the presenters demonstrated pounding on the table with his fist while loudly declaring: "I don't have to debate fluoridation any more than I have to debate that this table is flat!" as a technique to silence anyone who brought up science unfavorable to fluoridation. So much for framing scientific conversation for civil community discourse.

As this anthology illustrates, those of us who protest fluoridation policy are often targeted by aggressive fluoridationists who engage in smear campaigns, social media stalking, and worse. But I was not a scientist, doctor, or dentist. Neither was I a public figure. I was a free-lance consultant. Why would someone care so much about what I said or wrote? Yet, someone considered me dangerous enough to pay money to silence me—a criminal act.

The Hits

Perhaps I should feel flattered that the fluoridationists took me so seriously. When I first engaged on social media, I was challenged with, "Are you a woo-hoo doctor or water salesman?" The trolls dropped that ad hominem approach when I responded that I was an analyst from Corporate America. However, they obviously didn't realize the extent of my talents or tenacity.

I was able to trace the hack on my Disqus account to the Facebook account of a Romanian freelance software developer. It took some effort on the part of the Disqus team to undo that hack, a hack which cleverly prevented me from directly contacting Disqus myself. Facebook figured it out in short order, but the software team for the social media platform used by my local paper struggled. That team told me they had never seen anything like it. Eventually, they engineered a fix that allowed me to comment again. However, the Halloween joke photo I used in October persisted for years—evidence of the original date and lingering traces of the sophisticated hack.

Incredibly, that was not the end of it. In 2022, I discovered that none of the emails I sent to either my local paper or anyone at the Boston State House were being received. This was a second hack. I developed work-arounds. Eventually, those hacks cleared on their own.

Someone, somewhere in the fluoridationist world, paid good money to silence my voice, again.

City Hall Schemes

A 2019 public records request to my city hall revealed that the chairman of my Board of Health (BOH) was working with notable fluoridationist players off-line to figure out how to silence me with not-so-subtle intimidation. None of that back and forth was available in the public records; they had apparently communicated by phone and shared drafts via private email accounts. However, the chair had sent the Director of Public Health a short email, which was a public record, informing her of his behind-the-scenes activities and advising her that his dental co-conspirator would send me and city leaders an email the next day that would intimidate me into silence. It didn't.

This same BOH chairman gave a presentation to the BOH in a neighboring town that shares our newspaper. It was a hit job on my presentation to my City Council. I have a copy of his PowerPoint and listened to the recorded audio of the event. He began by thanking a group of out-of-town fluoridationists by name for helping him with his presentation. Given that one slide implied some nefarious intent on my part for only emailing "six of the nine city councillors" when I had emailed a City Council subcommittee plus the Mayor and a couple of others in city government, I suspect he did little to nothing to create that presentation as he certainly knew who was who in City Hall.

This careless, ethically-challenged, and tone-deaf chairman once told me that "they knew" fluoridation was harmful to some consumers, but it was the "greater good" that counted. He told other residents with thyroid disease whose doctors advised them to avoid fluoridated water that they were "collateral damage." He subsequently denied making those comments or ever hearing of any thyroid doctors recommending fluoride avoidance, but there are a half dozen of us who know otherwise.

The chair of my BOH was a non-practicing medical doctor who earned his living through his non-profit and its relationship with pharmaceutical companies.

I read once that the value of a person can be measured by the enemies he or she makes. I certainly didn't set out to make enemies. I only wanted to spare my friends and neighbors the misery I experienced that began during my second pregnancy and resulted in my almost losing my child, a now adult child who still experiences neurotoxic effects consistent with prenatal fluoride poisoning.

Dental Deception

It has been eleven years since I became an environmental health activist, and the same dental players continue with their entirely disingenuous, frequently dishonest, and occasionally criminal behavior.

In January 2025, I attended a Board of Health meeting in Newburyport, MA, at the request of a couple of residents. It was the first BOH meeting I'd physically attended on this topic because, in my state at this time, the BOH does not have local authority to end fluoridation once begun. But my contacts promised me that this BOH was going to vote fluoridation out that night with a two to one vote. That was one of several oddities about what was and was not going on that piqued my interest. I told the organizer that the fluoridationists might seem quiet, but she could be sure they were active behind the scenes and the meeting would not proceed as expected.

It is important to know that Newburyport is a seaport community with many million- and multimillion-dollar homes. The median family income is above $100k. As I understand it, essentially everyone buys bottled water because of the general poor quality of city tap water. Residents routinely complain about brushing their teeth with smelly tap water.

When I signed into the meeting, I saw the name above mine belonged to one of the dental players mentioned in my 2016 letter. I settled in for the show.

The fluoridation agenda item was introduced by the chairman announcing that it had never happened before, but the Mayor had asked the BOH to not take any action. The Mayor advised waiting 60 days for a public hearing on fluoridation before making any decision. Then the chairman informed the room that a former member of the BOH would deliver a presentation representing the 'other side' in order to provide the sitting BOH with balance.

After an emotional outburst from the attendees, my dental adversary launched into a twenty-minute PowerPoint presentation where he established his credentials and experience and then treated us to the usual American Dental Association (ADA) fluoridation mythology and rhetoric. He claimed every bit of science unfavorable to fluoridation had been debunked, including the 2024 Systematic Review and 2025 Meta-analysis from the National Toxicology Program (NTP, 2024; Taylor et al., 2025). The NTP validated individual fluoride exposure, as measured in maternal urine in a significant portion of pregnant women living in 'optimally' fluoridated communities, resulted in lower offspring IQ on a dose-response trend line. He also cavalierly dismissed science associating fluoridation with other health conditions before lionizing several studies which, in fact, were all scientifically refuted.

For example, the NTP toxicologists went out of their way to explain why they did not consider the sloppy New Zealand study in their systematic review. Reasons for identifying it as low-quality and high-bias include: flawed assumptions and significant omissions. It seems many of the "unfluoridated" children identified by postal code had been taking prescribed fluoride supplements.

The problem was I was one of perhaps two of the forty attendees who understood the references, but confusing his audience was his intent and this was just his warm up. The dentist then launched into the meat of his presentation, a complicated series of slides with lots of graphs and jargon that he claimed proved that fluoridation reduces the risk of cavities for middle-class teenagers with dental insurance by up to 26%, which predicts more cavities for local teens above the five or more cavities they currently have in their adult teeth if Newburyport stops fluoridating its water, regardless of topical fluoride use.

I know the fluoridation literature. I had never seen this study. I knew it was unpublished and unlikely to pass a credible peer-review. So, in the moment of stunned silence when he ended, I called out, "Is that published?" He replied, "It's been submitted for publication."

That dentist, who was sitting next to the exit, then grabbed his coat and slipped out the door as the room erupted. I was told later by the organizer who invited me that my open challenge was the "drop mic" moment of the evening.

Moral Resolve

I guess the fluoridationist trolls were right in trying to silence my voice. If I hadn't been there and willing to insert myself at the appropriate time, it was unlikely that the BOH or attendees would have realized that they were the victims of a sophisticated con by a respected local dentist.

When I subsequently looked up his practice, I saw he not only offers fluoride treatments to children, but also to adults. He is the owner of the practice which employs two other dentists, eight dental hygienists and two administrative staff. My dental colleagues who oppose fluoridation tell me fluoride treatments in successful practices like this typically generate hundreds of thousands of dollars in gross income.

This brings me to the root of the matter: The seductive magic potion narrative about fluoridation is very profitable to dentists who market fluoride treatments and repair dental fluorosis. The American Dental Association which is a consumer group that lobbies on behalf of its dental membership knows this.

I'm not overly interested in topical fluoride applications; and I don't feel I need to convince every person with whom I engage that fluoridation policy is harming people and planet.

However, I, like the many wonderful people with whom I have collaborated over the past decade, feel a moral responsibility to speak out against this optional program that uses municipal water to systematically poison consumers from womb to tomb. Fluoridation policy is a scheme foisted on us by profiteers who don't care a whit for the pain and suffering they impose on others in order to enable their comfortable lifestyles.

It's that personal integrity that launched me into the fluoridation milieu with the 2015 "Erin Brockovich letter," the first of two she signed at my request (Spencer, 2015; Spencer, 2016b). That letter addressed to the Institute of Medicine (IOM) and my subsequent efforts with other professionals (Spencer, 2016a) garnered me an invitation to be listed as a Food & Water Watch member harmed by fluoridation in its 2016 petition to the EPA and subsequent 2017 lawsuit. That lawsuit, filed in federal court, found in our favor with a September 2024 determination that fluoridation policy is a hazard that poses an unreasonable risk to the developing brains of infants. The "Findings of Fact and Conclusions of Law" (Chen, 2024) are legal and scientific realities that should compel the EPA to take action to protect people like my son and me.

I may not be able to undo the damage done to my bones or to my family, but I can look at myself in the mirror knowing I've done my best to protect naïve victims who have been drinking deception for decades.

The Fluoridegate Scandal

By: Daniel G. Stockin, MPH

ABOUT: *Daniel G. Stockin MPH worked in the public health, health care, and environmental health fields. He worked at two large universities and two large integrated health care systems in southern California. His background and experience include work in toxics assessment and hazardous materials management, and he served as the manager of the EPA Western Regional Lead Training Center. He became involved in the work to end water fluoridation in 2004. His fluoride expertise is a sought-after resource for members of the media, law firms, citizen groups, public officials, and legislators. His work at The Lillie Center included numerous projects with the goal of ending water fluoridation.*

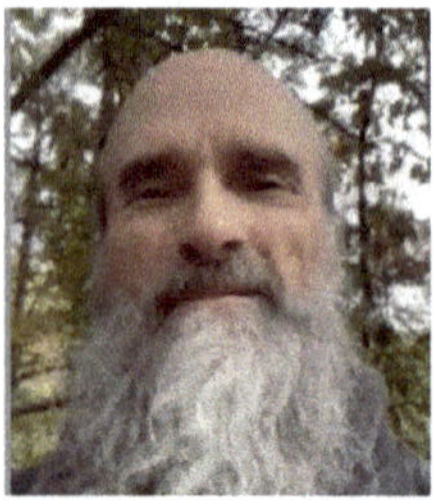

CHAPTER 36

"I am most deeply concerned for poor families who have babies. If they cannot afford unfluoridated water for their babies' milk formula, do their babies not count? Of course they do. This is an issue of fairness, civil rights, and compassion."

—Ambassador Andrew Young (2016)

I WAS JUST a quiet, nerdy scientist.

I worked with biological agents, hazardous chemicals, and radioactive materials. People trusted me to advise them about nerve poisons, shock sensitive explosive chemicals, and a lot of very dangerous environments and exposures. My background was in toxics assessment and hazardous materials management. I believed in the system of universities, government agencies, and other organizations with which I interacted on a daily basis.

I found out that my faith in this system was misplaced when I made the egregious mistake of starting to ask questions about fluoride safety in drinking water.

My peers were acting strangely. In fact, when it came to examining fluoride issues, their actions were more than disturbing. Scandalous even. This is why I eventually coined the phrase "Fluoridegate scandal," and published the first news of the scandal in a Juneau, Alaska newspaper.

What became clear to me was that otherwise rational and educated people were often unwilling to relook at fluorides in drinking water. Doctors were parroting fluoridation talking points, and were making unbelievably basic, fundamental errors in their statements about how fluorides affected the body. It was obvious to me that there was already enough science to have ended water fluoridation. Yet, fluoridation was continuing and groups were actually pushing for it to be expanded. And the fluoride supporters were working to put pressure on those who opposed fluoridation.

Federal agency publications clearly showed that certain groups were more at risk from fluoride exposure. Blacks, Hispanics, kidney patients, diabetics, babies, and outdoor workers were acknowledged to be especially vulnerable or susceptible (Doull et al., 2006; Beltrán-Aguilar et al., 2005). But constituent and health advocacy groups were not actively being shown the science.

So, I decided to start contacting various groups such as the American Water Works Association and the National Kidney Foundation to ask if they knew about disproportionate harm from fluorides for minority groups and those with certain specific diseases. My colleagues and I also filed an ethics complaint with the joint CDC ethics committees, showing how CDC's work to promote fluoridation was violating its own ethics policies. The CDC Director of Public Health Policy followed us out after our presentation, shouting and reprimanding us for describing fluoridation ethics concerns to a room full of bio-ethicists.

Our CDC fluoridation ethics complaint circled the globe via the internet. After the ethics meeting, I received a call from an attorney. That call affected me. After having read our ethics complaint, the attorney called to comment that our allegations "look like the basis of civil and criminal charges to me." So then we began speaking with law firms. It became clear that lawyers in the know believed that fluoride harm at some point was going to dwarf tobacco in the courts.

Dr. Lillie of The Lillie Center, my colleague, suggested contacting leaders in minority communities. It was a compassionate, brilliant strategy that is still paying dividends to this day. She said it was not morally right that low-income and minority groups not be told the facts. I respected her character and strength in supporting this approach. I was white, but my wife was Hispanic and I knew firsthand how environmental poisons affected Hispanics. I had also worked on the issue of lead poisoning affecting low-income communities as manager of the EPA Western Regional Lead Training Center.

We coordinated a series of Freedom of Information Act requests (FOIA), working with various citizens around the country who submitted the requests under their own names, not mine. They asked for documents inside CDC and other government agencies with information about how the agencies were addressing the issues of kidney harm, harm to minority communities, etc.

All of this rattled some cages. Some of the Freedom of Information Act documents that we finally received (after a long delay) were heavily redacted. It appeared that around one-third of all the pages were whited-out. This was surprising: after all, why the secrecy, if fluoride in water was all-American, safe, mom's apple pie, and good for everyone? What was the substance of the emails and communications that needed to be hidden from the public? Fluoridegate was unraveling.

In the un-redacted portions of the FOIA documents we found how public health and dental officials were working overtime to shut down the issue of harm to minority groups. Statements issued by civil rights leaders Andrew Young, Gerald Durley, Bernice King, and Alveda King, opposing fluoridation and calling for Fluoridegate hearings, caused great anxiety in government agencies and dental trade association representatives. The fluoride promoters were worried that the rapidly expanding fluoride knowledge in minority groups and their church groups had the potential to "gain traction." The worry was that an accelerating growth of awareness might pose a real risk to the public perception that water fluoridation was safe and effective in preventing cavities.

I was stunned at the sheer number of consultants and government officials who were working to help contain the spread of news about disproportionate fluoride harm to kidney patients and low-income and minority communities. What also surprised me was the fact that fluoride promoters apparently actually thought they could keep the news from becoming widely known. Were they really that foolish?

I'll never forget how their foolish thinking manifested in Atlanta in 2011. Key national dental and public health officials, with help from The Pew Charitable Trusts, convened a meeting at historically black Morehouse College in Atlanta to speak with civil rights leaders Andrew Young and Dr. Gerald Durley. These two men had spoken against fluoridation publicly and had called for Fluoridegate hearings to be held. But much to their dismay, Dr. Durley had invited me to attend the meeting. So, I drove down to Atlanta. I was a few blocks away from the campus when I received a phone call. It was Dr. Durley. He told me not to come, that the group did not want me in the room.

The meeting was set up by the pro-fluoride side. It was their meeting. The National Dental Association, government agencies, and others flew in and brought in a number of attendees. I respected Dr. Durley and I trusted his judgment. So, I turned around my car. I knew there was nothing the fluoride promoters were going to say to the two civil rights leaders that would change their mind. Durley and Young were smart and ethical men who would not fall for half-truths and tools of misdirection. I also found out later, in the FOIA documents, that attendees signed a non-disclosure document. Me being in the room would certainly have poked a hole in the idea of non-disclosure of what was being said or what occurred!

I was a trouble-maker in the eyes of fluoridation promoters. Bill Maas, former head of CDC Oral Health who then worked with Pew Trusts as a consultant, said in a post-meeting email that Pew was "aware of the problems Dan Stockin has created, the terrible 2-part story by the Atlanta CBS affiliate, etc." (More about the TV station story later.)

Dr. Leon Stanislav, of the ADA National Fluoridation Advisory Committee, after the meeting wrote, "The initial tone was one of distrust and I think this was generated by Dan Stockin... Although I did not use it by name, I contrasted the Lillie Center with Pew...I indicated that Pew's reputation and due diligence was impeccable and that I would trust them far more than some organizations (unnamed)." He concluded his email, "this becoming a very large picture with a movement through the black ministries and, possibly, even as high as the administration. Maybe this is an opportunity for both sides."

Bill Maas sent Dr. Stanislav's summary to CDC officials, with this telling statement: "I trust you will keep this summary from Dr. Stanislav in confidence."

Wow. Why did it need to be kept in confidence? I suspect they did not realize the information would later come out in a FOIA document.

And why did Dr. Maas also say in his email, "Pew worked behind the scenes to ensure that the recent meeting...would occur, even though no one from Pew was present."?

Another thought-provoking comment.

Why the "behind the scenes" and "keep it in confidence," non-disclosure statements, and redacted emails? Why did FOIA documents show that over decades of support for fluoridation, the Oral Health Division at CDC was the only part of CDC involved in deciding to endorse fluoridation? No one from the CDC who had expertise in kidney disease, diabetes, toxicology, etc. was ever included.

And why did the office of even the U.S. Assistant Secretary for Health become involved in coordinating efforts to respond to the issue of harm to minorities? Was this a conspiracy? Given all the machinations that occurred before and after the meeting, it sure looked like it. This was Fluoridegate on full display.

My not being in that meeting room wasn't just that I had real-world, hands-on experience in chemical risk assessment and toxics handling and sampling. Fluoridation promoters needed to keep a lid on their strategies and statements. They hoped to convince Young and Durley that CDC's dental-oriented viewpoint negated my direct professional experience in toxics and the clear statements of the NRC report and other research. I would have been able to easily dispute their defenses of fluoridation and would have exposed fluoridation endorsers straight to their face. So, they pushed to keep the trouble-maker out of the room and hoped to contain the efforts of two honorable civil rights leaders.

As I began the drive home, I had an inner knowing that the tactics and secrecy before and after the meeting were going to work to our advantage. The developments were going to be added to the list of bizarre actions taken by fluoridation promoters that would one day help cause the collapse of fluoridation.

On this list of disturbing actions is what occurred in the Georgia state capitol. The fear about the issue of fluoridation harm to minorities manifested in a meeting of the 2011 Legislative Black Caucus in the Georgia state legislature. The American Dental Association had coincidentally elected its first ever black President, who decided it was time to meet with Georgia's large number of black legislators. He called out our organization, The Lillie Center, by name, and reassured them that "the best available scientific evidence" indicated that Black kidney patients and diabetics could consume fluoridated water "without negative health consequences."

I winced when I read the ADA's press release about the gathering and the President's comments. ADA had elected a Black President who was helping further the fluoride narrative that was harming members of the Black community. This was not going to age well.

There were a number of key points we kept bringing up to leaders and advocacy groups. If fluoridation was "extensively researched" as to its safety, as the dental organizations and CDC claimed, why was the 2006 National Research Council (NRC) report from the National Academies of Science on fluorides calling for literally volumes of basic research to be done? This proves that whole-body fluoride safety had not been "extensively researched".

Why had susceptible subpopulation groups described in the NRC report not been proactively contacted to tell them of risks to their constituents? And why were normal risk assessment protocols and procedures not being followed by EPA when assessing fluoride safety? Fluoridegate was growing as untruths about fluoride safety were being exposed on many fronts.

Why had the National Kidney Foundation (NKF) allowed its name to be on a list of fluoridation endorsers assembled by the American Dental Association? I discovered that the Kidney Foundation's position paper on fluoridation was so old, it was actually still in a document typed on a typewriter! After receiving key correspondence about fluoride risks, why did NKF quietly withdraw its endorsement of fluoridation, but decide kidney patients "should be notified of the potential risk of fluoridation exposure" by burying the news of NKF's new stance deep within the NKF website? It appeared the only way a kidney patient would see the information was if they knew enough already to do a search for fluoride on the website. What about the millions of kidney patients who had no idea about fluoride risks and did not know enough to go looking for fluoride information deep within the NKF website?

Fluoride accumulate in the kidneys as the body tries hard to expel it. In the total population of Americans, one in nine American adults were going to be kidney patients. Surely openly advising this large group about fluoride risks would seem important, I reasoned. And what about Black, Hispanic, and other groups that suffered disproportionate amounts of kidney disease?

It also seemed a useful idea to start telling people that CDC information showed Blacks and Hispanics have significantly more harm from dental fluorosis, a permanent disfiguring of teeth from early childhood exposure to fluorides. So, we printed up large photos of the teeth staining from "very mild" and "mild" to "moderate" and "severe" fluorosis, and I began walking the streets of Atlanta and on college campuses, showing passersby the photos. Strangely, it appeared no one had ever done such a basic thing before: showing the public the pictures, and how even "very mild" fluorosis could be devastating to those affected by it. I thought that it only made sense to show parents of young children, adults, seniors, and people of different demographic groups pictures of what has disfigured the teeth of so many in their communities.

Channel 10 in Atlanta learned we were showing dental fluorosis photos to average citizens. The TV station aired a piece on fluorosis and our work. I set up a website where people could see photos of fluorosis and submit their own photos. The FOIA documents showed how upset officials were that the TV station had aired the fluorosis project story. I smiled. This was happening in CDC's backyard, in Atlanta. The world's foremost promoter of fluoridation was having to deal with people in its backyard finding out that fluoride was not so benign after all.

The oldest and largest group of Hispanics in the nation, the League of United Latin American Citizens (LULAC), adopted a national resolution opposing fluoridation in 2011. Telemundo Atlanta aired a three-part television expose on fluorosis in Hispanics, "Agua Potable o Veneno" in late 2015. I was one of those interviewed, along with the CDC. The series won an Emmy.

Dr. David Kennedy, a brilliant man, a dentist, and a longtime fluoridation opponent, called to ask if he could use the term Fluoridegate in the title in a movie he wanted to produce. *Fluoridegate: An American Tragedy* was a compelling movie which featured experts speaking about fluoride toxicity. We distributed the movie on discs to the offices of senators and congressional representatives in Washington, DC, and in the Georgia state capitol building in Atlanta. I felt the discs were seeds that would over time—along with the efforts of so many others—grow to help bear the fruit of an end to fluoridation.

The Truth is Now Coming to Light

So why has fluoridation continued for so long? It's not because we didn't have enough science to have ended it. We do want more science; I support that goal. But we have had sufficient knowledge to have ended the practice for a very long time.

Group think and group inertia, fear of lawsuits against fluoridation promoters, and fear of loss of income, reputation, and credibility—these all played a role in keeping the public in the dark about the harm caused by fluoridation. But the fluoridation house of cards is now wobbling; it is about to collapse. We have more information than ever before, and not just scientific studies. We have also learned about the cover-up that is Fluoridegate. The deception was foisted upon a trusting public, but the truth is now coming to light.

Dr. Lillie had a unique way of saying it: "There's a funny thing about the truth. Even if no one believes it, the truth needs no one to support it. It will still be standing after everything else has all fallen down around it."

EPILOGUE

Co-editor: Karen Favazza Spencer

"He who does not bellow the truth when he knows the Truth makes himself the accomplice of liars and forgers."

-Charles Péguy (1873-1914)

NO ONE WAKES up one day and decides to take an unpopular position that will alienate family and friends. Becoming an activist, as several stated in the preceding chapters, is more of an accidental occurrence. It often happens when there is a realization that an injury that they or someone in their family experienced was predictable and preventable, and that those with the power to prevent that injury chose to look the other way and let it happen.

Nevertheless, taking action to address controversial issues often leads to alienation and more psychological trauma. That is certainly the case with fluoride opposition.

So, who are these people who risk ridicule and repudiation by speaking the truth to power? They are a retired Army Corps of Engineers whistle-blower living in Alaska and they are a personal chef living in Texas, both of whom are willing to stand up in front of their city council year after year. They are a network of nurses stretching across Tennessee and Kentucky who reach out to state politicians as often as they can, given their family and professional commitments. They are horse ranchers in Colorado and they are an audiologist, dentists, and doctors specializing in environmental health in New York City hospitals. They are mothers, they are fathers, they are daughters, they are brothers. They are us. We couldn't possibly mention all the wonderful people who have spoken the truth to politicians over the years and we couldn't possibly have gathered all of their stories in even a dozen volumes (see Appendix A). We hope we've gathered stories from enough of a cross-section of these courageous individuals to let you know that opposing fluoridation is not crazy. It is perhaps the sanest action any of us has taken in our life.

Some of the people who initially agreed to submit to this collection of essays withdrew because they're writing their own personal books or are involved in litigation. A few declined to participate in print because they fear retaliation. A couple experiencing post-traumatic stress syndrome, or ongoing traumatic stress, withdrew because they found writing about the actions taken against them for speaking out was too stressful. These people include doctors, dentists, and scientists.

I once wrote that many fluoridationists are ignorant of the science of fluoride harm while others are willfully blind to that science, but that some fluoridationists are dishonest. At this point in time, I truly believe there are very few who can claim ignorance—at least not among the dental and medical ranks. So, the question is: how do they maintain their willful blindness to the science documenting harm? Are they just lazy or are they dishonest? There is certainly evidence that the studies that defend fluoride use are fraudulent, but this is not the time or place to go into that detail. The question is why do fluoridationists of all stripes behave the way they do despite the evidence and ethics against even low-dose fluoride exposure?

One of the most ironic injustices of fighting fluoridation is that the fluoridationists accuse us of the actions of which they themselves are guilty, such as omitting and misrepresenting facts. This behavior is consistent with gaslighting, aka psychological manipulation. It is also a trait of narcissistic and psychopathic personalities—one possible explanation for persistent fluoridation promotion.

I'm sure a few of the arrogant fluoridationists truly believe that what they're doing is the right thing, but what is that belief based on? Is it based on a sense of tribal loyalty—ideology? Is it based on some financial incentive, of which there are many? Is it a result of indoctrination or confabulation? Is it cognitive distortion? Is it criminality? Or are they just grown-up schoolyard bullies?

One example of outrageous behavior that I'll share involves Dr. Phyllis Mullenix, PhD, and the founding and current VP of the American Fluoridation Society (AFS), Boston dentist Myron Allukian. They each presented at a 1997 Natick, MA, town meeting. Dr Mullenix was supporting the recommendation to not start fluoridation in an exceptionally well-done special town committee report (Gallo et al., 1997). Dr. Allukian argued the opposite. As they were leaving the meeting, the dentist cornered the scientist in the lobby. He shouted at her that the evidence of harm she presented couldn't possibly be true. She invited him to come to her home to look at the data for himself. He retorted something to the effect of 'was she too cheap to mail him photocopies?' And at that, he pulled a handful of change from his pocket and threw it at her. At this point, she had her back against the wall, and a small crowd was frantically urging her apoplectic adversary to back off. Dr. Mullenix's husband, seeing the altercation from across the room, rushed over to insert himself between the irate dentist and his diminutive wife.

According to a water worker who was present that night and was still employed by Natick twenty years later, Natick fluoridated in spite of the recommendation not to fluoridate from its special committee and the brilliant presentation from Dr. Mullenix at that public town meeting. It was an executive decision that was the result of political pressure from a local dentist exerted in a private meeting that occurred after the public meeting.

The same arrogance and backroom politics continue to fuel unfathomable bad behavior today. The FDA has proposed the withdrawal of pediatric fluoride supplements from the market because not only have they never been FDA approved, but also there is scientific evidence of damage to the intestinal microbiome, thyroid function, and immunity in children from low-dose early-life fluoride exposure—in addition to the evidence of developmental neurotoxicity.

Dental associations sent out alerts to their membership with a template of sample language for submitting a public comment to the FDA in opposition to the FDA proposal. Over 4,000 dentists submitted comments following that template. Moreover, when in-person comments and presentations were made in July 2025, the audience of mostly pro-fluoride dentists and pediatricians applauded rhetoric, untruths, and *ad hominem* attacks from their side. Their side included an oral comment from the garrulous president of the AFS as well as the pro-fluoride argument of an American Academy of Pediatricians (AAP) representative who previously had testified under oath that she regarded a 5-point lower IQ in 10% of children as an appropriate trade-off for fluoride use.

This same audience refused to acknowledge the learned and detailed presentations of harm from medical doctors and scientists with expertise in toxicology and environmental health that compared the effect of fluoride with the effect of lead (Reagan-Udall, 2025). Are fluoride devotees so closed-minded that they are incapable of either compassion or critical thought? Or are they exhibiting the cultish loyalty that has periodically resulted in human horrors?

From another quarter, the American Chemistry Council (ACC), which represents the interests of industry profiteers, seems to have exerted pressure on the EPA and DOJ to appeal the 2024 verdict that requires the EPA to take action to protect the public from the unreasonable risk posed by fluoride exposure consistent with fluoridation policy (Chen, 2024). The appeal is not arguing the facts of harm but is attempting to manufacture a technical legal argument for why the EPA should not protect consumers as directed—an action that instead would protect the profits of various stakeholders.

The media has had almost as much of a field day with blasting that FDA recommendation for banning pediatric fluoride supplements as they have with defending fluoridation and maligning states and communities that have taken action to ban water fluoridation. Those news stories always include denials of science and gratuitous libel against HHS Secretary Robert F. Kennedy, Jr. Those propaganda pieces frequently include interviews with personable ADA dentists who stick to the sanctioned script with practiced skill. The ADA partners with the AAP and AFS, all of whom are well-funded in their efforts. They collectively present public-relations-crafted talking points and logical fallacies engineered to manipulate opinions. Is the media virtue-signaling or protecting the interests of its corporate sponsors?

This brings me back to my central question: Why do some people refuse to acknowledge scientifically documented harm and even work to continue that harm, while others, like the authors of the chapters in this anthology, have stayed the course in an attempt to protect consumers despite the personal and professional cost to themselves?

Yes, hubris, greed, and self-interest versus empathy, integrity, and courage explain the two groups, but there has to be something more. Perhaps it is because those of us who oppose the 'magic potion' mythology harbor a core belief that an imperfect and corrupted world does not have to be the way it is, that we can each exert our personal agency to change the world for the better.

ACKNOWLEDGEMENTS

Thank you to all chapter contributors for their patience, cooperation, advice, and encouragement.

Special thanks to Lynne Campbell for copyediting suggestions, to Brenda Staudenmaier for helpful marketing suggestions, and to Kevin Limeback, a teacher and graphic designer, for his cover design.

AFTERWORD

JUST AS THIS COLLECTION of essays was about to go to press in September 2025, dental, medical, and scientific dogma experienced an assault which brings to mind the opening salvos of the great world revolutions. None of us can predict the future, and large organizations like governments are notoriously resistant to change. However, the events in Washington, DC, this month that signal what, we hope, will spell the end of the pollution of foods, water, and medicines with fluoride and other toxins began with the release of the Make America Healthy Again (MAHA) Report. It contained 128 recommendations. According to the report, the CDC, NIH, and EPA will update regulations for fluoride and "forever chemicals" in water based on gold-standard science and the FDA has taken the first steps to remove pediatric fluoride supplements from the market based on evidence of harm to the microbiome.

A live-streamed meeting hosted by Health and Human Services Secretary Robert F. Kennedy, Jr., and Vince Haley, the Director of the White House Domestic Policy Council and executive director of the MAHA Commission, showcased leadership commitment to MAHA goals. Speakers included HHS second-in-command Jim O'Neill; NIH Director Jay Bhattacharya, MD, PhD; EPA Administrator Lee Zeldin, JD; FDA Commissioner Martin Makary, MD, MPH; Vice Chair of the White House Council of Economic Advisers Pierre Yared, PhD; and Secretary of Agriculture Brooke Rollins, JD. Several of these leaders mentioned their commitment to investigating the harmful effect of fluoride exposure on health.

Two Senate hearings, so far, were consistent with the underpinnings of the MAHA report. One of the September hearings addressed the government cover-up of Covid-vaccine injuries and the other exposed the suppression of "inconvenient science" by individuals and institutions committed to their narratives.

On the same day, the *New York Times* released a sophisticated video as an Opinion Editorial, "You Might Have Already Fallen for MAHA's Conspiracy Theories," which explains why, in its opinion, smart health-conscious people are fooled—in other words, the propagandists will not go quietly into the night.

—The Editors

APPENDICES

APPENDIX A:

UMass Fluoridation Collections

The following is a list of collections on water fluoridation in the Robert S. Cox Special Collections & University Archives Research Center at the W.E.B. DuBois Library, University of Massachusetts Amherst. The DuBois Library's special collections department preserves archives on movements for social change of all kinds. Each entry contains information on the size of the collections, the types of materials contained, and the description of each collection as written by Rob Cox. As of this writing, there are many more fluoride collections pending processing. Used with permission of the library. See library website at http://scua.library.umass.edu/?s=fluoridation

Contact: Michael F. Dolan PhD, editor of the Fluoride Action Network's Fluoridation Review. He can be reached at mdolan.ecsn@outlook.com

Martha Bevis Papers ca.1960-2007
100 boxes 150 linear feet
Call no.: MS 737
An important figure in building a network of antifluoridation activists, Martha Bevis was born in North Carolina in 1927 and lived most of her adult life in Houston, Texas. She worked on the staff of Senator Lyndon Johnson beginning in the early 1950s, remaining with him through his period as Vice President. Always energetic, she was involved in a number of political and civic organizations, including those promoting natural childbirth and breastfeeding, but from the mid-1970s, she was especially associated with the antifluoridation movement. A founder of the Safe Water Foundation of Texas, she became a key litigant in a case seeking to block fluoridation of the water supply in Houston, and although the court ruled in 1980 that fluoride was harmful, it permitted the city council to proceed with fluoridation. From that point forward, she played a key role regionally and nationally as an organizer, researcher, propagandist, and funding source for the antifluoridation movement. Bevis died in Houston on April 22, 2007.

This massive archive stems from Martha Bevis's role as a connector and mediator of information for the antifluoridation movement. Beginning in the 1970s, Bevis gathered, copied, and distributed huge quantities of information on the health effects of fluoride, legal strategies and cases opposing fluoridation of public water supplies, and the antifluoridation movement generally. Bevis maintained a regular correspondence with other activists and antifluoride organizations and played an important role in gathering and preserving the papers of other activists.

Norman B. Blumenthal Collection 1999-2005
30 boxes 45 linear feet
Call no.: MS 951
A native of Washington, D.C., and graduate of the University of Wisconsin (1970) and Loyola University of Chicago Law School (1973), Norman Blumenthal moved to La Jolla, Calif., in 1976 to accept a position as Chief Operating Officer and General Counsel for an oil and gas exploration company. After twelve years in the corporate sector, Blumenthal entered private practice, shifting focus to the protection of employees, consumers, and securities buyers from unfair business practices and pursuing both class action and individual cases. Among other notable cases, Blumenthal led a class action suit against the city of Escondido, Calif. (Coshow v. City of Escondido, 132 Cal. App. 4th 687), arguing that their decision to fluoridate the city water supply in 2001 amounted to "mass medicating the entire community" without consent using chemicals that were known to be carcinogenic. In 2005, the court upheld the City's fluoridation plan.

The Blumenthal collection represents the extensive legal and research files employed by the plaintiffs in Coshow v. Escondido and the appeals that ensued, including correspondence, litigants' files, depositions, exhibits, "expert documents," research materials and drafts, "extras."

Christopher Bryson and Joel Griffiths Papers 1997-2010
6 boxes 9 linear feet
Call no.: MS 810
In the spring of 1997, the investigative journalists Christopher Bryson and Joel Griffiths were commissioned by the *Christian Science Monitor* to investigate the connections between the Manhattan Project and the origins of fluoridation of drinking water supplies. Using reclassified documents obtained through Freedom of Information requests and deep archival research, Bryson and Griffiths uncovered a powerful story that connected the rise of fluoridation to the rise of atomic weapons production in the early Cold War era. Although the *Monitor* elected not to publish the article, it appeared in the anti-fluoridation journal *Waste Not* in 1998, and was cited as the year's 18th most censored story in the 1998 Project Censored Series. Bryson continued his work on the military-industrial roots of fluoridation in a later book, *The Fluoride Deception* (2004), which received that year's Project Censored Award.

The Bryson-Griffiths collection consists of materials compiled by the authors during the course of their research, representing the intellectual work of a decade of study on the politics and science of fluoridation. The collection includes a range of correspondence, transcripts of original interviews, memos between Bryson and Griffiths, and archival material gathered from the Manhattan Project and Kettering Laboratory archives. Noteworthy among these materials is a series of suppressed, unpublished, industry-funded studies that found fluoride harmful.

Albert W. Burgstahler Papers ca.1956-2007
75 boxes 120 linear feet
Call no.: MS 798
The chemist and ardent opponent of fluoridation of drinking water, Albert W. Burgstahler was born in Grand Rapids, Mich., in 1928. After receiving degrees from Notre Dame (BS 1949) and Harvard (PhD 1953), he embarked on a productive career of over forty years at the University of Kansas. His research in the synthesis and chemistry of natural products and the biological properties of fluorinated amino acids, led Burgstahler to a keen interest in environmental pollutants, particularly fluorides, and from the mid-1960s on, he enjoyed a reputation as one of the most prominent and prolific scientific voices opposing fluoridation. His efforts and long service as editor and chief of the International Society for Fluoride Research's quarterly journal, Fluoride, was formally recognized by the Fluoride Action Network in 2006, which awarded him its Scientific Integrity Award. Burgstahler retired from KU in 1998 and died on Oct. 12, 2013.

A large and diverse assemblage, the Burgstahler collection reflects the career of a stalwart in the anti-fluoridation movement. Spanning nearly five decades, the correspondence, publications, and research offer a perspective on Burgstahler's activism in science and public policy and documents his association with other anti-fluoridation activists, including George Waldbott and Paul Connett.

Robert J. Carton Papers 1935-2002 *Bulk*: 1983-2002
3 boxes linear feet
Call no.: MS 643
The environmental scientist Robert J. Carton emerged in the mid-1980s as one of the leading scientific critics of fluoridation of the water supply. After receiving his doctorate in Environmental Science from Rutgers University, Carton accepted a position in 1972 with the Office of Toxic Substances in the Environmental Protection Agency, assessing the risks associated with a range of toxic substances from asbestos to arsenic and hexachlorobenzene. By 1985, Carton became concerned about EPA standards for fluoride in drinking water, taking a public stance against undue political influence in framing those standards and insisting that there was no scientific evidence that fluorides prevented tooth decay and that any level of fluoride exposure presented a significant health hazard. In 1992, Carton left the EPA to work for as Chief of Environmental Compliance for the U.S. Army Medical Research and Materiel Command in Fort Detrick, Maryland.

Consisting primarily of research, notes, and some correspondence relating to the health effects of fluoridation of drinking water, the collection documents Robert Carton's nearly two-decade long struggle against the EPA and federal government. Also included are transcripts of filings relating to various legal challenges against fluoridation during the mid-1980s.

Elaine Marie Chesley Papers 1975-2002
1 box 1.5 linear feet
Call no.: MS 717
A resident of Brainerd, Minn., Elaine Chesley (1927-2011) was a woman of strong convictions and an activist in several causes, particularly the antifluoridation movement. As a member of Minnesotans Opposed to Forced Fluoridation in the mid-1970s, Chesley and the more strident Irene Johnson successfully prevented fluoridation of the water supply in Brainerd, and she remained active in the movement as a researcher and activist. She was also involved in several civic, environmental, and peace groups, including the League of Women Voters, the Green Party, Women Against Military Madness, the Women's International League for Peace and Freedom, Brainerd Coalition for Peace, and Save Our Northland. Chesley died at the age of 84 on May 25, 2011.

The Chesley Papers consist of materials collected in relation to antifluoridation activism. In addition to copies of a handful of historic documents on fluoride toxicity, the collection includes selective publications and correspondence.

Paul, Ellen, and Michael Connett Anti-Fluoridation Collection, 1950-2016 *Bulk*: 2000-2015
6.5 boxes, 8 linear feet
Call no.: 1170
In 1996, Paul Connett was persuaded by his wife Ellen to investigate the controversial practice of water fluoridation. In 2000, he was one of the founders of the Fluoride Action Network which he directed for 15 years (2000-2015). In 2003, Paul gave an invited presentation to a panel appointed by the US National Research Council, which published a landmark review of fluoride's toxicity in 2006.

In 2010, with two other authors, James Beck, MD, PhD and Spedding Micklem, DPhil (Oxon), Connett published The Case Against Fluoride (Chelsea Green 2010).

Paul Connett is recognized as one of the most important anti-fluoride activists of the early 21st century. The collection consists of material generated during his work with the Fluoride Action Network, which includes the contributions of his wife Ellen and their son Michael. Michael is now a lawyer who has brought a case against the EPA over fluoride.

The collection contains newsletters, correspondence, scientific papers, legal documents, clippings, publications, photographs, audio and video recordings, and a collection of 3/4" videotaped oral histories with leaders of the anti-fluoridation movement. Also contains material from Paul and Ellen's involvement with Work on Waste, USA, the environmental group opposed to municipal solid waste incineration (see MS 767, Work on Waste USA, Inc. Records).

Stephen A. Dean Collection 1983-2016 *Bulk*: 2013-2016
1 box 0.25 linear feet
Call no.: MS 979
Since the 1960s, the chiropractor Stephen Dean has been one of the leading activists in Massachusetts opposing fluoridation of the water supply. Based in Springfield, he has been an effective organizer in antifluoridation campaigns in communities around the state, arguing against fluoridation both as a medical hazard and a violation of individual choice. In 2005, he led the successful effort to strike down a state mandate to fluoridate all civic water supplies.

This small collection contains a handful of articles and clippings collected by the activist Stephen A. Dean regarding fluoride and the fluoridation of water supplies, and a note offering his expert perspective to journalists writing about the controversy.

Frederick B. Exner Collection 1952-1969
1 box 1.5 linear feet
Call no.: MS 924
The radiologist Frederick Exner settled in the Pacific Northwest after receiving his MD from the University of Minnesota in 1927. Concerned about proposals to fluoridate water in Seattle, he and his collaborator George Waldbott became national figures in opposing fluoridation by the early 1950s and for decades, were considered among the most effective scientific voices in the movement. A prolific writer and lecturer, Exner is particularly remembered for his influential book, The American Fluoridation Experiment (1957), co-written with Waldbott.

The Exner collection contains a number of mimeographed and printed articles by Exner on the environmental dangers and toxic effects of fluoride, dating from the early years of the antifluoridation movement.

John Remington Graham Collection 1978-1982
3 boxes 4.5 linear feet
Call no.: MS 724
As the principal attorney representing the plaintiffs in two lawsuits to prevent the fluoridation of civic water supplies, John Remington Graham had a profound impact on the antifluoridation cause. In November 1978, Graham convinced Allegheny County (Pa.) Judge John P. Flaherty to prohibit fluoridation in the borough of West View, Pa., with the judge writing that it was "simple prudence" to do so in the face of evidence that fluoride was a carcinogen. Four years later, Judge Anthony Ferris ruled similarly in the case of Safe Water Foundation of Texas v. city of Houston, citing not only the

carcinogenicity of fluorides, but their toxicity and inefficacy in reducing dental decay.

Consisting of the trial transcripts of Paul Aitkenhead v. Borough of West View (No. GD-4585-78) and Safe Water Foundation of Texas v. City of Houston, District Court of Texas (151st Judicial District, No. 80-52271), the Graham collection documents two high-profile, successful attempts to use the legal system to prevent the fluoridation of public water.

Jeffrey L. Green Papers ca.1990-2014
17 boxes 25.5 linear feet
Call no.: MS 877
The founder and director of Citizens for Safe Drinking Water, Jeffrey Lee Green (1946-2014) was a national organizer in the anti-fluoridation movement. A management consultant specializing in the health professionals, Green was adept at using the legal and legislative process to raise awareness of the potential toxicological dangers of fluorides. In 1996, Green helped his colleague David Kennedy facilitate a ballot measure to stop fluoridation in California, and they were instrumental in initiating a congressional investigation into fluoride between 1998 and 2000. Green later contributed to the 2006 National Research Council report on fluoride. Green died suddenly on Nov. 5, 2014.

The collection documents Jeff Green's work with Citizens for Safe Drinking Water, providing strategic advice for grassroots legal and political challenges to fluoridation. Of particular note are legal files relating to two important cases in California: one challenging the city of Escondido's decision to use hydrofluosilicic acid and the second leveling a constitutional objection to fluoridation without public consent.

Isabel Jansen Papers ca.1950-1985
12.5 boxes 19 linear feet
Call no.: MS 613
A Registered Nurse and surgical assistant at Marquette University Medical and Dental Schools, Isabel Jansen was a long-time opponent of fluoridation of drinking water. In 1949, her hometown of Antigo, Wisconsin, became one of the first in the state to put fluorides in its water supply. Jansen emerged as a prominent voice in opposition, arguing that fluorides had a cumulative toxic effect when ingested over a long period, and using public health data, she concluded that fluoridation was strongly correlated with an increase in mortality from heart disease and with a variety of other deleterious health effects. In 1960, she succeeded in ending fluoridation, however after a follow up survey showed a dramatic rise in tooth decay, Antigo residents voted five years later to reintroduce fluoride. Jansen has continued a vigorous resistance, publishing a series of articles on the public health impact and *Fluoridation : A Modern Procrustean Practice* (1990) .

The Jansen Papers include a range of correspondence, news clippings, articles, and notes regarding Isabel Jansen's long struggle against the fluoridation of drinking water.

David Kennedy Papers, ca. 1975-2016
5 boxes, 7.5 linear feet
Call n.: 1094
The son and grandson of dentists, David Kennedy earned degrees from the University of Kansas (BS 1967) and University of Missouri at Kansas City Dental School (DDS 1971) before establishing a practice in preventive dentistry in San Diego, Calif. During a successful career in which he served as President of the International Academy of Oral Medicine and Toxicology, Kennedy emerged as a prominent critic of fluoridation and the use of mercury amalgams, and was a consistent scientific voice of opposition to civic fluoridation of the water supply. He retired in 2000 to devote his efforts fully to improving the dental profession and to improve public understanding of oral health.

Along with the papers of his long-time associate Jeff Green, the Kennedy papers are a major resource for study of the anti-fluoridation movement in California and grassroot efforts there to repeal water fluoridation. The collection contains a thorough record of legal efforts to prevent water fluoridation, files relating to his activism, and audio recordings from professional meetings and other forums.

Malcolm G. Kennedy Papers 1967-1983
3 boxes 4.5 linear feet
Call no.: MS 678
Malcolm G. Kennedy became active in the antifluoridation struggle in 1954 when the possibility of fluoridating the water supply in his native Portland, Maine, was first proposed. Kennedy was a well-known figure in antifluoridation circles for over three decades and was the first president of the Greater Portland Citizens Against Public Fluoridation.

Centered on activities in Portland, the Kennedy Papers document antifluoridation activism during the height of the controversy in the late 1960s and early 1970s. A relatively rich body of correspondence with regional and national colleagues in the movement is accompanied by supporting materials and some newspaper clippings relating to efforts to fluoridate water supplies in Maine.

Hardy Limeback Papers 1977-2002
2 boxes 3 linear feet
Call no.: MS 776
A Professor of Preventive Dentistry at the University of Toronto from 1983 until his retirement in 2012 and a former President of the Canadian Association of Dental Research, Hardy Limeback was among the most prominent supporters in Canada of fluoridation of the water supply. However in 1999, Limeback reversed course, apologizing publicly for his role in promoting fluoridation and arguing

both that the therapeutic benefits of fluoridation had been greatly inflated and that the toxicity of fluorides had been ignored, leading to impacts ranging from dental fluorosis to lowered IQ and embrittlement of bones.

The Limeback collection contains a series of studies of the impact on health caused by fluoridation of public water supplies and a box of videotapes featuring Limeback and others discussing fluoridation.

Norman and Mary-Louise Meyer Papers 1942-1984
Bulk: 1960-1980
3 boxes 4 linear feet
Call no.: MS 778
Opposition to fluoridation of public water supplies in Massachusetts swelled in the 1950s, culminating in passage of a law in 1958 mandating that towns that wished to fluoridate would first put the proposal to public referendum. The primary force advocating for this law was the Massachusetts Citizens Rights Association, an organization founded and directed by Norman and Mary-Louise (Shadman) Meyer of Wellesley and which remained the leading anti-fluoridation group in the Boston area for twenty years. Having met and married while students at Harvard (1943) and Wellesley, respectively, the Meyers were tireless supporters of civic activities ranging from educational and environmental causes to public television (through the Citizens for Public Television in Boston), and disability (Norman served as director of the Protestant Guild for the Blind in Watertown), and they were stalwart members of the Wellesley town meeting. Norman Meyer died in Tortola in 1986, with Mary-Louise following in 1999.

The Meyer collection is a rich assemblage of letters and other materials documenting the Massachusetts Citizens Rights Association and the struggle against fluoridation in Wellesley, Newton, and other communities in eastern Massachusetts. Central figures in the movement, the Meyers maintained a wide correspondence with other activists throughout the region and published and disseminated information on the dangers of fluorides in the water supply.

Robert J. H Mick Papers 1950-1991
1 box 1.5 linear feet
Call no.: MS 677
Originally a proponent of fluoridating the water supply, the dentist Robert J.H. Mick became an ardent opponent following animal studies he conducted in the late 1940s. Although he alleged that he was threatened with court martial for his views while serving in the Army in Germany between 1953 and 1956, Mick has remained a high profile professional critic of fluoridation, famously offering a $100,000 prize to any one who could prove that fluoridation of water was healthy. The prize remained unclaimed. Mick ran as a Republican for congress in New Jersey in 1970, largely as an antifluoridation crusader.

The Mick Papers contain a small quantity of correspondence, talks, and affidavits relating to a decades-long career in the antifluoridation movement, as well as publications and other materials relating to fluoridation of water supplies.

New York State Coalition Opposed to Fluoridation Records, ca. 1975-2005
12 boxes, 18 linear feet
Call no.: MS 663
Founded in 1977, the New York State Coalition Opposed to Fluoridation is a non-partisan policy making and political action organization devoted to informing the public about the deleterious physiological effects of fluorides. With a membership comprised of professionals and non-professionals, physicians, scientists, and environmentalists, the Coalition works to raise awareness among elected officials at all levels of government about the need for environmental protection and works with an international network of similar organizations with the ultimate goal of ending the fluoridation of public water supplies.

The NYSCOF collection documents two decades of an organized, grassroots effort to influence public policy relating to water fluoridation in New York state and elsewhere. In addition to 7.5 linear feet of subject files relating to fluoridation, the collection includes materials issued by and about NYSCOF, several audio and videotapes, and documentation of their work with elected officials.

Carol Patton Papers 1956-2009.
7 boxes 10.5 linear feet
Call no.: MS 672
Born in Allentown, Pa., on Jan. 19, 1938, Carol Lazo Patton became an ardent activist in the antifluoridation movement, and one of its great supporters. After studying at the Allentown Hospital School, Patton became a registered nurse at Columbia Presbyterian Medical Center in New York city. Both professionally and personally concerned about health issues and the environment, Patton became involved in the antifluoridation movement by the mid-1970s, and became a major supporter of the Fluoride Action Network and other antifluoridation groups, playing a particularly important role in the struggle in her home states of Florida and Pennsylvania. Patton died on March 17, 2009, at her home in Jupiter, Florida.

The Patton Papers contain a record of over 35 years of antifluoridation activism, including valuable correspondence between Patton and other antifluoridation activists, publications and correspondence on fluoride toxicity and public policy, legal challenges to fluoridation, and materials issued by antifluoridation groups. Of particular significance is approximately 1.5 linear feet of material on the early antifluoridation fight in Virginia that Patton, probably associated with Landon B. Lane, apparently acquired as a result of her own work in that state.

Ionel Florian Rapaport Papers 1948-1971
7 boxes 10.5 linear feet
Call no.: MS 642
Born into a Jewish family in the town of Buzau, Romania, the endocrinologist and psychopathologist Ionel Florian Rapaport entered the University of Paris in 1937 to study under the eminent psychologists Maxime Laignel-Lavastine and Charles Blondel. Surviving the war by posing as a Christian, he completed a dissertation on ritual castration, *Les Faits de castration rituelle, essai sur les formes pathologiques de la conscience collective* (1945), which was published three years later as *Introduction à la psychopathologie collective : la secte mystique des Skoptzy*. In 1953, Rapaport emigrated to the United States and joined the faculty at the Psychiatric Institute of the University of Wisconsin, where he became noted for research into the social aspects of mental disorders and juvenile delinquency. It was there in 1956, that he discovered a statistical correlation between the incidence of Down Syndrome and exposure to fluorides, a study that became widely cited by opponents of fluoridation of the water supply and widely criticized by proponents. Rapaport died of cancer in 1972.

The Rapaport Papers contain a large quantity of raw data, research notes and correspondence relating to over two decades of research into mental disorders, centered largely upon his study of the link between Down Syndrome and fluoridation. Due to the potential sensitivities of some material in the collection, researchers must agree not to reveal the names of any patients before gaining access.

Ellie Rudolph Papers ca.1975-2002
25 boxes 37.5 linear feet
Call no.: MS 680
A resident of Oakmont, Pa., near Pittsburgh, Ellie Rudolph has worked with a number of grassroots organizations to oppose fluoridation of the water supply. One of the activists in the landmark 1978 case that prevented fluoridation in the borough of West View, Pa., Rudolph has worked with the Pennsylvania Environmental Network, was a founding member of the Fluoride Action Network, and a former director of the Pennsylvania Chapter of Health Alliance International.

The Rudolph Papers document almost three decades of grassroots antifluoridation activism, primarily in western Pennsylvania. The collection includes a wide array of material relating to the antifluoridation struggle, including several feet of topical files, some correspondence, reprints of scientific and popular articles on the subject and videotapes.

Myrtle K. Sapora Papers, 1966-1994
7 boxes, 10.5 linear feet
A life-long resident of Illinois, Myrtle Sapora was born on February 14, 1916, the daughter of William and Jeanie Kenney. After marrying Allen I. Sapora, a member of the teaching staff in leisure studies at

the University of Illinois, in 1948, and settling in Champaign-Urbana, Myrtle became an ardent activist in the antifluoridation movement, working a both the state and national levels. She was a member of the Illinois Pure Water Committee for many years and died on August 3, 1995 at the of 79.

The depth of Sapora's commitment to the antifluoridation movement is reflected in this rich collection, which includes research materials, newsletters and ephemera from antifluoridation groups, informational handouts, news clippings, and a few audiotapes of meetings. Concentrated in the later 1970s through early 1990s, Sapora's correspondence is particularly revealing, with interesting exchanges with politicians, letters to the editor, and other lobbying targets, as well as a number of important figures in the movement, including Albert Burgsthaler, Ellie Rudolph, and John Yiamouyanis.

Jean Thielman Papers ca.1960-1980
1 box 1.5 linear feet
Call no.: MS 676
As Secretary for the Citizens Committee Against Fluoridation for Western Pennsylvania, Jean Thielman was one of the key litigants in the landmark 1978 case that halted fluordiation of the water supply in the borough of West View, near Pittsburgh. Having become involved in opposition to fluoridation of the water supply in the 1960s, Thielman was part of a network of activists that included Ellie Rudolph, Eugene Albright, and Martha Bevis.
The Thielman Papers consist of a small assemblage of correspondence and supporting materials pertaining to antifluoridation activism in western Pennsylvania during the mid-1970s.

George L. Waldbott Papers 1930-1989 *Bulk*: 1957-1982
7 boxes 10.5 linear feet
Call no.: MS 609
After receiving his medical degree from the University of Heidelberg in 1921, George L. Waldbott accepted a residency at Henry Ford Hospital in Detroit, and embarked on a pioneering career in the study and treatment of allergic diseases. He is noted for his fundamental research on human anaphylaxis and penicillin shock, allergy-induced respiratory problems, and later in his career, the health impact of air pollutants. In 1955, Waldbott began conducting research in fluoride toxicity, becoming one of the first physicians to warn of the health effects of mass fluoridation. A founder of the International Society for Fluoride Research, he was considered one of the key figures in the antifluoridation movement for over two decades, contributing dozens of books and articles, including the influential *The American Fluoridation Experiment* (1957) and *Fluoridation :The Great Dilemma* (1978). He died in Detroit on July 17, 1982, from complications following open heart surgery.

The Waldbott Papers document one physician's long struggle against the fluoridation of the American water supply. In addition to a considerable quantity of correspondence with other leading antifluoridation activists, the collection includes an array of subject files relating to fluoridation, air pollution, and allergens, as well as drafts of articles and offprints, news clippings, and notes.

John Yiamouyiannis Papers 1967-1999
22 boxes 33 linear feet
Call no.: MS 645
One of the most prominent and vocal scientific critics of fluoridation, the biochemist John Yiamouyiannis (1943-2000) spent over three decades fighting the professional and political establishment. A graduate of the University of Chicago with a doctorate in biochemistry from the University of Rhode Island (1967), Yiamouyiannis became interested in the health effects of fluoride while employed as an editor with the Chemical Abstracts Service. His growing opposition to fluoridation, however, led to conflict with his employers and after being placed on probation in 1972, he resigned. Becoming a key organizer in the antifluoridation movement, he served at various times as the Executive Director of Health Action, the Science Director of the National Health Federation, founder and president of the Safe Water Foundation, and editor of the journal Fluoride. He also ran for the Senate from Ohio and twice for the U.S. Presidency on small party tickets, never garnering more than a handful of votes. Yiamouyiannis died of cancer at his home in Delaware, Ohio, on Oct. 8, 2000, at the age of 53.

Offering important insight into the antifluoridation movement in the 1970s through 1990s, the papers of John Yiamouyiannis offer a perspective on an unusually prolific and determined activist. The collection contains a large quantity of research material and correspondence relating to Yiamouyiannis's antifluoridation work, and perhaps most importantly an extensive series of transcripts relating to civil cases in which he was involved.

Philip E. Zanfanga Papers, 1966-1994
1 box, 1.5 linear feet
The physician Philip E. Zanfagna was a prominent early opponent of fluoridation of the public water supply. Born in Lawrence, Mass., in January 1909, Zanfagna earned his MD at Boston University and spent the bulk of his professional career as a specialist in allergic diseases at Lawrence General Hospital. Placed in command of a military hospital in Tennessee during the Second World War, he became immersed in pharmaceuticals research, through which he became aware of the health effects of fluoride. Over the next three decades, he emerged as a prominent opponent of fluoridation of the public water supply and of the suppression of debate over the topic within the scientific community. He published widely on the topic during the 1960s and 1970s and was recognized as an important antifluoridation activist, becoming a founder and first president of the International Society for Fluoride Research and a leading figure in the Massachusetts Citizens Rights Association. Zanfagna died in June 1982 at the age of 73.

A small but interesting collection, the Zanfagna papers contain a small quantity of correspondence relating to antifluoridation activism and research, 1969-1972; a set of audiotapes of the Frankfurt Conference of the International Society for Fluoridation Research, October 1967; and a handful of research reports of fluoride toxicity. The collection also includes a paperback copy of Zanfagna's best known book (co-authored with Gladys Caldwell), *Fluoridation and Truth Decay* (1974).

APPENDIX B:

Letters to the UK Parliament

This series of four letters (mailed with extensive addendums and attachments) were co-authored by UK scientists, Drs Howard and Paul Connett et al. Also included, the dismissive response from Stephen Kinnock MP, Minister of State for Care, dated 15th November 2024.

1st Letter to 10 Downing Street. 5th September, 2021

The Right Honourable Boris Johnson,
Prime Minister,
10 Downing Street
London

Dear Prime Minister:

SUBJECT: **Leading Scientific researchers concur that fluoridated tap water has the potential to damage the fetal and infant brain.**

We are writing to you because we believe that neither you nor your chief advisers are aware of the recent serious findings that fluoride, at the doses people experience living in fluoridated communities, has the potential to damage the brains of children. We are concerned that this compelling new evidence has not triggered any warnings from any health department in the UK, especially warnings to pregnant women.

The following key scientific research forms the basis for our concerns:

- Well-designed prospective cohort studies funded by both the National Institute of Environmental Health Sciences [NIEHS] in the USA as well as Health Canada, have shown a loss of IQ and increased symptoms of ADHD in offspring when pregnant women are exposed to fluoride **at doses commonly experienced in fluoridated communities in Canada** (Bashash, 2017, 2018 and Green, 2019). The consequences are very serious. According to Dr Philippe Grandjean, from Harvard University, *"Fluoride is causing a greater overall loss of IQ points today than lead, arsenic or mercury"*, (https://doi.org/10.1111/risa.13767)

- In addition, Till et al., 2020 have shown a large reduction in IQ when children were bottle-fed as babies in communities which were fluoridated, compared with babies who were bottle-fed in non-fluoridated communities.

- According to Linda Birnbaum, Ph.D., former Director of the U.S. NIEHS (2009-2019) and two leading public health researchers (Bruce Lanphear, MD, MPH, and Christine Till, PhD) who authored two key fluoride-IQ studies (Green, 2019 and Till, 2020), ingestion of fluoride during pregnancy confers no dental benefit to the fetus, so this is a situation where risks are being taken for no proven benefit (see their editorial published in Environmental Health News, Oct 7 2020 - https://www.ehn.org/fluoride-and-childrens-health-2648120286/costs-outweigh-benefits).

- In addition, an important well-conducted study from Sweden has shown an increased prevalence of hip fracture in post-menopausal women associated with long-term exposure to natural fluoride **at levels in water in the same range as the UK fluoridates its water** [Helte et. al. 2021]. This is very serious because, as you probably know, hip fractures in the elderly are debilitating, costly to treat, lead to a loss of independence and often shortens the life of those impacted. This finding also underlines the fact that fluoride, which accumulates in the bone and other calcifying tissues, can impact our health over a whole lifetime of exposure.

Given the extensive evidence that ingesting fluoride does little to reduce tooth decay and that fluoride is harmful to both the young and the old, please cancel plans to expand the water fluoridation programme and seek an end to existing fluoridation schemes. Until that end is achieved please make sure that a) pregnant women be warned to avoid ingesting fluoride and b) parents be warned not to use fluoridated water to make up infant formula.

While we recognize that right now the UK, along with many other countries, is being forced to deal with the health risks imposed upon us by the pandemic, we should not be imposing unnecessary risks on our population via the water supply.

In summary, Prime Minister, we sincerely hope that your health advisers will acknowledge the strong scientific evidence of fluoride's neurotoxicity (and other ill health effects) and put the health of our people above promoting what appears to be a well-intended but clearly outdated practice of water fluoridation. This would not be the first time that a well-entrenched medical or dental practice has had to give way to advances in scientific understanding of unexpected side effects.

Your sincerely,

Emeritus Professor Vyvyan Howard MB. ChB. PhD. FRCPath.
Retired pathologist. Past President, International Society of Doctors for the Environment (ISDE)

Professor Paul Connett, PhD,
Retired professor of chemistry, Director of the Fluoride Action Network, www.FluorideALERT.org

Dr H.S. Micklem, D.Phil (Oxon) Edinburgh, Scotland.

Note: both Connett and Micklem are co-authors of the book *The Case Against Fluoride* (Chelsea Green, 2010)

References

Bashash et al, Prenatal Fluoride Exposure and Cognitive Outcomes in Children at 4 and 6-12 Years of Age in Mexico, *Environmental Health Perspectives*, Sept. 19, 2017

Bashash et al, Prenatal Fluoride Exposure and Attention Deficit Hyperactivity Disorder (ADHD) Symptoms in Children at 6-12 Years of Age in Mexico City, *Environment International*, Dec. 2018

Green et al, Association Between Maternal Fluoride Exposure During Pregnancy and IQ Scores in Offspring in Canada, *Journal of the American Medical Association Pediatrics*, Aug. 19, 2019

Till et al, Community Water Fluoridation and Urinary Fluoride Concentrations in a National Sample of Pregnant Women in Canada, *Environmental Health Perspectives*, Oct. 10, 2018

Helte et al, , Fluoride in Drinking Water, Diet, and Urine in Relation to Bone Mineral Density and Fracture Incidence in Postmenopausal Women, Environmental Health Perspectives , 6th April, 2021. Vol. 129, No. 4

2nd Letter to 10 Downing Street. 27th December 2021

The Right Honourable Boris Johnson
Prime Minister,
10, Downing Street
London SW1A

27 December 2021

Ref: **Leading scientific researchers critique the Government's Water Fluoridation Policy Paper (Health & Care Bill 2021), threat to the developing brain.**

Dear Prime Minister:

Further to our letter dated 5th September 2021, we have not yet received any acknowledgement of its receipt or any reply from your office despite it being sent by recorded delivery. We enclose a copy with this current letter and trust that you and your health advisors will respond as a matter of urgency, regarding the very serious issues we present. Sadly, we have to report that one of our co-signers, Professor Spedding Micklem, passed away October.

As you may be aware, the Health and Care Bill 2021, is now in the House of Lords but what is very concerning is the apparent lack of thorough diligence performed by the Department of Health & Social Care (DHSC) in presenting its Policy Paper in support of mandatory water fluoridation, with its bias towards oral health and grossly inadequate review of the literature pertaining to the health risks posed by fluoridation, particularly its threat to the developing brain.

It is important to bring to your attention and that of the Health Secretary, the scientific evidence and reasoning why we believe the various references footnoted in the Policy Paper, lacked real scrutiny and failed to deal adequately or accurately with the very serious neurotoxicity studies funded by US government agencies (Bashash, 2017, 2018; Green, 2019 and Till 2020).

The whole debate on water fluoridation changed irrevocably in 2017 with the publication of a 12-year, prospective mother-child cohort study by Bashash et al. This was funded by the US Government and published in a high impact journal (Environmental Health Perspectives published by the National Institute of Environmental Health Sciences). It showed a 4 to 5 point loss of IQ in offspring, associated with maternal fluoride intake, typical of a fluoridated community.

The results of this study were so startling it would be helpful to add some detail here. 300 mother/baby pairs were followed for 12 years. The mother's fluoride exposure was measured directly via urinary fluoride level and the paired offspring's IQ was measured (again individually) at 4 and 6-12 years of age. All the previous criticisms of the 60 or so prior cross-sectional studies, showing lowered IQ associated with fluoride, were addressed in the Bashash 2017 study. Since then, three (3) more similarly robust US Government funded studies (Bashash, 2018, Green, 2019 and Till 2020) have been published. All point in the same direction - infant IQ loss (or increased ADHD symptoms) associated with fluoride exposure at the doses experienced in artificially fluoridated communities.

It appears that the UK's four Chief Medical Officers have already concluded Water Fluoridation is safe, citing the footnoted references made in the Policy Paper. However, many of these references are either misquoted or based on outdated science and the many, newer peer-reviewed studies are either misrepresented or not referenced at all.

To raise one glaring error in the section: 'Evidence of potential harm', the Policy Paper's authors state:

> *"There have also been some more recent studies reporting associations between exposure to fluoride and adverse developmental neurological effects [18, 19]. However, the evidence does not support this and various authoritative expert evaluations from different international organisations all agree that there is no convincing evidence that fluoride in drinking water at levels used in fluoridation schemes or at concentrations below the regulatory drinking water limit is harmful to general health [20, 21, 22 23, 24].*

However, three (3) of the five cited footnoted references [21, 23 & 24], claiming that "*the evidence does not support*" the US-funded Bashash 2017 and Green 2019 studies, were published before 2017 and thus it is absurd to use them to dismiss such important findings. Furthermore, even though the CADTH report [footnote ref. 20] was published after 2017, incredibly it did not review the Bashash 2017 study nor the Green 2019 study. The NZ Review [footnote ref 22] published in 2021, claims that these four key US government-funded studies (Bashash, 2017, 2018; Green 2019 and Till 2020) were undertaken at fluoride concentrations much higher than used in NZ (average F 0.85 ppm). That is simply not true and is an egregious error of statement.

We must, therefore, urge the DHSC and the Policy Paper's authors, to review again, these four US studies listed above. In doing so, they will find that these were either conducted in communities fluoridated at 0.7 ppm or lower (Green, 2019 and Till 2020), or, in the case of Bashash (2017 and 2018), involved pregnant women who were receiving equivalent doses to pregnant women in fluoridated communities based upon their urine levels.

Moreover, in addition to the failure of the authors of the Policy Paper to adequately review the IQ studies that they footnote /cite, they somehow managed to miss 17 other IQ studies, finding lowered IQ in children exposed to fluoride in utero or infancy published between

2017 and 2021. A complete annotated list of all 19 IQ studies is provided in the addendum, herein.

There is also an absence of reference to many recent studies showing fluoride's association with other health effects at doses experienced in fluoridated communities. These include: Hypothyroidism (Peckham, 2015; Malin, 2018): ADHD (Malin and Till, 2015; Bashash, 2018 and Riddell, 2019); Interference with sleep patterns (Malin, 2020); Increase in biomarkers of damaged kidney function (Wei, 2021, Malin, 2019, Jiménez-Córdova, 2018), and, an increased prevalence of hip fracture in post-menopausal women (Helte et al., 2021). More details and references on these omitted studies are given in the addendum.

The Childsmile Programme

Turning to benefits, another major omission in the Policy Paper (upon which the Health and Care Bill relies for its promotion of water fluoridation) is any reference to the **Childsmile** programme (NHS Scotland) which has had very successful results without the need to fluoridate the drinking water supply. Importantly, because it focuses on the child's education, both dental hygiene and diet, Childsmile helps to reduce obesity which causes many costly health problems. Also, because of early access to parents, it helps to fight the prevalence of baby bottle tooth decay, which often leads to operations under anaesthesia for children under 5, which is very costly for the NHS dental service.

In summary, Prime Minister, the inclusion of water fluoridation clauses in the Health and Care Bill 2021, appears to be a poorly researched endeavour, flawed in its lack of balanced scientific references within the Policy Paper, with many key studies omitted and rushed through by the DHSC.

In our view, it is essential that the clauses endorsing fluoridation be withdrawn from the Bill. Not to do so will not only cause unnecessary harm to our children and others but it will also cause your government acute embarrassment in the future. Our concerns are based on high quality science. The issue of fluoride's neurotoxicity at low doses is not going to go away –and in fact, gets stronger on a nearly monthly basis. Indeed, as we were writing this letter news came through of a new IQ study, from Indonesia, and a major review on fluoride's neurotoxicity and possible mechanism of action from the University of Cincinnati, both published within the last few days (links to these given in the addendum).

Furthermore, since the US National Toxicology Program has been engaged since 2016 in a systematic review of all the neurotoxicity studies, it would be prudent to wait for the publication of its final report, expected in early 2022, in order to aid the SC's anticipated and much needed reassessment of this issue. In any event, with such a major intervention proposed by the Bill, the Government needs to

consider how it will warn expectant mothers and parents who bottle-feed their infants, to avoid fluoridated water, and how low-income families will be able to manage this.
Finally, over and beyond the Health and Care Bill, we urge you to put the need to protect the development of the infant brain above any further effort to promote (or protect) what appears to be a well-intended but clearly outdated practice of water fluoridation. This would not be the first time that a well-entrenched medical or dental practice has had to give way to advances in scientific understanding of unexpected and very serious side effects.

We await your reply.

Yours sincerely,

Emeritus Professor Vyvyan Howard MB. ChB. PhD. FRCPath.
Retired pathologist. Past President, International Society of Doctors for the Environment (ISDE)

Professor Paul Connett, PhD,
Retired professor of chemistry, Director of the Fluoride Action Network www.FluorideALERT.org

cc. The Secretary of State for Health & Social Care; the Rt Hon. Sajid J Avid MP
cc. The four UK Chief Medical Officers.
cc. The Chair and members of The Health Select Committee.

Addendum: The addendum to this letter is available from the authors.

3rd Letter to 10 Downing Street.

The Right Honourable Rishi Sunak MP
Prime Minister
10, Downing Street
London SW1A

16 June 2023

Ref: UK Government's Water Fluoridation Policy (Health & Care Bill 2021), poses a serious threat to the developing brain.

Dear Prime Minister,

We are writing to you following the recent public release of the US National Toxicology Program (NTP) review of fluoride toxicology, particularly concerning developmental toxicity in the fetus and infant. We also attach copies of two earlier letters sent to your predecessor, Boris Johnson, in 2021, concerning this topic. These letters were prompted because of two clauses in the Health and Care Bill 2022, allowing for water fluoridation ('WF') to be mandated by central government, without any local government intervention being permitted. The timing of this move to central government control of WF is, in our opinions, very unfortunate. The scientific information underpinning the basis of the US NTP review has been in the public domain from 2017 onwards. And yet, the recent UK Policy Paper on WF (a 4-yearly review) failed to take any of this into consideration, which is a serious and puzzling omission. The purpose of this letter is to bring this matter to the attention of the Prime Minister by two experienced scientists (one a medical doctor and one a chemist), who are predominantly interested in the wellbeing of UK children.

The US NTP Report.

There is now an urgent reason to hesitate the introduction of any further steps towards extending water fluoridation in the UK. We have described previously the findings of several high-quality US Government funded peer-reviewed studies, showing that exposure to fluoridated water during pregnancy and baby-bottle feeding leads to a substantial loss of IQ in the offspring (and also an associated increase in the incidence of ADHD). The NTP review, made by the leading toxicologists in the US, has confirmed that the loss of IQ seen in these studies is valid and real. The pro-fluoridation lobby both inside and outside of the US Government did its best over several years to dilute, delay and even suppress the NTP review's findings, for fear of its impact on the US fluoridation program, but eventually what was deemed the "final" version by the NTP science team was published on the NTP website on March 15, 2023. The NTP report was provided to the Judge in a TSCA hearing on April 11th 2023, following which he ordered that it should enter the public domain.

Comments by NASEM being used by UK Government respondents to attempt to nullify the NTP report.

We understand that the dental lobby supporting WF within the NHS has made claims, similar to those of the American Dental Association (ADA), in stating that that NASEM (National Academies of Sciences, Engineering, and Medicine) had noted that the NTP failed to provide adequate scientific evidence for its conclusions regarding fluoride's neurotoxicity. This is **totally incorrect**. What NASEM in fact did was to call on the NTP to explain its methodology and findings with greater clarity and transparency (a procedural matter) which is completely distinct from stating that the underlying science did not support the findings that fluoride is a neurotoxicant (a substantive matter).

Importantly, NASEM's committee explicitly stated that it did NOT independently evaluate the underlying scientific evidence and was not charged with reaching any conclusion regarding the hazard rating the NTP has given to fluoride's neurotoxicity. We would therefore ask that the UK's Health Ministry retracts such irresponsible false claims and does not continue to perpetuate them in its responses to those questioning the Policy.

Note should be taken that in the documents released by the NTP on March 15, 2023, the NTP science team stated that: "*Several of the highest quality studies showing lower IQs in children were done in optimally fluoridated (0.7 mg/L) areas...*"

Additionally, the NTP also stated that there was "*no obvious threshold*" for these findings. They cited a graph in their report that showed "*a steep drop in IQ of about 7 points over a fluoride range from 0.2 to 1.5 mg/L.*"

The CATFISH Study.

The recent CATFISH study in the North West of England, costing £1.6 million, has failed to show any real benefit in reducing children's dental inequality. Therefore, the whole basis of WF is undermined through lack of efficacy. More importantly, the UK has never conducted toxicological studies to the quality and magnitude of those conducted in the US and around the world, many of which were peer reviewed and the subject of the NTP's review. How, therefore, can the Health Ministry mandate a Policy which flies in the face of current, high quality scientific data which clearly and unequivocally demonstrates that fluoride is a developmental neuro-toxic substance? On public health grounds alone, this should lead to the cessation of water fluoridation altogether in the UK. Setting aside the enormous costs that would be associated with extending WF in the UK, public knowledge of this research is inevitably going to lead to pressure for complete cessation of the practice. No parent will be prepared to risk their child's intelligence, i.e. brain damage which is irreversible, in order to save a fraction of a filling, which is easily repairable.

Finally, Prime Minister, we sincerely hope that you will be able to devote some attention to this matter, affecting the future intellectual well-being of the UK's children. We also mention here the problems caused by fluoride to thyroid function and bone density, leading to hip fractures, mentioned in our 2nd letter to Boris Johnson. We hope to hear from your scientific advisors with a response which is up to date on the current scientific literature. This would need to include expertise in developmental neuro-toxicology.

We would be happy to meet and discuss these matters with you and your delegated experts. We would appreciate it if your Office could confirm that this letter and the two previous letters to Boris Johnson have been lodged with House of Commons Library.

Yours sincerely

Emeritus Professor C. Vyvyan Howard. MB. ChB. PhD. FRCPath.
Emeritus Professor Paul Connett. MA. PhD.

CC: The Secretary of State for Health, Rt Hon Stephen Barclay MP.

4th Letter to 10 Downing Street.
27th September 2024
The Right Honourable Sir Keir Starmer MP
Prime Minister
10, Downing Street
London SW1A

27/09/2024
Ref: UK Government's Water Fluoridation Policy (Health & Care Bill 2021), poses a serious threat to the developing brain.

Dear Prime Minister,

We are writing to you following the recent judgement in the California High Court following a case under the Toxic Substances Control Act. Judge Edward Chen has declared fluoridated drinking water to pose an unacceptable risk to public health because of damage to the fetal and infant brain, resulting in loss of IQ. The likely outcome of the judgement is that US Environmental Protection Agency will have to mandate the cessation of artificial water fluoridation. We attach a copy of the judgement.

We have written in the recent past to Boris Johnson and Rishi Sunak, bringing to their attention the science underlying the outcome of Judge Chen's judgement. We were exercised by the
inclusion in the Health and Care Bill of two clauses transferring the responsibility of implementing water fluoridation from local to central government. It appears that the UK government is now on the cusp of extending water fluoridation, just as incontrovertible proof of damage to the developing brain has been published in the U judgement.

Furthermore, two recently published studies, funded by the UK taxpayer, have shown that water fluoridation is not efficacious. The CATFISH study was published in 2023 and studied the effect of fluoride on dental health in children. The LOTUS study was published in 2024 and studied adults. Apart from a virtual total lack of efficacy, the studies did not demonstrate any benefit for socially deprived population.

In the light of this new information, we would urge you to halt any current and future proposals to extend water fluoridation in the UK while the implications of this new information is considered. We would be happy to contribute to such a debate.

Yours sincerely

Professor Stephen Peckham
Professor Paul Connett
Professor Vyvyan Howard

Response:
Transcript of the letter to Gregory Campbell CBE MP (Vyvyan Howard's MP who submitted the above letter to Sir Kier Starmer, on behalf of his constituent) from Stephen Kinnock MP, Minister of State for Care, dated 15th November 2024.

Dear Gregory,

Thank you for your correspondence of 3 October (2024) to the Prime Minister on behalf of your constituent Professor Vyvyan Howard about water fluoridation. I apologise for the delay in replying.

I appreciate Professor Howard's concerns.

We are aware of recent decisions and publications in the United States, particularly the US National Toxicology Program's (NTP) *Monograph on the State of the Science Concerning Fluoride Exposure and Neurodevelopment and Cognition: A Systematic review*. As Professor Howard may be aware, the earlier evaluation and draft documents were peer reviewed by the US National Academy of Science, Engineering and Medicine and other external experts. The NTP concluded that there is *moderate confidence* that fluoride exposure was associated with lower IQ in children, where drinking water concentrations are greater than the World Health Organisation (WHO) drinking water guideline value of 1.5 milligrams per litre (mg/l). All UK water fluoridation schemes have fluoride levels in line with the WHO's recommended levels.

The NTP's *moderate confidence* indicates that there is evidence to suggest an association between exposure and outcomes, but some limitations exist. These include factors such as potential publication bias, indirectness, imprecision or unexplained inconsistent results across studies. The evidence is not enough to support high confidence, but the findings are supported by multiple studies.

There is no convincing evidence, including the NTPs systematic review, that fluoride levels below 1.5mg/l carry a risk of adverse neurodevelopmental effects in children.

The NTP also reported that there is insufficient evidence on fluoride exposure and adverse effects on cognition in adults. Conclusions could not be drawn from the conducted studies, as they were too heterogeneous and limited in number. Further information is available at https://ntp.niehs.nih.gov/research/assessments/noncancer/completed/fluoride

Water fluoridation schemes are in place in 25 countries, including Australia, New Zealand, Canada and Ireland. Professor Howard may be interested in Australia's systematic review on water fluoridation, which can be found at www.nhmrc.gov.au/health-advice/public-health/fluoridation

and Ireland's *Impact of community water fluoridation on systemic health excluding oral health: An evidence review*, which can be found at
www.hrb.ie/wp-content/uploads/2024/06/Impact of community water fluoridation on systemic health.2022.pdf.

The Secretary of State is required by legislation to monitor the effects of water fluoridation schemes on health, and to produce reports at least every four years. The reports are available at
https://assets.publishing.service.gov.uk/media/622ee4518fa8f56c1d3113dd/water-fluoridation-health-monitoring-report-2022.pdf
the 2022 report compares data on the health of people living in different areas of England with the concentration of fluoride in their drinking water supply. The next report is due in 2026.

Yours sincerely,

Stephen Kinnock

APPENDIX C:

The 2013 *National Assembly Commission on Fluoridation*

QUEBEC, CANADA: On February 2013, the *Regroupement des citoyens pour une eau saine à Richmond* had the idea of launching a petition on the website of the National Assembly of Quebec to demand a parliamentary commission to shed light on fluoridation, which it considered ineffective, dangerous for health and the environment, and a waste of public funds. A parliamentary commission on the fluoridation issue was held on April 22 and 23, 2013, at the Parliament of Quebec. Confirmation of the Commission's date was not given until three weeks before the event, requiring a superhuman organizational effort to find experts and people able to prepare and submit detailed briefs at the last minute. Of the 31 briefs presented, 27 opposed fluoridation, including some from prominent opponent experts. All briefs are archived and can be viewed on the National Assembly of Quebec website. Here is the list in chronological order of submission, as provided by the National Assembly. We have added their positions in favor of or opposed to fluoridation in parentheses to the official list.

Réseau environnement (Association des techniques de l'eau du Québec) (**Opposed**)
The Green Party of Quebec (**Opposed**)
Dr James S. Beck, MD, physician and author (**Opposed**)
Dr Roger Master, Ph.D. (**Opposed expert**)
Kathleen S. Thiessen, Ph.D. and member of the 2006 NRC Report on Fluoride in Drinking Water (**Opposed**)
Gaëtan Ruest, Mayor of Amqui (**Opposed**)
Richard Arseneault, Denturist of Richmond (**Opposed**)
Dr Pierre Larose, DDS, Dentist (**Opposed**)
David Veileux, Engaged Citizen (**Opposed**)
Coalition québécoise pour une gestion responsable de l'eau, Coalition Eau Secours (**Opposed**)
Dr Christian Linard, Ph.D. in Biochemistry, Professor at the University of Quebec in Trois-Rivières (**Opposed**)
Dr Paul Connett, Ph.D. in Chemistry, Founder of Fluoride Action Network (FAN) (**Opposed**)
Citizens' Group for Clean Water in Richmond (**Opposed**)
Nick Fonda, Citizen of Richmond (**Opposed**)
Monique Meunier, Citizen of Richmond (**Opposed**)
The Common Front for Clean Water, represented by Gilles Parent, ND.A. and Pierre Jean Morin, and a contribution to two chapters by Dr Poonam Mahajan, DDS, of India, and Dr Richard D. Sauerheber, B.A. Biology, Ph.D. Chemistry, University of California. (**Opposed**)

Friends of the Earth of Quebec, environmental organization (**Opposed**)
Sylvie Paquet, citizen of Quebec (**Opposed**)
Association des médecins spécialistes en médecine communautaire, med.specialists assoc. (**for**)
Maître James Robert Deal, lawyer working on the legal issue in USA (**Opposed**)
La coalition trifluvienne pour une eau très saine (**Opposed**)
Dr Eve-Marie Arcand, holistic dentist (**Opposed**)
Qualité de vie écodurable, environnemental group (**Opposed**)
L'institut national de la santé publique, a governmental agency (**for**)
National Pure Water Association Ltg (**Opposed**)
L'Ordre des dentistes du Québec, (**for**)
Le Ministère de la santé et des Services sociaux du Québec (**for**)
Deborah E, Moore, collection of studies on fluorides and fluoridation (**Opposed**)
Robert Duchesne, Citizen of Trois-Rivières (**Opposed**)
Marie-Ève Dubé-Legault, Citizen de Trois-Rivières (**Opposed**)
Anna Zeliszcak, Chantal Coté, Jean Dupont, and Josée Grenon, Regroupement de citoyens contre (**Opposed**)

APPENDIX D:

Email to the BBC

March 28, 2025
Tim Davie CBE, Director-General, BBC
c/o Siân Berry, MP
House of Commons
London SW1A 0AA
Email: sian.berry.mp@parliament.uk

Re: **The BBC and misinformation about the dangers posed by water fluoridation**:

Like many others who have grown up in the UK, the undersigned have trusted the BBC to tell the truth when it comes to controversial issues. However, in recent times this trust has been found wanting in the case of water fluoridation and science of fluoride's toxicity.

In recent years (since 2017) the BBC has failed to report on major scientific findings on fluoride's neurotoxicity (Bashash 2017,[28] Green 2019,[29] Till 2020[30]) even while a bill was going through parliament which would essentially make water fluoridation mandatory.

More recently the BBC has paid little attention to a major 7-year governmental review of fluoride's neurotoxicity by the US National Toxicology Program (NTP 2024[25]) and failed even to mention a lawsuit in which a US federal judge ruled on Sept 24, 2024, that water fluoridation posed an "**unreasonable**" risk to the developing brains of America's children (link to 80-page Ruling[26]).

Instead, BBC listeners have been treated to a Kindergarten level treatment of the issues in an 11-minute piece, March 25, 2025, on the BBC World Service (Fluoride: What you need to know)[31]. This program was unprofessional, biased and inaccurate. For example, no effort was made to get comments from scientific opponents of fluoridation, and the claim that lowering of IQ has only occurred at levels of fluoride **much higher** than those used in water fluoridation programs worldwide (0.6 - 1.2 ppm) is absolutely untrue.

The three US government-funded studies[28-30] cited above were conducted in either fluoridated communities in Canada (F =0.6 ppm) or in Mexico City where the fluoride levels in mothers 'urine were almost identical to the levels found in fluoridated cities in Canada and the USA (approximately 0.8 ppm).

Moreover, the NTP review - the most comprehensive governmental review of the issue to date - identified a lowering of IQ at 1.5 ppm - which leaves absolutely no margin of safety to protect all children drinking water at 1.0 ppm (the level used in the UK). For this protection one would normally use a margin of safety of 10. In other words, to minimize the neurotoxic threat to children, including the most vulnerable, you would not want children drinking water with a fluoride level greater than 0.15 ppm (1.5 ppm divided by 10). This would make water fluoridation unthinkable, unless one holds the view that protecting children's teeth is more important than protecting their brains.

Even the latter assumes that water fluoridation, as opposed to topical treatment with fluoridated toothpaste, actually does reduce tooth decay. In this regard a professional review of this controversial issue would have looked closely at evidence presented by two recent UK government funded studies (Lotus-2022[5] and Catfish-2024[6]) and the most recent Cochrane review of the matter (Cochrane 2024[7]) rather than rely on a long history of poorly controlled studies (see chapters 6-8 in our book[3])

What disturbs us about the BBC treatment of this issue, is that among ourselves, we have done many years of research on this matter, and so we know how bad this BBC report was. But what about other issues in which we do not have the luxury of our own research. Can we trust the BBC on these other issues? Once trust is lost it is very hard to get it back.

In conclusion, we call upon the Director General of the BBC to investigate the BBC's bias on this issue and to check into the testimony of a BBC correspondent who informed us that, when he went to file a story on this issue, he was told by his "superiors" that he could not include a discussion of the NTP Review or the Federal Lawsuit discussed above. Because of this he has resigned his position at the BBC. We hope the Director General will show the same level of integrity...

Sincerely,

Paul Connett, PhD
Vyvyan Howard, MB, ChB, PhD, FRCPath

APPENDIX E:

Certificates of Analyses

These Tulsa, OK, documents are from 2013. The arsenic concentrations are highlighted. Notice the variation for each batch, up to 60.1 in the snapshots below.

Division
Location **Riverview**
Product **FSA**

Mosaic

Element	Cd	Hg	Se	Co	Mo	V	Ba	W	Cu	Pb	As
Units	ppm	ppm	ppm	ppm	ppm	ppm	ppm	ppm	ppm	ppm	ppm
Sample Period											
01/11 06/11	<0.20	<0.07	<0.50	<0.35	<1.00	0.37	<0.10	<1.00	0.14	<0.27	47.5
07/11 12/11	<0.20	<0.07	<0.50	<0.35	<1.00	<0.36	<0.10	<1.00	<0.37	<0.27	43.8
01/12 06/12	0.01	<0.09	<0.27	<0.04	<0.22	0.24	0.05	<1.11	<0.10	0.02	44.0
07/12 12/12	0.01	<0.09	<0.27	<0.04	<0.22	0.28	0.07	<1.11	<0.10	0.01	47.8
01/13 06/13	0.01	<0.04	<0.04	0.01	0.09	0.28	0.06	<0.07	0.08	0.01	60.1

Element	Ni	Sb	B	Zn	Bi	Mn	Cr	U	Be	Ag	Tl	Fe	Al	Na	SO_4
Units	ppm	ppm	ppm	ppm	ppm	ppm	ppm	ppm	ppm	ppm	ppm	ppm	ppm	ppm	ppm
Sample Period															
01/11 06/11	<0.45	<0.12	<3.24	<0.92	<0.01	<0.24	<0.54	<0.30	<0.03	<0.01	<0.01				
07/11 12/11	<0.45	<0.12	<3.24	<0.92	<0.01	0.72	<0.54	<0.30	<0.03	<0.01	<0.01				
01/12 06/12	<0.15	<0.22	<1.70	<0.29	<0.02	0.56	0.17	0.23	<0.03	<0.01	<0.01	13.7	13.5	50.3	457
07/12 12/12	<0.15	<0.22	<1.70	<0.29	<0.02	0.73	0.22	0.28	<0.03	<0.01	<0.01	17.3	18.4	85.6	680
01/13 06/13	0.12	0.03	0.24	0.27	0.001	0.89	0.27	0.25	0.002	<0.001	0.0004	20.3	19.4	108	713

/28/2013 3:10 PM   T1ITPFAX01 -> 9187421253   Page 2 of 2

Page 1 of 1

Mosaic

8813 Hwy 41 South
Riverview, FL
Telephone: (813) 677-9111 - TELX52666
Fax: (813) 671-6283 ACCOUNTING

This product was produced at the Production Plant - Riverview facility

CAR NO: GATX011210

Deliveries: 5001084843

Material: Our / Your reference
200011 FLUOROSILICIC ACID /

Quality Certificate
Date
03/20/2013
Purchase order item/date

Delivery item/date
5001084843 000010 / 03/08/2013
Order item/date

Customer number
2445

Inspection lot 110000002967 from 03/20/2013

Chemical Analysis		
Net H2SiF6	24.20	%
P2O5	0.04	%
Free Acid	0.35	%
Lead	0.00	ppm
→ Arsenic	→ 52.00	ppm
Physical Analysis		
Density	1.2230	g/cm3
APHA	30	CU

"We certify that product shipped with this Certificate of Analysis meets AWWA B703-11"

NSF

Kwasi Sakyi-Amfo
QC Lab Supervisor - Riverview

APPENDIX F:

Complaint Letter Sent to Dr Christine Till's University

Editors' note: The libelous attempts by credentialled parties to discredit the research efforts led by Dr Till in order to disappear the inconvenient science uncovered by her team, and similar teams, reaches new heights of boldness and mis/disinformation with this letter suggesting possible actions against the authors.

International Group of Fluoridation Experts
<interntl.fluoridationexperts@gmail.com>

September 21, 2020

Mr. Paul Tsaparis
Chair, York University Board of Governors
1050 Kaneff Tower, Keele Street
Toronto, ON Canada M3J 1P3

c/o Pascal Robichaud
Secretary, Executive Committee
pascalr@yorku.ca

Dear Mr. Tsaparis and Members of the Board of York University, Toronto, Canada,

As governors of York University, you are entrusted with managing potential risk to the reputation of the University.

Therefore, we call upon you to establish an independent international committee to evaluate the quality of academic research which has engendered significant concern about public health in communities in Canada and the United States. We refer to the work of Associate Professor Dr. Christine Till, who has co-authored many papers, including with York University students, purporting to find that community water fluoridation is associated with significant harm.

The public health and scientific communities have already forcefully critiqued at least two of Dr. Till's studies (please see Appendix One). Nevertheless, Dr. Till's work continues to have sway in the political and public decision making process because it asserts a "possibility" that water fluoridation is dangerous, however dubious the work's methodology and conclusions.

That "possibility" frightens some elected officials and administrators. We are advised that several United States boards, which oversee water quality, are currently deciding whether to cease community water fluoridation because of concerns advanced by Dr. Till, her students and associates, including that fluoride harms the developing brain. This "possibility" also featured in debate about fluoridation reinstatement in Calgary, Alberta, Canada in October, 2019.

Dr. Till's fluoride research conclusions diverge significantly from current research on the safety of community water fluoridation (CWF). Numerous national reviews have found that fluoridation has an acceptable safety profile (such as Australia, 2017; Ireland, 2018; and Canada, 2019). Indeed, the recent Canadian review concluded:

> "There is consistent evidence that CWF protects against dental caries [decay] in children and adults and leads to improved oral health outcomes **with very uncommon and minor side effects**, and that CWF programs are cost saving from a societal perspective." [emphasis added]

More recently, a German Senate Commission on Food Safety review (Guth et al., 2020) concluded that:

> "based on the totality of currently available scientific evidence [which explicitly includes Dr. Till's maternal fluoride study], the present review does not support the presumption that fluoride should be assessed as a human developmental neurotoxicant at the current exposure levels in Europe."

Moreover, scientists have been unable to attempt to replicate Dr. Till's 2019 maternal fluoride study. Repeated requests to Dr. Till, to her funder, the United States *National Institute of Environment Health Sciences* and to the data repository, *Maternal-Infant Research on Environmental Chemicals* have not been met with a complete data set.

We understand that some Canadian professors have brought similar concerns to the York University Board of Governors, and note that the Board delegated the matter to the York University President, who dismissed the concerns as a matter of academic freedom. We agree with the Canadian professors' concerns. We disagree that the question is whether Dr. Till has academic freedom to publish her fluoride work. Dr. Till has exercised such freedom. **The question is whether ideology is being misrepresented as science, affecting public health and harming the reputation of York University**. Similar concerns were expressed about Andrew Wakefield's publication that purported to find an association between the measles, mumps and rubella vaccine and autism. A high volume of criticism about Dr. Till's fluoride work and the noted expertise of the critics make the nature of Dr. Till's fluoride publications a serious question for York University's Board to help resolve.

Fluoride research has great significance to public health in many nations. Dental decay is the most common chronic disease of childhood. Untreated dental decay prevents children from eating, sleeping, playing, concentrating and learning and so can delay brain development. Untreated dental decay has led to death in the United States. Community water fluoridation (CWF) reduces dental decay by approximately 25%.

For these reasons, we call upon York University to establish an international, independent committee to determine whether the published work of Dr. Christine Till on the subject of fluoride meets the international criteria by which publications are known as "science". An international, expert, arms-length committee should review all Dr. Christine Till's published research reports related to fluoride and fluoridation to determine whether these reports:

1. properly review the existing literature;
2. rely upon articles only from credible journals;
3. use sound, internationally accepted research methods;
4. use sound, internationally accepted statistical methods;
5. make conclusions based on the data; and
6. receive peer review by arm's length and objective expert reviewers.

Numerous publications by Dr. Christine Till report Dr. Gideon Koren as a co-author. While some of Dr. Koren's articles were subject to scrutiny, these are not related to fluoride. We do not propose that the articles Dr. Till co-authored with Dr. Koren (and others) be subject to the scrutiny of the committee.

We further request that this committee of international independent experts examine the public and media statements (please see Appendix Two) made by Dr. Till about her publications to determine whether:

- Dr. Till's public comments on her publications and the video she co-produced fairly report the studies' outcomes; closed caption available here
- Her public health recommendations are appropriate and consistent with her study findings; and
- Her public statements are characterized by truthfulness.

If the video is determined not to represent fairly Dr. Till's research reports, then we call upon York University to conduct a forensic audit to determine whether the video was financed with public funds entrusted to the oversight of York University for scholarly research and reliable research dissemination, and if so, to require that Dr. Till repay such funds.

This investigation is urgent because the first wave of pandemic restrictions limited people's access to routine preventive dental care, including dental hygiene and in-school dental screening; a second wave could well do the same. Moreover, pandemic-induced unemployment has caused many people to lose their employment-based dental health coverage. Consequently, the oral health of people in many countries depends more than usual on the preventive health measure of fluoridation, which dubious York University-associated publications are putting at risk.

Given that York University does not have schools of dentistry, medicine or nursing, we recommend that the international experts be chosen by the Royal Society of Canada, in collaboration with similar societies in other countries that offer the benefit of water fluoridation: the United States (the National Academies of Science, Engineering, and Medicine), United Kingdom (The Royal Society) and Australia (Australian Academy of Science). The committee should include experts in statistics, epidemiology and research ethics, as well as public health, toxicology, dentistry, medicine, psychology and nursing.

The committee's members' names and email address ought to be published so that documents might be sent directly to the committee by interested parties by a determined date (perhaps by October 15, 2020). The outcome of the review must be made public in whole on the York University website within five working days of its receipt by the York University Board (it is hoped by December 15, 2020). Time is of the essence.

Science advances when researchers follow the rules and prudential customs of science. Whether Dr. Till has done so is the essential question which we ask you to help resolve through the transparent process we have outlined above. We appreciate that this letter comes during a pandemic that strains all institutions' resources and, therefore, regret that our request comes at this time. Nevertheless, we note that dental decay is likely to affect many more children and adults around the world than COVID-19.

We look forward to hearing from you at your earliest convenience.

Thank you for your attention to this matter, which is having a significant effect on public health

Yours sincerely,

Michael Lennon OBE, MDS, DPD, FDSRCS(Ed),. FFPH.
John F Beal MBE, PhD, BDS, MFDS, MFPH(Hon), FRSPH
Myron Allukian Jr. DDS MPH
Scott Tomar, DMD, DrPH*
Michael Foley BDSc MPH MEpi
Josefine Ortiz Wolfe, PhD, RDH, CHES
Mairead Harding, BDS, MFGDP (UK), MDPH, PhD, FDS
Sergio Uribe, DDS, PhD
Alice M. Horowitz, PhD, MA, RDH
Ken Perrott, PhD
Thomas W. Hennessy, MD, MPH
Denice Curtis, DDS, MPH, DHS

Jennifer Meyer PhD, MPH, CPH, RN
Ruby L. Fried, PhD

/Accompanying

Appendix One: Expressions of Concern about Dr. Till's Maternal Fluoride Paper

Appendix Two: Dr. Till's Public Commentary on her Published Reports

Appendix Three: Dr. Christine Till's Research Reports Related to Fluoride or Fluoridation

Cc. various media outlets

***EDITORS' NOTE:** Scott Tomar denied during a podcast that he signed this letter. He subsequently tried to downplay his denial (see Chapter 25 for details).

Undark Podcast: *"during our fact-check of this episode we found out that there were several with his signature. I followed up with him and he said that he misspoke here. He said, in part and I quote from an email: "I do not believe that there was fabrication of data, and I think that's what I had in mind when I answered your question.* ***I was mistaken when I said that I did not sign letters alleging research misconduct."***

APPENDIX G:

National Post (Canada) Article Calling for an Investigation of Dr Christine Till's work

An example of an article from one of the "various media outlets" referenced as carbon-copied in the letter in the previous appendix.

International experts call for independent probe of Canadian research linking fluoride and lower IQ

An arm's-length review is needed to determine whether 'ideology is being misrepresented as science,' the group of academics and health officials says in a letter

By **Tom Blackwell**

Published Sep 22, 2020

Last updated Sep 22, 2020

Several international experts have taken the unusual step of urging a Canadian university to arrange an independent investigation into research that controversially linked fluoride in drinking water to lower intelligence in children.

The academics and public health officials from six countries say studies by York University's Christine Till have been widely criticized, yet are still influencing often-emotional debates over fluoridation in American and Canadian cities.

An arm's-length review is needed to determine whether "ideology is being misrepresented as science," the group says in a letter sent to York's board Monday.

The fact Till is using an animated video and public comments to advocate against pregnant women drinking fluoridated water, despite shortcomings in her research, makes this more than a simple scientific debate, said Myron Allukian Jr., one of the signatories.

"It's bothersome that an academic goes around yelling 'Fire, fire,' when there's no fire," said Allukian, former president of the American Public Health Association and Harvard dental professor. "She is misleading the public and others by distorting the data and not doing the proper analyses."

The letter is also signed by professors and other experts in the U.S., the U.K., Ireland, Australia, New Zealand and Chile.

Till, a neuropsychologist, strongly refuted the group's arguments Tuesday.

Some of the scientific critiques of her work have themselves been riddled with error, she said, while the U.S. National Toxicology Program is expected to come out with a report this week that backs up her findings on the neurological effects of fluoride.

Till said her public interventions on the topic have chiefly been to correct others who have misrepresented her words or research.

A commentary Till published earlier this year suggested she is being confronted by "overt cognitive biases" in a polarized debate over fluoride.

"I think there's a lot of fear that the evidence, the scientific evidence, is mounting that fluoride is an environmental neuro-toxicant," she said in an interview Tuesday. "It's raising doubts ... The science doesn't support deep-held, entrenched belief."

Till also stressed that she is not calling into question the wisdom of fluoridated water overall, just suggesting pregnant women should cut their fluoride intake, noting that infants get no benefit from the chemical until their teeth have erupted.

In fact, the prominent journal that published Till's key study of fluoride and IQ said it subjected the paper to added scrutiny and peer review because of its implications. The JAMA Pediatrics editor has said he would tell his wife not to drink tap water if she were pregnant.
And separate studies from China, Mexico and other places, though also criticized and generally considered less rigorous, have had similar findings.

Barbara Joy, a university spokeswoman, said York has policies in place to deal with such requests and "we will be responding fully once we have carefully reviewed the concerns."
The U.S. Centers for Disease Control has declared fluoridation of drinking water one of the 10 greatest public health achievements of the 20th Century, reducing cavities by an estimated 25 per cent.

But it has long been a contentious issue. Opposition once veered int conspiracy-theory territory, though now relies more on published research into possible harms. The movement still has links to the scientifically dubious anti-vaccination lobby.

The fact Christine Till is advocating against pregnant women drinking fluoridated water, despite shortcomings in her research, makes this more than a simple scientific debate, one critic says.

Till's study last year on IQ and fluoridation thrust her into the centre of the fray. It examined maternal consumption of the chemical, both by looking at fluoride in urine and mothers' reports of their fluoridated-water consumption.

Of the 500 mothers from six Canadian cities included in the study, those with 1 part per million more fluoride in their urine had boys whose IQ was an average of 4.5 points lower between ages three and four. Their girls had slightly higher IQs, and there was no difference when the sexes were combined.

Those who reported higher fluoridated-water consumption had children of both sexes with an average 3.7 points lower IQ, the study concluded.

Till has also published a paper linking fluoridated water and ADHD, and one that concluded baby formula made with fluoridated water was associated with lower IQs.

The letter cites critiques that largely dismissed the results of the IQ paper on various grounds.

A detailed report by Canada's CADTH, the independent, government-funded agency that evaluates new drugs and other health issues, said Till's conclusions were simply "not supported by the data."

The report cited "multiple weaknesses," including potentially wrong estimation of the mothers' fluoride exposure and variables like parental IQ and diet after birth that weren't considered but could have skewed the results.

A review by Germany's Leibniz Research Centre for Working Environment and Human Factors raised similar concerns and concluded the study did not justify calling fluoride a "human developmental neurotoxin."

But Till said she had catalogued three pages of factual errors in the CADTH report, which she said the German review relied on extensively.

The letter also points to an animated video produced by Till and colleagues that leaves out much of the nuance in her findings. It states flatly that her study and one in Mexico found "fluoride led to IQ deficits in children." Till's work suggested there was an association between the two, not a proven cause-and-effect relationship.

She defended the video as an accurate representation of the totality of research on the issue.

"We're talking about an exquisitely sensitive developing brain (and) mounting evidence that fluoride is toxic to the developing brain," said the York professor. "How much more evidence do we need before we start protecting the fetus and young infants?"

Meanwhile, Till also wrote to the city council of Green Bay, Wis., in July as it debated fluoridation, suggesting that, based on her results and others, pregnant women should decrease their fluoride consumption.

She said she did so to correct an inaccurate report of her comments to the council earlier, and would love to just concentrate on science.

But another of the letter's signatories accused her of propagating "junk science."

"Dr. Till wrote on York University stationery to undermine public health recommendations, during a pandemic, in another country based on her research which her own national agency CADTH has fully discredited," said Jennifer Meyer, a population health sciences professor at Alaska's College of Health.

APPENDIX H:

Dr Dickson's Email to the Mayor of Calgary

January 14, 2021
Good day, Mayor Nenshi,

I know you and many on council have been subjected to harsh and often unfair attacks and criticisms in the media. We need media to be more objective, fair, open-minded and balanced.

This is an important subject for all of us, that of media bias and irresponsibility. It is particularly flagrant on the contentious topic of artificial water fluoridation.

The most recent case of brazen bias from the Calgary Herald came last month when they refused an opinion piece, in response to 2 very poorly written and factually and scientifically bereft articles by Juliet Guichon and Catherine Ford, who collectively have a minuscule amount of knowledge on the topic. Ours is co-authored by Dr. Hardy Limeback, PhD/dentist, now retired from Head of Preventative Dentistry at the University of Toronto and is the most knowledgeable person in Canada on fluoride, and by myself, a Calgary doctor who has led or co-led the safe water campaign in Calgary for over 2 decades.

Here is the opinion piece that we submitted, which is science based and with links to pertinent new studies and literature.

You be the judge. We in the safe water and anti-fluoridation movement have the science, common sense, and the ethics and morality on our side.

Thanks.

Dr Bob

Robert C Dickson, MD, CCFP, FCFP
Founder SAFE WATER CALGARY

OpEd accepted then rejected by the Calgary Herald:

May 2021 will mark an auspicious anniversary—Calgary public water will be free of toxic hydrofluosilicic acid from Florida industry waste stacks for an entire decade!

Many local dentists note no major differences in the oral health of children. Similar to when our city was fluoridated, the poorer socioeconomic groups have more dental decay. Unfortunately, we have not made significant advances in oral nor whole body health for our most disadvantaged.

Proponents of this failing practice cite a questionable 25% cavity reduction rate. The Cochrane Collaboration, the gold standard of evaluating medical effectiveness, cited the low quality of the vast majority of studies finding effectiveness, and couldn't find significant evidence of fluoridation reducing cavities in adults or in reducing cavity disparities for the poor. (https://www.cochrane.org/CD010856/ORAL_water-fluoridation-prevent-tooth-decay)

25%, even if accurate, is less than one cavity per child, hardly the efficacy that prevents emergency dental surgery or justifies mass medication. Even supporters such as the CDC admit fluoride acts mainly topically, not through ingestion. World Health Organization data shows fluoridated nations have essentially the same cavity rates as non-fluoridated countries. (http://fluoridealert.org/wp-content/uploads/FAN-Fluoride-Efficacy-Flyer-Print-FINAL-1.pdf)

A recent opinion piece in the Herald stated the Calgary study from 2016 found cavity rates increased after the city council voted to stop fluoridating in 2011. The study lead is on record stating cavity rates were increasing just as much before 2011 as after, and that stopping fluoridation made no statistical difference. (http://www.caphd.ca/sites/default/files/MosaicNewsletter_FALL17_final.pdf)

The strongest scientific evidence is neurotoxicity - simply put, brain damage. Several recent studies, with major Canadian input and funded by the U.S. National Institutes of Health, found higher fluoride levels can lower IQs and increase ADHD rates in children. After publishing one, the editor of the Journal of the American Medical Association Pediatrics, a Seattle physician, concluded "I would not want my wife to drink fluoridated water" if she was pregnant. (https://fluoridealert.org/articles/jamacriticsims/)

He's just one of numerous leading professionals emphasizing neurotoxic risks. After analyzing 92 IQ studies, the U.S. National Toxicology Program's draft report concluded " fluoride is presumed to be a cognitive developmental hazard to humans." (http://fluoridealert.org/content/overview-ntp/)

Toxicologist Steven Gilbert, PhD, director of the Institute of Neurotoxicology & Neurological Disorders, said "This is another in a long line of studies over the past three decades that have found fluoride's neurotoxicity. The science clearly indicates that water fluoridation should be ended as soon as possible." (https://safewaterspokane.org/ntp-fluoride-statement)

Linda Birnbaum, PhD, former Director of the National Institute of Environmental Health Sciences, said
"Fluoride offers no benefits to the fetus and infant and . . . new evidence suggests that fluoride is toxic to the developing brain at levels routinely found in the general population." (https://www.ehn.org/fluoride-and-childrens-health-2648120286.html)

Philippe Grandjean, MD, PhD, Harvard researcher, co-author of over 500 studies and advisor to the Danish National Board of Health, asserted "The IQ losses associated with community water fluoridation are substantial and of significant public health concern." (http://fluoridealert.org/wp-content/uploads/EPA-trial-Grandjean-Declaration.pdf)

The science is now so strong that it's the focus of a historic lawsuit in federal court in the USA against the EPA for allowing fluoridation. The judge has already said "there is serious evidence" of fluoridation's neurotoxicity, and EPA should "take a second look" to reexamine-fluoridated-water-risks. (https://fluoridealert.org/news/epa-should-reexamine-fluoridated-water-risks-judge-says/)

And it's not just brain damage. Numerous studies have shown that fluoride is an endocrine disruptor and increases risk of dental fluorosis, hypothyroidism, diabetes and kidney disease, among others. The identification of both the known risks and need for further research strongly contradicts proponent's mantra that fluoridation is safe for everyone. (https://www.nap.edu/catalog/11571/fluoride-in-drinking-water-a-scientific-review-of-epas-standards)

The pattern is common. The government declared DDT, DES, asbestos and lead in paint and gasoline safe, refusing for decades to acknowledge the accumulating robust studies documenting their harm. By the time the government finally banned them, millions had suffered diminished quality of life, needless suffering and disease, and death. Fluoridation is following precisely that same path.

The possible prevention of 1/2 to 1 cavity simply cannot justify causing so many health harms

Supporters of fluoridation stubbornly refuse to accept or acknowledge the new science. 95% of our world has chosen not to fluoridate its water. Calgary should not fall victim to the blinded refusal to acknowledge fluoridation's well documented health risks.

Dr. Robert C Dickson, MD, CCFP, FCFP is a Calgary Family Physician and the founder of Safe Water, Calgary www.safewatercalgary.com

Dr. Hardy Limeback, PhD, DDS, Professor Emeritus, Faculty of Dentistry, University of Toronto

APPENDIX I:

EPA Letter Authorizing Using Pollution Chemicals for Fluoridation

UNITED STATES ENVIRONMENTAL PROTECTION AGENCY
WASHINGTON, D.C. 20460

MAR 30 1983

OFFICE OF
WATER

Leslie A. Russell, D.M.D.
363 Walnut Street
Newtonville, Mass. 02160

Dear Dr. Russell:

Thank you for your letter of March 9, 1983, in regard to the fluoridation of drinking water.

The information available to the Environmental Protection Agency is that fluoridation is a safe and effective means for reducing the occurrence of dental caries. The fluoridation process has been endorsed by several Presidents of the United States and by several Surgeons General, including the current Surgeon General, Dr. C. Everett Koop. A copy of Dr. Koop's statement on fluoridation is enclosed.

Water treatment chemicals, including fluosilicic acid, have been evaluated for their potential for contributing to the contamination of drinking water. The Water Treatment Chemicals Codex, published by the National Academy of Sciences, prescribes the purity requirements for fluosilicic acid and other fluoridation chemicals.

In regard to the use of fluosilicic acid as a source of fluoride for fluoridation, this Agency regards such use as an ideal environmental solution to a long-standing problem. By recovering by-product fluosilicic acid from fertilizer manufacturing, water and air pollution are minimized, and water utilities have a low-cost source of fluoride available to them. I hope this information adequately responds to your concern.

Sincerely yours,

Rebecca Hanmer

Rebecca Hanmer
Deputy Assistant Administrator
for Water

Enclosure

APPENDIX J:

Fluoride Fumigants in Foods

According to the EPA, Sulfuryl Fluoride breaks down rapidly in the human body to fluoride. And because of that, EPA approved two tolerances: one for fluoride and the other for Sulfuryl Fluoride. They were the highest tolerances ever set by the government for fluoride. A few examples of the two tolerances:

EPA Tolerances for SULFURYL FLUORIDE as a post-harvest fumigant		
Food commodity	**Fluoride residue levels (ppm)**	**Sulfuryl Fluoride residue levels (ppm)**
Egg, dried	900	1
Milk, powdered	5	2
Cheese	5	2
Coconut, postharvest	40	1
Pistachio, postharvest	10	3
Vegetable, legume, group postharvest-includes: Chickpea, Fava, Kidney, Lima, Mung, Navy, Pea, Pinto, Runner, Snap, Soy)	70	0.5
Ginger, postharvest	70	0.5
Oat, groats/rolled oats	75	0.1
Wheat flour, postharvest	125	0.05
Wheat, germ, postharvest	130	0.02
All processed food commodities not otherwise listed	70	2

BIBLIOGRAPHY

Adair SM, Bowen WH, Burt BA et al. Recommendations for using fluorides to prevent and control caries in the United States. *CDC MMWR*. August 17, 2001 / 50(RR14);1-42

Agency for Toxic Substances & Disease Registry. Toxicological profile for Fluorides, Hydrogen Fluoride and Fluorine. U.S. Department of Health and Human Services Public Health Service Agency for Toxic Substances and Disease Registry, 2003

Agricultural Act of 2014 – Sec. 10015 Regulation of Sulfuryl Fluoride. Page 806.

Alimam W, Auvinen A. Cancer risk due to ingestion of naturally occurring radionuclides through drinking water: A systematic review. *Sci Total Environ*. 2025 Mar 10;968:178849.

American Academy of Environmental Medicine, Fluoride Action Network, Food & Water Watch et al. "Petition to the U.S. Environmental Protection Agency to ban the addition of fluoridation chemicals to water pursuant to section 21 of the Toxic Substances Control Act." November 22, 2016. Available from: http://fluoridealert.org/wp-content/uploads/epa-petition.pdf

American Dental Association: Council on Dental Health and Health Planning. "White Paper on Fluoridation" 1979.

American Dental Association (ADA). Infants formula and fluoride. *J Amer Dent Assoc* 2007;Vol. 138;132. Available from: https://jada.ada.org/article/S0002-8177(14)61101-6/pdf

Armed Forces Institute of Pathology, Department of Veterinary Pathology. Wednesday Slide, 2002.

Arnold FA Jr, Dean HT, Knutson JW. Effect of fluoridated public water supplies on dental caries prevalence. *Public Health Rep* (1896). 1953;Feb;68(2):141-8.

ASPCA Animal Poison Control Center. Grapes, raisins, and renal failure: mystery or myth? *ASPCA Animal Watch*. 2004;24(1):14-15. Available from: https://web.archive.org/web/20090205172006/http://www.aspca.org/site/DocServer/grapes.pdf?docID=189

Atomic Accidents. Manhattan Project History: The Philadelphia Incident. Atomic Heritage Foundation. June 4, 2014. Available from: https://ahf.nuclearmuseum.org/ahf/history/atomic-accidents/

Australian Democracy Network. Confronting State Capture. 2022. Available from: https://australiandemocracy.org.au/

Bailey R. Impurifying our precious bodily fluids. *Reason Magazine*, December 5, 2001.

Baletti B. Profanity-laced Emails, Misuse of CDC Funds: How Big Fluoride Tries to Prevent Towns From Removing Fluoride. *The Defender,* April 15, 2025a.

Baletti B. Florida Becomes Second State to Ban Fluoride in Public Drinking Water. *The Defender*, May 6, 2025b.

Baletti B. Critics Slam Fluoride Study by Researchers With Ties to Pro-Fluoride Lobby. *The Defender*, June 2, 2025c.

Barbier O, Arreloa-Mendoza L, Del Raza, LM. Molecular mechanisms of fluoride toxicity. *Chemico-Biological Interactions*. 2010;188(2):319-333.

Barr A. A short account of tuberculosis in Ireland 1850–1900. *Ir J Med Sci* 1956; 31, 58–67.

Bashash M, Thomas D, Hu H, Martinez-Mier EA, Sanchez BN, Basu N, Peterson KE, Ettinger AS, Wright R, Zhang Z, Liu Y, Schnaas L, Mercado-García A, Téllez-Rojo MM, Hernández-Avila M. Prenatal Fluoride Exposure and Cognitive Outcomes in Children at 4 and 6-12 Years of Age in Mexico. *Environ Health Perspect.* 2017 Sep 19;125(9):097017.

Bassin E. Association Between Fluoride in Drinking Water During Growth and Development and the Incidence of Osteosarcoma for Children and Adolescents. PhD Thesis 2001 p.75.

Bassin, E, Wypij D, Davis RB, Mittleman MA. Age-specific fluoride exposure in drinking water and osteosarcoma (United States). *Cancer Causes Control* 2006;17:421–428.

Bates A. Recorded proceedings of the Senate Committee on Health and Human Services, Oregon State Legislature, 71st session (April 11, 2001).

BBC. Hannah Gelbert and Phoebe Hopson. BBC World Service (Fluoride: What you need to know) March 25, 2025. Available from: https://www.bbc.co.uk/sounds/play/w3ct67zk.

Begley S. Fluoridation, Cancer: Did Researchers Ask the Right Questions? *Wall Street Journal*. 22 July 2005.

Beltrán-Aguilar ED, Barker LK, Canto MT, Dye BA, Gooch BF, Griffin SO, Hyman J, Jaramillo F, Kingman A, Nowjack-Raymer R, Selwitz RH, Wu T; Centers for Disease Control and Prevention (CDC). Surveillance for dental caries, dental sealants, tooth retention, edentulism, and enamel fluorosis—United States, 1988-1994 and 1999-2002. *MMWR Surveill Summ.* 2005 Aug 26;54(3):1-43.

Bennett CL, Champigneulle O, Bennett A, Witherspoon B, Bove C. Fluoroquinolone-Associated Disability and Other Fluoroquinolone-Associated Serious Adverse Events: Unexpected Toxicities Have Emerged in Recent Years. *Cancer Treat Res.* 2022;184:1-39.

Beresniak A, Duru G, Berger G, Bremond-Gignac D. Relationships between black tea consumption and key health indicators in the world: an ecological study. *BMJ Open*. 2012;2:e000648

Berg J, Gerweck C, Hujoel PP, King R, Krol DM, Kumar J, Levy S, Pollick H, Whitford GM, Strock S, Aravamudhan K, Frantsve-Hawley J, Meyer DM; American Dental Association Council on Scientific Affairs Expert Panel on Fluoride Intake From Infant Formula and Fluorosis. Evidence-based clinical recommendations regarding fluoride intake from reconstituted infant formula and enamel fluorosis: a report of the American Dental Association Council on Scientific Affairs. *J Am Dent Assoc*. 2011 Jan;142(1):79-87.

Boyd AE. Tuberculosis and pauperism in Ireland. *Br. J. Tuberc.* 1908,2(3),159-166

Boyer S. Executive Director, Washington State Board of Pharmacy. Letter to Dr Osmunson. May 7, 2009.

Breaker R. First person: How we discovered fluoride riboswitches. Yale School of Medicine. December 21, 2011.

Brothwell DJ, Limeback H. Fluorosis risk in grade 2 students residing in a rural area with widely varying natural fluoride. *Commun Dent Oral Epidemiol*. 1999;27:130-6.

Brothwell DJ, Limeback H. Breastfeeding is protective against dental fluorosis in a nonfluoridated rural area of Ontario, Canada. *J Human Lactation*. 2003;Nov;19(4):386-90.

Broze D. #FluorideTrial: Scientist Says He Was Threatened Because of Fluoride Study - Week 1 In Review. The Last American Vagabond. June 12, 2020.

Broze D. "Dr. Paul Connett on the Historic Trial That Could End Water Fluoridation." The Conscious Resistance, 24 February 2020. Available from: https://theconsciousresistance.com/dr-paul-connett-on-the-historic-trial-that-could-end-water-fluoridation

Bryson C, Griffiths J. Fluoride, Teeth and the Atomic Bomb. Project Censored. *Waste Not* #414 September 1997. Available from: https://fluoridealert.org/content/wastenot414/

Bryson C. *The Fluoride Deception*. Seven Stories Press, 2006.

Budnick N. 'The F Word: Fluoridation Controversy in Oregon: A Federal Agent is Lobbying Salem to Spike Our Water Supply With Poison. Who Needs a Conspiracy?' *Willamette Week*, 2001; February 21, pp. 22-28.

Burgstahler AW, Spittle B. Medline again rejects Fluoride. [editorial]. *Fluoride*, 2009;42(4):256-259.

Burk D, Dean Burk Foundation, Yiamouyiannis J. "Fluoridation Linked Human Cancer Based on Time-Trend Mortality Data." Abstract: Seventh Annual Conference of the International Society for Fluoride Research. February 8-10, 1976.

Buzalaf MAR, Whitford GM. Fluoride metabolism. *Monogr Oral Sci*. 2011;22:20-36.

Caldwell G, Zanfagna PE. Fluoridation and Truth Decay. *Top-Ecol Press,* 1974.

California EPA. Sulfuryl Fluoride (Vikane®). Risk Characterization Document. Volume 1. Health Risk Assessment. Medical Toxicology Branch. Department of Pesticide Regulation, *California Environmental Protection Agency*. July 2006. Available from: https://fluoridealert.org/wp-content/uploads/2025/07/sf-ca.epa_.hra_.july-2006.pdf

Calvert GM, Mueller CA, Fajen JM, Chrislip DW, Russo J, Briggle T, Fleming LE, Suruda AJ, Steenland K. Health effects associated with sulfuryl fluoride and methyl bromide exposure among structural fumigation workers. *Am J Public Health*. 1998 Dec;88(12):1774-80.

Canton Stops Fluoridation - Spurred by College Faculty, Staff & Students. Press release by the NY State Coalition Opposed to Fluoridation. February 21, 2003; Available from: https://fluoridealert.org/news/canton-stops-fluoridation-spurred-by-college-faculty-staff-students/

Carton RJ, Hirzy WJ. Inside the Fishbowl. *Heads Up Newsletter*, November 1985

Carton RJ. Review of the 2006 United States National Research Council Report: Fluoride in Drinking Water. *Fluoride* 39(3)163–172. July-September 2006.

Carvalho JG, Leite AL, Yan D, Everett ET, Whitford GM, Buzalaf MAR. Influence of genetic background on fluoride metabolism in mice. J Dent Res, 2009;88(1):1054-8. [Abstracted in Fluoride, 2009:42(4):303-4.]

CDHP. Fluoridation Advocacy: Pew's Contributions and Lessons that Emerge. Children's Dental Health Project. July 2015. Available from: https://s3-us-west-2.amazonaws.com/cdhp-fluoridation/CDHP_FlouridationAdvocacyReport_FINAL.pdf

Centers for Disease Control and Prevention (CDC). Achievements in public health, 1900-1999: fluoridation of drinking water to prevent dental caries. *MMWR*. 48(41): 933-940. 1999.

Centers for Disease Control and Prevention (CDC). Volcanoes and your safety. 2024. Available from: https://www.cdc.gov/volcanoes/about/index.html#:~:text=in%20volcanic%20ash.-,Gases,volcanic%20eruption%20to%20the%20next.

Chachra D, Limeback H, Willett TL, Grynpas M. The Long-Term Effects of Water Fluoridation on the Human Skeleton. *J Dent Res.* 2010 Nov;89(11):1219-23.

Chen EM. Findings of Fact and Conclusions of Law. Case No, 17-cv-02162-EMC. United States District Court, Northern District of California. Food & Water Watch, Inc., et al., Plaintiffs v. United States Environmental Protection Agency, et al., Defendants. 24 September 2024. Available from: https://www.courtlistener.com/docket/6201332/445/food-water-watch-inc-v-environmental-protection-agency/

Choi AL, Sun G, Zhang Y, Grandjean P. Developmental fluoride neurotoxicity: a systematic review and meta-analysis. *Environ Health.* 2012; 120(10):1362-8.

Christakis D, Rivara F. JAMA Pediatrics podcast of editors' summary of the 2019 study by Green et al.: Association Between Maternal Fluoride Exposure During Pregnancy and IQ Scores in Offspring in Canada. Available from: https://fluoridealert.org/fan-tv/jama-pediatrics-podcast-on-fluoride-iq/

Clement International Corporation. Toxicological profile for fluorides, hydrogen fluoride, and fluorine. Prepared for: Agency for Toxic Substances and Disease Registry U.S. Public Health Service, Atlanta, GA: Page 112. 1993. Available from:http://www.fluoridealert.org/uploads/atsdr-1993.pdf

Cohn PD. "An Epidemiologic Report on Drinking Water and Fluoridation." New Jersey Department of Environmental Protection and New Jersey Department of Health. November 30, 1992. Available from: https://www.nj.gov/health/ceohs/documents/eohap/haz_sites/regional_state/drinking_water/drinkingwater_fluoridation.pdf

Colombini S. Ladapo advises communities to stop adding fluoride to water supplies. *Health News Florida*, November 22, 2024. Available from: https://health.wusf.usf.edu/health-news-florida/2024-11-22/ladapo-advises-communities-to-stop-adding-fluoride-to-water-supplies

Colquhoun J. Disfiguring dental fluorosis in Auckland. *Fluoride* 1984;17(4):234-242.

Colquhoun J. Child dental health differences in New Zealand. *Community Health Studies* 1987;11:85-90.

Colquhoun J. Is there a dental benefit from water fluoride? *Fluoride* 1994;27:13-22.

Colquhoun J. Why I changed my mind about water fluoridation. Perspectives in Biology and Medicine, 1997;41:29-44. Reprinted with permission in *Fluoride*, 1998;31(2):103-18.

Colquhoun J, Mann R. The Hastings fluoridation experiment: science or swindle? *The Ecologist*, 1986;16:243-248.

Colquhoun J, Mann R. The Hastings fluoridation experiment: postscript. *The Ecologist,* 1987;17:125-126.

Connett E. 2001. Sulfuryl Fluoride. Comments submitted to US EPA from Ellen Connett on the proposed tolerances of Sulfuryl Fluoride.

Connett E. The Childsmile program. Fluoride Action Network. Nov. 5, 2017.

Connett M. Petition to the U.S. Environmental Protection Agency to ban the addition of fluoridation chemicals to water pursuant to section 21 of the Toxic Substances Control Act. November 22, 2016.

Connett PH and Connett MP. A safe drinking water standard for fluoride: LOAELs and protecting the most vulnerable. Submission to the National Research Council, Subcommittee on Fluoride in Drinking Water, National Academy of Sciences, Washington DC. August 12, 2003.

Connett PH, Beck J, Micklem S. *The Case Against Fluoride: How Hazardous Waste Ended Up in Our Drinking Water and the Bad Science and Powerful Politics That Keep It There.* Chelsea Green Publishing, 2010.

Connett, EM. "Part 2. IQ-Studies Reporting 'No Effect'; and one study that shows a large increase in IQ." Fluoride Action Network. April 10, 2025. Available from: https://fluoridealert.org/studytracker/iq-studies-reporting-no-effect-and-one-study-that-shows-a-large-increase-in-iq-part-2/

Cook HA. Fluoride and tea. *Lancet*. 1969 Aug 9;2(7615):329.

Coplan MJ, Patch SC, Masters RD, Bachman MS. Confirmation of and explanations for elevated blood lead and other disorders in children exposed to water disinfection and fluoridation chemicals. *Neurotoxicology*. 2007 Sep;28(5):1032-42.

Cordain L, Lindeberg S, Hurtado M, Hill K, Eaton SB, Brand-Miller J. Acne vulgaris: a disease of Western civilization. *Arch Dermatol*. 2002 Dec;138(12):1584-90.

Cox GJ, Matuschak MC, Dixon SF, Dodds ML, Walker WE. Experimental dental caries: IV. Fluorine and its relation to dental caries. *J Dent Res*. 1939;18(6):481-490.

Cragoe D. "Dr. Hans Moolenburgh- Fluoride Fighter of the Netherlands." YouTube, Doug Cragoe, 21 August 2014 Available from: https://www.youtube.com/watch?v=Jw3xbtS4vpM

Cragoe D. "Use non-fluoridated water when making infant formula." YouTube, Doug Cragoe, August 2009. Available from: https://www.youtube.com/watch?v=IhMuBiPeHTE

Cunningham J, McCaugh H, Malin A, Flora D, Till C. Fluoride exposure and duration and quality of sleep in a Canadian cohort. *Environmental Health*; 2021;20:16.

Dean, T. Endemic Fluorosis and Its Relation to Dental Caries. *Public Health Reports*, 1938. [Reprinted as a Classical Article, 2006.]

Diesendorf M. Is there a scientific basis for fluoridation? *Community Health Studies* 1980;4(3):224-230.

Diesendorf M. The mystery of declining tooth decay. *Nature* 1986a;322(6075):125-129.

Diesendorf M. A re-examination of Australian fluoridation trials. *Search* 1986b;17:256-262.

Diesendorf M. Is fluoridation effective? *Fluoride* 1987;20(2):51-53.

Diesendorf M. Anglesey fluoridation trials re-examined. *Fluoride* 1989;22:53-58.

Diesendorf M. Have the benefits of water fluoridation been overestimated?. *International Clinical Nutrition Review* 1990a;10(2): 292-303.

Diesendorf M. Health hazards of fluoridation: a re-examination. *International Clinical Nutrition Review* 1990b;10(2):304-321.

Diesendorf M. How science can illuminate ethical debates: a case study on water fluoridation. *Fluoride* 1995;28(2): 87-104.

Diesendorf M. Fluoridation: breaking the silence barrier. In: Martin B (ed.). Confronting the experts. New York: State University of New York Press, 1996;45-75.

Diesendorf M. A strategy for resisting the vested interests driving the collapse of the biosphere and civilization. *Ecological Civilisation* 2025;2:10005._Available from: https://doi.org/10.70322/ecolciviliz.2025.10005

Diesendorf M, Diesendorf A. Suppression by medical journals of a warning about overdosing formula-fed infants with fluoride. *Accountability in Research: Policies and Quality Assurance*. 1997;5(1-3):225-237. Available from: http://dx.doi.org/10.1080/08989629708573911

Diesendorf M, Sutton PRN. Fluoride: New Grounds for Concern. *The Ecologist*; 1986;16:237-242.

Diesendorf M, Taylor R The Path to a Sustainable Civilisation: Technological, socioeconomic and Political Change. Palgrave Macmillan, 2023. Available from: https://doi.org/10.1007/978-981-99-0663-5

Diesendorf M, Varney W. Fluoridation – politics and strategies. *Social Alternatives* 1986;5(2):48-53.

Diesendorf M, Colquhoun J, Spittle BJ, Everingham DN, Clutterbuck FW. New evidence on fluoridation. *Aust. J. Public Health* 1997;21:187-190.

Dossier technique sur la fluoration 1974," Ministère des Affaires sociales", 1974.

Douglass CW, Joshipura K.. Caution needed in fluoride and osteosarcoma study. *Cancer Causes & Control* 17(4):481-82. May 2006.

Doull J, Boekelheide K, Farishian BG, Isaacson RL, Klotz JB, Kumar JV, Limeback H, Poole C, Puzas JE, Reed N-MR, Thiessen KM, Webster TF, Committee on Fluoride in Drinking Water, Board on Environmental Studies and Toxicology, Division on Earth and Life Studies, National Research Council of the National Academies. Fluoride in drinking water: a scientific review of EPA's standards. Washington, DC: The National Academies Press; 2006. (NRC, 2006). Available from: https://nap.nationalacademies.org/catalog/11571/fluoride-in-drinking-water-a-scientific-review-of-epas-standards

Dow. Sentenced to Death. Advertisement for Dow Methyl Bromide Insecticide, 1938. Available from: https://digital.sciencehistory.org/works/26mzn00

Du L et al. The effect of fluorine on the developing human brain. Zhonghua Bing Li Xue Za Zhi21(4): 218-20. August 1992, Translated and republished in *Fluoride*, October 2008; Available from: https://fluoridealert.org/studytracker/the-effect-of-fluorine-on-the-developing-human-brain/

Ecclesiastes 9:10a, "Whatsoever thy hand findeth to do, do it with thy might." Esther 4:14b, "And who knoweth, whether thou art come to the kingdom for such a time as this?" Westminster Shorter Catechism 68. A., "The sixth commandment requireth all lawful endeavors to preserve our own life, and the life of others."

Emsley J, Jones DJ, Miller JM, Overill RE, Waddilove RA. An unexpectedly strong hydrogen bond: ab initio calculations and spectroscopic studies of amide-fluoride systems. *J. Am. Chem. Soc.* 1981;103(1):24–28.

Environmental Protection Agency (EPA). Sulfuryl Fluoride; Proposed Order Granting Objections to Tolerances and Denying Request for a Stay. A Proposed Rule by the Environmental Protection Agency. Published Document: 2011-917 (76 FR 3422). January 19, 2011; Available from: https://www.federalregister.gov/documents/2011/01/19/2011-917/sulfuryl-fluoride-proposed-order-granting-objections-to-tolerances-and-denying-request-for-a-stay

Environmental Protection Agency (EPA). Tolerances for residues: Cryolite and Sulfuryl Fluoride. Fluorine compounds. Code § 180.145. Available from: https://www.ecfr.gov/current/title-40/chapter-I/subchapter-E/part-180/subpart-C/section-180.145

Exner RF, Waldbott GL. The American Fluoridation Experiment. The Devin-Adair Company, 1957.

Fagin D. Second Thoughts About Fluoride. *Scientific American*. January 2008.

Federal Register. Proposed HHS Recommendation for Fluoride Concentration in Drinking Water for Prevention of Dental Caries. Federal Register 76(9):2383-2388, January 13, 2011.

Fluoride Action Network (FAN). Objectors' Consolidated Objections to Final Rules Establishing Tolerances for Residues of Sulfuryl Fluoride and Fluoride Anion. November 2006; Available from: https://fluoridealert.org/wp-content/uploads/sf-nov.2006.pdf

Fluoride Action Network (FAN). Fluoridated Water & Infant Formula, 2012. Available from: https://fluoridealert.org/content/science-watch09/

Farmus L, Till C, Green R, Hornung R, Martinez-Mier EA, Ayotte P, Muckle G, Lanphear B, Flora D. (2021). Critical windows of fluoride neurotoxicity in Canadian children. *Environmental Research*; 200:111315.

Farmus L, Till C, Green R, Hornung R, Martinez-Mier EA, Ayotte P, Muckle G, Lanphear B, Flora D. Critical windows of fluoride neurotoxicity in Canadian children – In Reply to Guichon. *Environmental Research*. 2023a;115201

Farmus L, Till C, Green R, Hornung R, Martinez-Mier EA, Ayotte P, Muckle G, Lanphear B, Flora D. Critical windows of fluoride neurotoxicity in Canadian children – In Reply to Wood. *Environmental Research*, 2023b;115299

Fein NJ, Cerklewski FL. Fluoride content of foods made with mechanically separated chicken. *J Agric Food Chem*. 2001;49(9):4284-4286.

Feltman R, Kosel G. Prenatal and postnatal ingestion of fluorides—Fourteen years of investigation—Final report. *J Dent Med*. 1961;16:190-199

Feltman R. Prenatal and postnatal ingestion of fluorides - A Progress Report. *Dental Digest*. August 1956.

Fiore G, Veneri F, Di Lorenzo R, Generali L, Vinceti M, Filippini T. Fluoride Exposure and ADHD: A Systematic Review of Epidemiological Studies. *Medicina (Kaunas).* 2023 Apr 19;59(4):797.

Florida Department of Health. 2024. Guidance for Community Water Fluoridation. November 22, 2024. Available from: https://www.floridahealth.gov/_documents/newsroom/press-releases/2024/11/GUIDANCECommunityWaterFluoridation.pdf

Fluoride Action Network (FAN). The Deepwater Documents: Lawsuit Against the US Bomb Program Over Fluoride Poisoning. June 11, 2012a. Available from: https://fluoridealert.org/content/deepwater/

Fluoride Action Network (FAN). The Manhattan Project's Secret Wartime Conference on Fluoride Toxicity. June 11, 2012b. Available from: https://fluoridealert.org/content/1944-conference/

Fluoride Action Network (FAN). Interview with Gary Owen Pittman. 2022. Available from: https://www.youtube.com/watch?v=CkGNCpaPhVA

Fluoride Action Network (FAN). The Phosphate Fertilizer Industry: An Environmental Overview. June 11, 2012c. Available from: https://fluoridealert.org/content/phosphate01/#:~:text=1.,US%20and%20other%20wealthy%20countries).

Fluoride: How Much is Too Much? CBC 1999. Available from: https://www.cbc.ca/player/play/video/1.3593971

Fluoridegate: An American Tragedy. YouTube, uploaded by David Kennedy DDS, 13 May 2013. Available from: https://www.youtube.com/watch?v=rVQwgsjTjbA

Foulkes RG. Thirty-five years of Fluoride [Guest Editorial]. *Fluoride* 2002;35(4 Pt 1):213-27.

Gaeta, D.C., Mühle, J., Vimont, I.J. et al. California dominates U.S. emissions of the pesticide and potent greenhouse gas sulfuryl fluoride. *Commun Earth Environ* 5, 161 (2024). Available from: https://www.nature.com/articles/s43247-024-01294-x

Galetti PM, Joyet G. Effect of Fluorine in Thyroidal Iodine Metabolism in Hyperthyroidism. Journal of Clinical Endocrinology, 1958;18,10,1102–1110.

Gallico M. How to keep your dentist from killing your Labrador retriever (and other pets). *Medium*. Published June 28, 2016. Available from: https://medium.com/@MelissaGallico/how-to-keep-your-dentist-from-killing-your-labrador-retriever-and-other-pets-9777e3bdab68

Gallico M. The Hidden Cause of Acne: How Toxic Water Is Affecting Your Health and What You Can Do About It. Healing Arts Press. 2018.

Gallo BJ, Kupperschmidt JB, Mancuso MR, Murray AJ, Strauss HS. Should Natick Fluoridate? A Report to the Town and Board of Selectmen. Natick Fluoridation Study Committee. Oct. 14, 1997.

Geier DA, Geier MR. Tooth decay prevention and neurodevelopmental disorder risk following childhood fluoride exposure. *BMC Pediatr*. 2025;Apr 2;25(1):265.

Gluckman P, Skegg D. "Health effects of water fluoridation: A review of the scientific evidence A report on behalf of the Royal Society of New Zealand and the Office of the Prime Minister's Chief Science Advisor." August 2014.

Goodman C, Bashash M, Green R, Song P, Peterson KE, Schnaas L, Mercado-García A, Martínez-Medina S, Hernández-Avila M, Martinez-Mier A, Téllez-Rojo MM, Hu H, Till C. Domain-specific effects of prenatal fluoride exposure on child IQ at 4, 5, and 6-12 years in the ELEMENT cohort. *Environmental Research*; 2022;211:112993.

Goodman C, Hall M, Green R, Hornung R, Martinez-Mier EA, Lanphear B, Till C. Maternal fluoride exposure, birth outcomes and fertility: The MIREC cohort. *Environmental Advances*; 2022b;7:100135. Available from: https://doi.org/10.1016/j.envadv.2021.100135

Goodman I, Hall M, Green R, Chevrier J, Ayotte P, Martinez-Mier A, McGuckin T, Krzeczkowski J, Flora D, Hornung R, Lanphear B, Till C. Iodine status modifies the effect of fluoride exposure in pregnancy on preschool boys' intelligence. *Nutrients*; 2022c;14(14)

Goodwin M, Emsley R, Kelly MP, Sutton M, Tickle M, Walsh T, Whittaker W, Pretty IA. Evaluation of water fluoridation scheme in Cumbria: the CATFISH prospective longitudinal cohort study [Internet]. Southampton (UK): National Institute for Health and Care Research; *Public Health Res*. 2022;10(11).

Gordonoff T, editor. The toxicology of fluoride. Basel/Stuttgart: Schwabe & Co. Verlag; 1964.

Graham HN. Green Tea Composition, Consumption, and Polyphenol Chemistry. *Preventative Medicine* 1992;21, 334-350.

Graham JR, Burk D, Morin P. A current restatement and continuing reappraisal concerning demographic variables in American time-trend studies on water fluoridation and human cancer. *Proc. Pennsylvania Academy of Sci*. 1987;61:138-146.

Graham JR, Morin PJ. "Highlights in North American Litigation During the Twentieth Century on Artificial Fluoridation of Public Water Supplies," Florida State University *Journal of Land Use and Environmental Law*: Vol. 14: No. 2, Article 1. 2018.

Grandjean P, Hu H, Till C, Green R, Bashash M, Flora D, Tellez-Rojo MM, Song PXK, Lanphear B, Budtz-Jørgensen E. A Benchmark Dose Analysis for Maternal Pregnancy Urine-Fluoride and IQ in Children. *Risk Anal*. 2022 Mar;42(3):439-449.

Grandjean P., Meddis A., Nielsen F., Hu H., Till C, Goodman C, Iben H. Beck, Tina K. Jensen, Niels Bilenberg, Budtz- Jørgensen E. Dose-dependence of prenatal fluoride exposure at low levels in relation to cognitive performance at school age. *Eur J Public Health*, 2024;34(1):143-149

Green R, Lanphear B, Hornung R, Flora D, Martinez-Mier A, Neufeld R, Ayotte P, Muckle G, Till C. Fluoride exposure during fetal development and intellectual abilities in a Canadian birth cohort. *JAMA Pediatrics;* 2019;173(10):940-948.

Griffiths J. "Fluoride Report Softened." *Medical Tribune*. 1989.

Griffiths J. "Fluoride: Commie Plot or Capitalist Ploy," *Covert Action Quarterly*, 1992.

Griffiths J, Bryson C. "Fluoride, Teeth and the Atomic Bomb." *Waste Not*. Sept. 1997.

Grimaldi D. Will heat treatment kill all insects? Entomology Blog, 2025. Available from: https://blog.entomologist.net/will-heat-treatment-kill-all-insects.htm

Grimbergen GW. A double-blind test for determination of intolerance to fluoridated water. Preliminary report. *Fluoride* 1974. 7(3):146-152.

Guan ZZ, Wang YN, Xiao KQ, Dai DY, Chen YH, Liu JL, Sindelar P, Dallner G. Influence of chronic fluorosis on membrane lipids in rat brain. *Neurotoxicol Teratol*. 1998; Sep-Oct;20(5):537-42.

Hall M, Hornung R, Chevrier J, Ayotte P, Lanphear B, Till C. Fluoride exposure and thyroid hormones in a Canadian pregnancy cohort, *Environmental International*, 2024;184, 108442.

Hall M, Lanphear B, Chevrier J, Hornung R, Green R, Goodman C, Ayotte P, Martinez-Mier A, Zoeller RT, Till C. Fluoride Exposure and Hypothyroidism in a Canadian Pregnancy Cohort. *Science of the Total Environment*, 2023;869, 61149.

Harrison MF. (a) Fluorine content of teas consumed in New Zealand. *Br J Nutr*. 1949; 3(2-3):162-6.

Harrison MF. (b) Urinary excretion of fluorine in some New Zealand subjects. *Br J Nutr*. 1949; 3(2-3):166-70.

He H, Cheng Z, Liu W. Effects of fluorine on the human fetus. *Chinese Journal of Control of Endemic Diseases*, 1989 4(3):136-8. [Translation published: 2008. *Fluoride*, Oct-Dec:41(4)321–326.]

Heller KE, Eklund SA, Burt BA. Dental caries and dental fluorosis at varying water fluoride concentrations. *J. Public Health Dentistry* 1997;57(3):136-143.

Helte E, Donat Vargas C, Kippler M, Wolk A, Michaëlsson K, Åkesson A. Fluoride in Drinking Water, Diet, and Urine in Relation to Bone Mineral Density and Fracture Incidence in Postmenopausal Women. *Environ Health Perspect*. 2021;Apr;129(4):47005.

Henry NL (Federal President, Australian Dental Association). Letter to Barry O. Jones, Minister for Science and Technology, dated 28 August 1985, with Minister's annotations.

Hileman B. Fluoridation of water: Questions about health risks and benefits remain after more than 40 years. *Chemical & Engineering News*.1988; 66:26-42.

Hirzy JW. United States EPA Scientists take stand against fluoridation of drinking water. 1999. Available from: https://actionpa.org/fluoride/nffe/

Hirzy JW, Connett P, Xiang Q, Spittle BJ, Kennedy DC. Developmental neurotoxicity of fluoride. A quantitative risk analysis towards establishing a safe daily dose of fluoride for children. *Fluoride*, 2016;*49*(4), 379.

Honicker CT. America's Radiation Victims: The Hidden Files. *New York Times.* Sunday Section 6, page 39 (9 pages). November 19, 1989. Available from: https://www.americanhealthstudies.org/nyt.1989.html

Hujoel PP, Zina LG, Moimaz SA, Cunha-Cruz J. Infant formula and enamel fluorosis: a systematic review. *J Am Dent Assoc*. 2009 Jul;140(7):841-54.

Husdan H, Vogl R, Oreopoulos D, Gryfe C, Rapoport A. Serum ionic fluoride: normal range and relationship to age and sex. *Clin Chem*. 1976 Nov;22(11):1884-8.

Ibarluzea J, Gallastegi M, Santa-Marina L, Jiménez Zabala A, Arranz E, Molinuevo A, Lopez-Espinosa MJ, Ballester F, Villanueva CM, Riano I, Sunyer J, Tardon A, Lertxundi A. Prenatal exposure to fluoride and neuropsychological development in early childhood: 1-to 4 years old children. *Environ Res*. 2022 May 1;207:112181.

Iheozor-Ejiofor Z, Worthington HV, Walsh T, O'Malley L, Clarkson JE, Macey R, Alam R, Tugwell P, Welch V, Glenny AM. Water fluoridation for the prevention of dental caries. Cochrane Database Syst Rev. 2015 Jun 18;2015(6):CD010856.

Iheozor-Ejiofor Z, Walsh T, Lewis SR, Riley P, Boyers D, Clarkson JE, Worthington HV, Glenny AM, O'Malley L. Water fluoridation for the prevention of dental caries. *Cochrane Database Syst Rev.* 2024 Oct 4;10(10):CD010856.

Iida H, Kumar JV. 2009. The association between enamel fluorosis and dental caries in U.S. schoolchildren. *JADA* 140:855-862.

Inkielewicz I, Krechniak J. Fluoride content in soft tissues and urine of rats exposed to sodium fluoride in drinking water. *Fluoride* 36(4):263-266. 2003; Available from: https://fluoridealert.org/wp-content/uploads/2025/07/inkielewicz-2003.pdf

Institute of Medicine (US) Standing Committee on the Scientific Evaluation of Dietary Reference Intakes. Dietary Reference Intakes for Calcium, Phosphorus, Magnesium, Vitamin D, and Fluoride. Washington (DC): National Academies Press (US); 1997. 8, *Fluoride*.

Institute of Medicine (US). Dietary Reference Intakes: The Essential Guide to Nutrient Requirements. Washington (DC): National Academies Press (US); 2006. *Fluoride*, pp. 312-319.

Institute of Medicine (US) Letter. From: by Erin Brockovich; Wm. A. Ingram, M.D.; David P. Matthews, J.D.; Daniel A. Eyink, M.D.; Jean Nordin-Evans, D.D.S.; Stephanie Seneff, Ph.D. April 27, 2015. Available from: https://fluoridealert.org/wp-content/uploads/brockovich-iom.april-27.2015.pdf

International Experts at Otago University, Dunedin September 2018." Fluoride Free, NZ, 22 May 2023. Available from: https://fluoridefree.org.nz/international-experts-at-otago-university-dunedin-september-2018/

Jaffe N, Caron M, Walsh L, Bierer B, Barnes M. Defamation Claims Arising from Research Misconduct Cases: Best Practices for Institutions. *Journal of Law, Medicine & Ethics*. 2025;53(1):47-54

Kavanagh D, Renehan J. Fluoride in tea—its dental significance: a review. *J Ir Dent Assoc*. 1998;44(4):100-5.

Kennedy D. How To Save Your Teeth: Toxic-Free Preventive Dentistry.1993.

Knapton S. Fluoride to be added to drinking water under new legal powers. *The Telegraph (U.K.).* Feb 7, 2024.

Ko L, Thiessen KM. A critique of recent economic evaluations of community water fluoridation. *Internat J Occup Environ Health* 2015; 21(2):91-120.

Koglin OH. (December 20, 2000) 'Oregon's top health officer tackles to-do list.' *The Oregonian*, p. B12.

Kopf C. Dentists Protect Fluoride Instead of Babies, 2012 blog. Available from: https://fluoridedangers.blogspot.com/search?q=Dentists+Protect+Fluoride+Instead+of+Babies%2C

Kopf C. Johnny Johnson's *Ad Hominem* Attack On Me. 2017 blog. Available from: https://fluoridedangers.blogspot.com/p/johnny-johnsons-ad-hominem-attack-on-me_35.html

Korfhage M. Fluoridation Opponents Gather More Than 20,000 Signatures. Willamette Week. October 4, 2012.

Krzeczkowski J, Hall M, St. Amour D, Oulhote Y, McGuckin T, Goodman C, Green R, Muckle G, Lanphear B, Till C. (2024). Prenatal fluoride exposure, offspring visual acuity and autonomic nervous system function in 6-month-old infants, *Environmental International*, 183:108336.

Kumpulainen J, Koivistoinen P. Fluorine in foods. *Residue Rev.* 1977;68:37-57.

Kurttio P, Pukkala E, Kahelin H, Auvinen A, Pekkanen J. Arsenic concentrations in well water and risk of bladder and kidney cancer in Finland. *Environ Health Perspect.* 1999 Sep;107(9):705-10.

Lakoff, G. Don't think of an elephant! Know your values and frame the debate: The essential guide for progressives. Chelsea Green Publishing Company. 2004

Les Fluorures, la fluoration et la qualité de l'environnement. Comité aviseur sur la fluoration des eaux de consommateur, Ministère de l'Environnement, Sainte-Foy, novembre 1979, 210 p. (The Red Book)

Leverett DH. Fluorides and the changing prevalence of dental caries. *Science* 1982; 217(4554):26-30.

Levy SM, Broffitt B, Marshall TA, Eichenberger-Gilmore JM, Warren JJ. Associations Between Fluorosis of Permanent Incisors and Fluoride Intake From Infant Formula, Other Dietary Sources and Dentifrice During Early Childhood. *J Amer Dent Assoc.* 2010; 141 (10): 1190-1201

Lévy M, Corbeil F, Fortin C, Lamarre J-R, Lavallière A, et al. Fluoration de l'eau : analyse des bénéfices et des risques pour la santé – un Avis scientifique l'Institut national de santé publique du Québec, juin 2007, p.42.

Li S, Smith KD, Davis JH, Gordon PB, Breaker RR, Strobel SA. Eukaryotic resistance to fluoride toxicity mediated by a widespread family of fluoride export proteins. *Proc Natl Acad Sci U S A.* 2013 Nov 19;110(47):19018-23.

Li X, Zhi J, Gao R. Effect of fluoride exposure on intelligence in children. *Fluoride.* 1995;28(4):189-192.

Limeback H, Ismail A, Banting D, DenBesten P, Featherstone J, Riordan JP. The Canadian consensus conference on the appropriate use of fluoride for the prevention of dental caries in children. *J Can Dent Assoc* 1998; 64:636-639.

Limeback H. A re-examination of the pre-eruptive and post-eruptive mechanism of the anti-caries effects of fluoride. Is there any anti-caries benefit to swallowing fluoride? *Commun Dent oral Epidemiol.*1999; 27:31-40.

Limeback H. Comprehensive Preventive Dentistry (H. Limeback ed.) John Wiley & Sons., 2012.

Limeback H. Fluoride Accumulation in Human Teeth and Bones: Is Dose Adjustment Now Required? *Canadian Journal of Public Health*, 1993;84(2),78–79.

Limeback H. Introduction to the Conference. *Commun Dent Oral Epidemiol.* 1999; 27:27-30.

Limeback H. Recent studies confirm old problems with water fluoridation. A fresh perspective. 2001, *Fluoride* 34(1): 1-6.

Liu JL, Xia T, Zhang M, He WH, He P, Chen XM, et al. Screening of environmental response genes related to dental fluorosis. *Fluoride*, 2006;39(3):195-201.

Long H, Jin Y, Lin M, Sun Y, Zhang L, Clinch C. Fluoride toxicity in the male reproductive system. *Fluoride*, 2009;42(4):260-76.

Long YG, Wang YN, Chen J, Jiang SF, Nordberg A, Guan ZZ. Chronic fluoride toxicity decreases the number of nicotinic acetylcholine receptors in rat brain. *Neurotoxicol Teratol*. 2002 Nov-Dec;24(6):751-7.

Lu Y, Guo FW., Yang XQ. The fluoride content in tea and its relationship to tea quality. *J Agric Food Chem*. 2004 Jul 4;52(14):4472-6.

Maas RP, Patch SC, Christian AM, Coplan MJ. Effects of fluoridation and disinfection agent combinations on lead leaching from leaded-brass parts. *Neurotoxicology*. 2007.

Malin AJ, Eckel SP, Hu H, Martinez-Mier EA, Hernandez-Castro I, Yang T, Farzan SF, Habre R, Breton CV, Bastain TM. Maternal Urinary Fluoride and Child Neurobehavior at Age 36 Months. *JAMA Netw Open*. 2024 May 1;7(5):e2411987.

Malin AJ, Riddell J, McCague H, Till C. Fluoride exposure and thyroid function among adults living in Canada: effect modification by iodine status. *Environment International*. 2018;121(Pt 1):667-674.

Malin AJ, Till C. Exposure to fluoridated water and attention deficit hyperactivity disorder prevalence among children and adolescents in the United States: an ecological association. *Environ Health*. 2015 Feb 27;14:17.

Manji F, Kapila S. Fluorides and fluorosis in Kenya- An Overview. In S. Likimani, ed., Fluorosis Research.Strategies. *Afr Med Res Found.*, Nairobi Kenya, pp 11-21.

Marcus, Wm. L. Memorandum Office of Water, EPA, to Alan B. Hais: "Fluoride Conference to Review the NTP Draft Fluoride Report." 1990.

Marier JR, Rose D, The Fluoride content of some foods and beverages, - Brief Survey using a modified Zr-Spands method. *J Foods Science* 31, 1966, 941-946.

Marinho VCC. Cochrane fluoride reviews: an overview of the evidence on caries prevention with fluoride treatments. *FDJ*. 2015;5(2).

Marthaler TM. Salt fluoridation and oral health. *Acta Medica Academica*. 2013.

Martin B, Baker CMA, Manwell C, Pugh C (eds.), *Intellectual Suppression: Australian Case Histories, Analysis and Responses.* Sydney: Angus & Robertson, 1986.

Martin B. Scientific Knowledge in Controversy: The Social Dynamics of the Fluoridation Debate. Albany: State University of New York Press, 1991.

Martin B. The controversy manual. Sparsnäs, Sweden: Irene Publishing, 2014.

Martin B. The scientific straightjacket: the power structure of science and the suppression of environmental scholarship. *The Ecologist*. 1981; 11(1):33–43.

Masters RD, Coplan MJ. Water Treatment with Silicofluorides and Lead Toxicity. *Intern. J. Environ. Studies* 56: 435-449 1999.

Masters RD, Coplan MJ, Hone BT, Dykes JE. Association of silicofluoride treated water with elevated blood lead. *Neurotoxicology*. 2000 Dec;21(6):1091-100.

McFarland MJ, Hauer ME, Reuben A. Half of the US population is exposed to adverse lead levels in early childhood. *Proc Natl Acad Sci U S A*. 2022;Mar 15;119(11):e2118631119.

Mellon Institute of Industrial Research. Agreement for The Sugar Institute Inc Industrial Fellowship no 1, Mellon Institute Industrial Fellowship no 785. Buhl Records, Detre Library & Archives, Heinz History Center. 1930.

Mesh A. Fluoride Campaign Spent $889,000 to Lose by 20 Points. *Willamette Week*. May 31, 2013.

Michael Connett, Fluoride & The Brain. YouTube, Fluoride Action Network, 10 December 2016. Available from: https://www.youtube.com/watch?v=qu3HD-RtY3E.

Michaels D. Doubt is their product: how industry's assault on science threatens your health. Oxford, UK: Oxford University Press, 2008.

Moimaz SA, Saliba O, Marques LB, Garbin CA, Saliba NA. Dental fluorosis and its influence on children's life. *Braz Oral Res*. 2015;29:S1806-83242015000100214.

Moolenburgh HC. Fluoride: The Freedom Fight. Mainstream Publishing, 1987.

Moore D, Nyakutsikwa B, Allen T, Lam E, Birch S, Tickle M, Pretty IA, Walsh T. How effective and cost-effective is water fluoridation for adults and adolescents? The LOTUS 10-year retrospective cohort study. *Community Dent Oral Epidemiol*. 2024 Aug;52(4):413-423.

Morin, P.J., Graham, J.R. and Parent, G. Fluoridation: Autopsy of a Scientific Error, Editions Berger, Eastman, QC, 2010, 234 p.

Morin, P.J., Graham, J.R. and Parent, G. La Fluoration : Autopsie d'une erreur scientifique, Éditions Berger, Eastman, QC, 2005, 315 p.

Mullenix PJ, Denbesten PK, Schunior A, Kernan WJ. Neurotoxicity of sodium fluoride in rats. *Neurotoxicol Teratol*. 1995 Mar-Apr;17(2):169-77.

Mullenix PJ. A new perspective on metals and other contaminants in fluoridation chemicals. *Int J Occup Environ Health*. 2014 Apr-Jun;20(2):157-66.

Multiple Authors. First International Conference on Declining Prevalence of Dental Caries, *Journal of Dental Research 1982*; 61 (Special Issue).

National Institute for Dental and Craniofacial Research (NIDCR). The Story of Fluoridation. 2024. Available from: https://www.nidcr.nih.gov/health-info/fluoride/the-story-of-fluoridation

National Research Council (NRC). Fluoride in drinking water: a scientific review of EPA's standards. 2006. The National Academies Press. Washington DC. "Assessing the efficacy of fluoride in preventing dental caries is not covered in this report" (p. 14). "As noted earlier, this report does not evaluate nor make judgments about the benefits, safety, or efficacy of artificial water fluoridation" (p. 16).

National Whistleblower Center. 'Reich Orders EPA to Reinstate Scientist" by Herb Ettel. February 10, 1994.Available from: https://www.toxicteeth.org/health/cancer/ntp/marcus3.html

Neurath C, Limeback H, Osmunson B, Connett M, Kanter V, Wells CR. Dental Fluorosis Trends in US Oral Health Surveys: 1986 to 2012. *JDR Clin Trans Res.* 2019 Oct;4(4):298-308.

Neurath C. The sugar industry's efforts to manipulate research on fluoride effectiveness and toxicity: a ninety-year history. *Environ Health* 24, 62 (2025).

NH&MRC (National Health and Medical Research Council). Report of the Working Party on Fluorides in the Control of Dental Caries, Canberra: Australian Government Publishing Service, 1985.

Nigra AE, Bloomquist TR, Rajeev T, Burjak M, Casey JA, Goin DE, et al. ECHO Cohort Consortium. Public Water Arsenic and Birth Outcomes in the Environmental Influences on Child Health Outcomes Cohort. *JAMA Netw Open*. 2025 Jun 2;8(6):e2514084.

NRC (National Research Council). 2009. Emergency and Continuous Exposure Guidance Levels for Selected Submarine Contaminants: Volume 3. Washington, DC: National Academies Press.

NSF (formerly National Sanitation Foundation). Fluoridation Products and Fluoride Fact Sheet. 2024. Available from: https://nsfinternational.widencollective.com/assets/share/asset/ry9p1atrke

NTP (National Toxicology Program). NTP monograph on the state of the science concerning fluoride exposure and neurodevelopment and cognition: a systematic review. Monograph 08. August. Division of Translational Toxicology, National Institute of Environmental Health Sciences, Research Triangle Park, North Carolina, USA. 2024.

NZ Fluoride Feud: Paul Connett's Presentation to the New Zealand Parliament. YouTube, Fluoride Action Network, 20 June 2018. Available from: https://www.youtube.com/watch?v=cfTSc5T7CNY

O'Grady D. Blame City, Hospital in Boy's Death. New York Daily News. June 9, 1977. Available from: https://fluoridealert.org/content/kennerly/

Osmunson B, Cole G. Community Water Fluoridation a Cost–Benefit–Risk Consideration. *Public Health Challenges*. 27 November 2024.

Paduano, M. The Fluoridation of Water in Britain: Concerns over fluoride levels in drinking water as expert urges Britain to reassess dosage. *Independent*. September 14, 2025.

Paduano M, Mcghie J, Boulton A. Mystery of babies with no eyes. *The Observer*. 17 January 1993.

Parent G. L'Inconséquence de la fluoration, Les grandes éditions du Québec inc., Montréal, QC, 1975.

Peckham S, Lowery D, Spencer S. Are fluoride levels in drinking water associated with hypothyroidism prevalence in England? A large observational study of GP practice data and fluoride levels in drinking water. *J Epidemiol Community Health*. 2015 Jul;69(7):619-24.

Pesticide Temporary Tolerances that appeared in the September 5, 2001, Federal Register. Available from: https://fluoridealert.org/wp-content/uploads/2025/08/connett-e.sulfuryl-fluoride-submission-to-epa.sept-2001.pdf

Petrović B, Kojić S, Milić L, Luzio A, Perić T, Marković E, Stojanović GM. Toothpaste ingestion-evaluating the problem and ensuring safety: systematic review and meta-analysis. *Front Public Health*. 2023.

Pittman, GO. Phosphate: Fluorides Toxic Torts. Gary Owen Pittman. 2011.

Pittman, GO. Relentless. Gary Owen Pittman. 2017.

Price W. Nutrition and Physical Degeneration. *Price Pottenger Nutrition*. 2009.

Public Law 113–79 113th Congress, Agricultural Act of 2014'-Feb. 7, 2014 128 STAT. 649.

Reagan-Udall Foundation for the Federal Food and Drug Administration. Use of Orally Ingestible Unapproved Prescription Drug Products Containing Fluoride in the Pediatric Population. Hybrid Public Meeting, July 23, 2025. Available from: https://reaganudall.org/news-and-events/events/use-orally-ingestible-unapproved-prescription-drug-products-fluoride

Reed B. Eyeless children championed by Observer win $7m test case. *The Guardian*. 21 December 2003.

Reeves T. National Fluoridation Engineer, U.S. Center for Disease Control. The Manufacture of The Fluoride Chemicals, Refer: FL-143, Sept. 2000.

Riddell J, Malin A, Flora D, McCague H, Till C. Association of water fluoride and urinary fluoride concentrations with attention deficit hyperactivity disorder in Canadian youth. *Environment International*; 133 (Part B). 2022 Mar;161:107091

Roberts A. 2024. What's in the water? Long-run effects of fluoridation on health and economic self-sufficiency. J Health Econ.98:102934.

Ross D. Health Official Delayed Report Linking Fluoride to Brain Harm. *Capital and Main*. March 14, 2023.

Tuggeri A. These countries don't fluoridate their water: here's why. BBC article. 2025. Available from: https://www.bbc.com/future/article/20250528-why-some-countries-dont-fluoridate-their-water

Safe Water Foundation of Texas vs City of Houston, no 80-52271, Harris County District Court of Texas Registry, 151st Judicial District, 1982.

Schmidt B. New coalition lobbies to fluoridate Portland's drinking water. Oregonian/Oregon Live. August 9, 2012.

Scott P, Richards E, Martin B. Captives of controversy: the myth of the neutral social researcher in contemporary scientific controversies. *Science, Technology, & Human Values*. 1990; 15(4):474–494.

Sener Y, Tosun G, Kahvecioglu F, Gökalp A, Koç H. Fluoride levels of human plasma and breast milk. *Eur J Dent*. 2007 Jan;1(1):21-4.

Shiboski CH, Gansky SA, Ramos-Gomez F, Ngo L, Isman R, Pollick HF. The association of early childhood caries and race/ethnicity among California preschool children. *J Public Health Den*t. 2003 Winter;63(1):38-46.

Smith A. Health (Fluoridation of Drinking Water) Amendment Bill passes final reading in Parliament. RNZ. Nov 9, 2021.

Smith E. The food of the poorer labouring classes in England. Sixth report of the medical officer of the Privy Council. London, UK: House of Commons,1864, pp.216–329.

Spencer KF. IOM Letter, From: Erin Brockovich, Wm. A. Ingram, MD; David P. Matthews, JD.; Daniel A. Eyink, MD; Jean Nordin-Evans, DDS; Stephanie Seneff, PhD, To: Institute of Medicine, April 27, 2015. Available from: https://fluoridealert.org/wp-content/uploads/brockovich-iom.april-27.2015.pdf

Spencer KF. ATA Letter, From Richard L. Shames, MD; William J. Rea, MD; Nathan Becker, MD, FACE, FACP; Heather Gingerich, MSc; Ellie Phillips, DDS; Marcus L. Scott, Esq. To: American Thyroid Association. February 16, 2016a. Available from: https://iabdm.org/wp-content/uploads/2016/03/Letter-to-ATA_2016_02_11.pdf

Spencer KF. NGA Letter, From: Erin Brockovich; Robert W. Bowcock; Michael D. Kohn JD, To: National Governors Association. April 27, 2016b. Available from: https://fluoridealert.org/wp-content/uploads/brockovich-2016.pdf

Spencer KF. Salem State Letter. From: Karen Favazza Spencer, To: Prof. Jennifer Jackman. Sept. 7, 2016c. Available from: https://fluoridealert.org/wp-content/uploads/SalemState2016.09.07.pdf

Spencer KF, Limeback H. Blood is thicker than water: Flaws in a National Toxicology Program study. *Med Hypotheses*. 2018 Dec;121:160-163.

Spittle B. Choppy waters continuing for community water fluoridation [editorial]. *Fluoride*, 2025 Mar 15:e334.

Spittle B. Further Medline rejection of Fluoride [editorial]. *Fluoride*, 2014:47(1):2-8.

Standard Handbook for Civil Engineers, Third Edition, Frederick S. Merritt, Editor; 1983 McGraw-Hill, Inc.

Staudenmaier B. I am Suing the US EPA Over Fluoride Added to Our Drinking Water. *The Clarion*. May 5, 2021. Available from: https://www.theonlineclarion.com/opinion/2021/05/05/i-am-suing-the-us-epa-over-fluoride-added-to-our-drinking-water/

Stilwell WF, Edson NL, Stainton PVE. Fluoridation of public water supplies. Report of Commission of Inquiry. 1957. Wellington: By authority, RE Owen, Government Printer; 1962.

Sutton PRN. Are most fluoridation promoters neurotics? Medical Hypotheses. Volume 39, Issue 3, November 1992, Pages 199-200.

Sutton PRN. Fluoridation: Errors & Omissions in Experimental Trials. 2nd ed. Australia: Melbourne University Press, 1960.

Sutton PRN. The Greatest Fraud Fluoridation. A Factual Book, Kurunda Pty, Ltd. 1996.

Taylor KW, Eftim SE, Sibrizzi CA, Blain RB, Magnuson K, Hartman PA, Rooney AA, Bucher JR. Fluoride Exposure and Children's IQ Scores: A Systematic Review and Meta-Analysis. *JAMA Pediatr*. 2025 Mar 1;179(3):282-292.

Till C, Grandjean P, Martinez-Mier EA, Hu H, Lanphear B. Health Risks and Benefits of Fluoride Exposure During Pregnancy and Infancy. *Annu Rev Public Health*. 2025 Apr;46(1):253-274

Till C, Green R, Flora D, Hornung R, Martinez-Mier EA, Blazer M, Farmus L, Ayotte P, Muckle G, Lanphear B. Fluoride exposure from infant formula and child IQ in a Canadian birth cohort. *Environmental International*; 2020;134:105315

Till C, Green R, Grundy JG, Hornung R, Neufeld R, Martinez-Mier EA, Ayotte P, Muckle G, Lanphear B. Community Water Fluoridation and Urinary Fluoride Concentrations in a National Sample of Pregnant Women in Canada. *Environ Health Perspect*. 2018 Oct;126(10):107001.

Till C, Green R. The evolving science of fluoride: When new evidence doesn't conform with existing beliefs. Pediatric Research. *Commentary for special issue on Controversies in Pediatrics*. 2021 Nov;90(5):1093-1095.

Tomašek I, Mouri H, Dille A, Bennett G, Bhattacharya P, Brion N, Elskens M, Fontijn K, Gao Y, Gevera PK, Ijumulana J, Kisaka M, Leermakers M, Shemsanga C, Walraevens K, Wragg J, Kervyn M. Naturally occurring potentially toxic elements in groundwater from the volcanic landscape around Mount Meru, Arusha, Tanzania and their potential health hazard. *Sci Total Environ*. 2022 Feb 10;807(Pt 1):150487.

Undark, Entanglements Podcast. Is Fluoride Toxic at Low Levels? 23 December 2024. Available from: https://undark.org/2024/12/23/podcast-fluoride-toxic-low-levels/

U.S. Department of Agriculture. Air Pollutants Affecting the Performance of Domestic Animals. Agricultural Handbook No. 380. Rev ed. Washington, DC: U.S. Department of Agriculture; 1972.

U.S. Department of Health and Human Services Federal Panel on Community Water Fluoridation. 2015. U.S. Public Health Service Recommendation for fluoride concentration in drinking water for the prevention of dental caries. Public Health Reports Vol. 130.

United States District Court (2024), Northern District, Lanphear declaration Civ. No. 17-CV-02162-EMC p.14

United States District Court, Northern District, Hu Declaration. Document No. 17-CV-02162-EMC

United States District Court. Case No. 17-CV-02162-EMC. Food and Water Watch et al. v. United States Environmental Protection Agency et al. (2024).

USDHHS. U.S. Department of Health and Human Services Federal Panel on Community Water Fluoridation. 2015. U.S. Public Health Service Recommendation for fluoride concentration in drinking water for the prevention of dental caries. *Public Health Reports* Vol. 130.

USEPA (U.S. Environmental Protection Agency). 1988. Summary Review of Health Effects Associated with Hydrogen Fluoride and Related Compounds: Health Issue Assessment. Research Triangle Park, NC: Office of Health and Environmental Assessment, Report No. EPA/600/8-89/002F.

USEPA (U.S. Environmental Protection Agency). 1994. Summary Review of Health Effects Associated with Mercuric Chloride: Health Issue Assessment. Research Triangle Park, NC: Office of Health and Environmental Assessment, Report No. EPA/600/R-92/199.

USEPA (U.S. Environmental Protection Agency). 2010a. Fluoride: Dose-Response Analysis for Non-Cancer Effects. Washington, D.C., U.S. Environmental Protection Agency, Office of Water, 820-R-10-019.

USEPA (U.S. Environmental Protection Agency). 2010b. Fluoride: Exposure and Relative Source Contribution Analysis. Washington, D.C., U.S. Environmental Protection Agency, Office of Water, 820-R-10-015.

Vani ML, Reddy KP. Effects of fluoride accumulation on some enzymes of the brain and gastrocnemius muscle of mice. *Fluoride* 2000; 33:17-26. Available from: https://fluoridealert.org/wp-content/uploads/2025/07/vani-2000.pdf

Varney W. Fluoride in Australia: A Case to Answer. Sydney: Hale & Iremonger, 1986.

Velez-León E, Pacheco-Quito EM, Díaz-Dosque M, Tobar-Almache D. Worldwide Variations in Fluoride Content in Beverages for Infants. *Children (Basel).* 2023 Dec 7;10(12):1896.

Waldbott GL. Medical evidence against fluoridation of public water supplies. *Australian Dental Journal*, 1955a;59:13-20.

Waldbott GL. Chronic fluorine intoxication from drinking water. *International Archives of Allergy and Applied Immunology*, 1955b;7(2):70-74.

Waldbott GL. Incipient fluorine intoxication from drinking water. *Acta Medica Scandinavica* 1956;156(3):157-168.

Waldbott GL. A struggle with titans. New York: Carlton Press; 1965.

Walbott GL, Burgstahler AE, McKinney L. Fluoridation: The Great Dilemma. Coronado Press, 1978.

Walker G. Fluoridation: Poison on Tap. Melbourne: Glen Walker, 1982.

Walters CB, Sherlock JC, Evans WH, Read JI. Dietary Intake of Fluoride in the United Kingdom and Fluoride Content of some Foodstuffs. *J Sci Food Agric.* 1983;34:523-528

Water Fluoridation: US Attorney Michael Connett's Presentation - Landmark Court Case Against US Govt." Fluoride Free NZ, 28 February 2025. Available from: https://www.youtube.com/watch?v=rFeP0zw2c0Q

Waugh DT, Godfrey M, Limeback H, Potter W. Black Tea Source, Production, and Consumption: Assessment of Health Risks of Fluoride Intake in New Zealand. *J Environ Public Health*. 2017;2017:5120504.

Waugh DT, Potter W, Limeback H, Godfrey M. Risk Assessment of Fluoride Intake from Tea in the Republic of Ireland and its Implications for Public Health and Water Fluoridation. *Int J Environ Res Public Health*. 2016 Feb 26;13(3):259.

Welsome E. The Plutonium Files: America's Secret Medical Experiments in the Cold War. The Dial Press. Health Action Press, 1999.

Wei W, Pang S, Sun D. The pathogenesis of endemic fluorosis: Research progress in the last 5 years. *J Cell Mol Med*. 2019 Apr;23(4):2333-2342.

WHO (World Health Organization). Fluorides. Environmental Health Criteria 227. 2002. Available from: https://www.inchem.org/documents/ehc/ehc/ehc227.htm

Wiatrowski E, Kramer L, Osis D, Spencer H. Dietary Fluoride Intake of Infants Pediatrics (1975) 55 (4): 517–522.

Wilkinson-Jones R. Calls for the whole county to have fluoridated water. *BBC Online*. January 10, 2025.

Wise, K. (2004). Factors Influencing the Outcomes of Public Health Legislation in the 2001 Oregon Legislature. [Master's Thesis, Oregon State University], p. 77-97, 104-115.

World Medical Association Declaration of Helsinki: ethical principles for medical research involving human subjects. *JAMA*, 2000 Dec 20;284(23):3043-5.

World Nuclear Association. Nuclear Fuel Cycle. Uranium from phosphates. 2025. Available from: https://world-nuclear.org/information-library/nuclear-fuel-cycle/uranium-resources/uranium-from-phosphates

Yiamouyiannis JA. Fluoride the Aging Factor: How to Recognize and Avoid the Devastating Effects of Fluoride. Health Action Press, 1983.

Yiamouyiannis JA, Burk D. Cancer from our Drinking Water? Congressional Record. U.S. House of Repr., 94th Congress.1st Session, 1975.

Yiamouyiannis, JA, Burk D. Fluoridation on Public Water Systems and Cancer Death Rate (CDR's) in Humans, *Fed Proc*. no 35, 1976.

Yiamouyiannis, JA, Burk D. Fluoridation and Cancer Age Dependence on Cancer Mortality Related to Artificial Fluoridation, *Fluoride*, vol. 10, no 3, 1977.

Zhai JX, Guo ZY, Hu CL, Wang QN, Zhu QX. [Studies on fluoride concentration and cholinesterase activity in rat hippocampus]. *Zhonghua Lao Dong Wei Sheng Zhi Ye Bing Za Zhi* [Chinese journal of industrial hygiene and occupational diseases] 2003 Apr;21(2):102-4.

Zhang S, Zhang X, Liu H, Qu W, Guan Z, Zeng Q, Jiang C, Gao H, Zhang C, Lei R, Xia T, Wang Z, Yang L, Chen Y, Wu X, Cui Y, Yu L, Wang A. Modifying effect of COMT gene polymorphism and a predictive role for proteomics analysis in children's intelligence in endemic fluorosis area in Tianjin, China. *Toxicol Sci*. 2015 Apr;144(2):238-45.

Zhao L, Liang G, Zhang D, Wu X. Effect of high-fluoride water supply on children's intelligence. *Fluoride*. 1996; 29(4):190-192.

Żwierełło W, Maruszewska A, Skórka-Majewicz M, Wszołek A, Gutowska I. Is Fluoride Blameless? The Influence of Fluorine Compounds on the Invasiveness of the Human Glioma-like Cell Line U-87. *Int J Mol Sci*. 2024 Nov 27;25(23):12773.

Profits from the sale of this book, after expenses, will be donated to organizations dedicated to environmental health

Visit our website:

heronlodgepress.ca

www.ingramcontent.com/pod-product-compliance
Lightning Source LLC
Chambersburg PA
CBHW070903080126
37874CB00040B/337
* 9 7 8 1 0 6 9 8 0 2 2 0 0 *